NGOs: The New Lexicon of Health Care

About the Author

Asok Kumar Sarkar, an alumnus of Tata Institute of Social Sciences, Mumbai, is presently Reader and Head in the Department of Social Work, Assam (Central) University, Silchar. Also, he is associated in different capacities with several universities and institutes like Visva Bharati University, Vidyasagar University, Indira Gandhi National Open University, and Institute of Development Studies, Kolkata.

Dr. Sarkar has participated in many national and international conferences, and published research articles in the journals of repute. His areas of research activities include maternal morbidity, reproductive health, NGO management and social development through them.

NGOs: The New Lexicon of Health Care

Asok Kumar Sarkar
Reader and Head,
Department of Social Work,
Assam (Central) University,
Silchar-788011 (India)

CONCEPT PUBLISHING COMPANY, NEW DELHI-110059

Cataloging in Publication Data—DK
Courtesy: D.K. Agencies (P) Ltd. <docinfo@dkagencies.com>

Sarkar, Asok Kumar, 1971-
NGOs : the new lexicon of health care / Asok Kumar Sarkar.
p. cm.
Includes bibliographical references (p.)
Includes index.
ISBN 8180692027

1. Non-governmental organizations—India—West Bengal. 2. Medical care—India—West Bengal. I. Title.

DDC 361.770 954 14 21

ISBN: 81-8069-202-7

First Published 2005

Published and Printed by
Ashok Kumar Mittal
Concept Publishing Company
A/15-16, Commercial Block, Mohan Garden
New Delhi-110059 (INDIA)

Phones : 25351460, 25351794
Fax : 091-11-25357103
Email : publishing@conceptpub.com

To My Mother
and
Development Initiators
of
Motherland

Foreword

Non-governmental Organisations (NGOs) have gained popularity and have been posed as an alternative to the state since the mid 1970s in the welfare sector. The NGOs have been described as more responsive and accountable than the state which was characterised as bureaucratic and tortuous to the needs of people. The trend during this period was to present NGOs as a substitute to the state, in some cases supplementing and even supplanting the state. The Indian Health Policy document of 1982 reflected this trend by declaring the inability of the state in fulfilling its role and sought a more prominent role for the private and NGO sector in supplementing the delivery of health services. There has been little systematic research on the characteristics and distribution of NGOs in community health. The experiences of few large NGOs in community health have been documented and have been projected as models. Some of these projects have tried innovative approaches to health and health service delivery but one of the key concerns from a public health perspective is that they are limited in their operations to a specific geographical area. Hence they are neither replicable nor can they be upscaled, financially and geographically.

Another important issue that needs to consider regarding NGOs in health care is the plurality that they present in terms of size, distribution, source of funding, ideological positions and so on. The evidence of this plurality has been provided by an earlier study of Dr Sarkar of NGOs in Assam and more recently in his study of NGOs in West Bengal. The study of NGOs in Assam shows that they are skewed in favour of better developed districts rather than backward ones. This raises an important question regarding their concern and claim that they work in poorer areas where the state is supposed to be weak or even dysfunctional. The reason for this kind of distribution can be partly explained by the need for infrastructure support like transport, communication, roads and related inputs that are necessary for even locating an organisation.

Since there are very few studies available on characteristics of NGOs in terms of organisational structure, sources of funding, services offered and personnel, Dr Sarkar's study provides some very valuable insights.

He has done an indepth study of some selected NGOs in West Bengal, which were purposively selected to show the variations in institutional forms in this sector. The study shows a high degree of dependence on national and foreign funds that influences priorities of the organisations. It raises an important question regarding the extent of autonomy that organisations enjoy and how far the 'felt needs' and priorities of the community are addressed. As far as the organisational structure is concerned it reveals a hierarchy and bureaucracy which is assumed to be a characteristic of government organisations. Contrary to popular perceptions that NGOs are non-bureaucratic is contested by the evidence from this study. The range of services provided by NGOs is also extremely varied and it is interesting that when it comes to health care they focus primarily on preventive and promotive services with little emphasis on curative services. Thus their programmes generate 'demand' for care but there is little effort to provide services to address their needs. These institutions singularly lack a public health perspective when it comes to their programme. There is lack of a comprehensive view of health and this gets reflected in their inability to provide an integrated perspective to health and development work.

The importance of this book is in the context of increasing privatisation and globalisation where the non-state sectors, both private and voluntary, are playing an escalating role in health sector. The VOs or NGOs have assumed an important role in provisioning of services, advocacy and even research. Many of them receive foreign funding and are very closely associated with the government for policy formulation. It is convenient for the government to hand over its responsibilities to the NGOs who are seen as important constituents of civil society. There is an important question about accountability of NGOs–in the final analyses. Are they accountable to the people or agencies who fund them? Can the government abdicate its responsibility to NGOs? Can NGOs replace the government in the provisioning of welfare services? Dr Sarkar's book provides answers to some of these questions based on empirical research in an area that has been under-researched.

New Delhi
April 2004

Rama V. Baru
Associate Professor,
Centre of Social Medicine and Community Health
Jawaharlal Nehru University, New Delhi

Preface

'Development' is an umbrella concept. It has different connotations such as economic development, social development, sustainable development, participatory development, grassroots development, people's centred development and so on. The term 'Sustainable Development' implies the real meaning of development. This development is contingent on various aspects such as social and economic security of the people, social status of women, female literacy, adoption of new technology, work participation of women, the internalization of investments to generate resources and so on. Better health, income, information, education, communication, gender justice, etc. can improve these aspects and thereby lead to development. These preconditions of development cannot be superimposed. They have to be built on the expectations, aspirations and motivation of the people. Therefore, people's own organizations i.e. NGOs are emerging gradually and participating actively in the process of social and economic transformation. Since health is one of the important ingredients of a state's overall development, the present book intends to focus on NGOs in health care. This volume is, in fact, a celebration of the gigantic roles that NGOs can perform and a critical appraisal of the ability of same organizations in the field of health care.

In an explicit manner, this book is an outcome of my long drawn research experience in NGO sector. Prof. Swapan Garain, my teacher, developed my research interest in this area and Dr. Rama V. Baru, my research guide set the direction to take up and carry out this work. Review of studies on NGOs shows there are diversity among the research initiatives. For instance, a few are individual case studies, few are related to programme activities, few deal with the organizational structure and the remaining studies relate to the beneficiaries. These studies are largely from a management or sociological perspective. A public health perspective, which has an interdisciplinary approach and can examine the social basis of these NGOs, their growth and distribution, their contribution, etc. is lacking in this area of research. It is also found that there are only two state level studies on NGOs in health care. Those were conducted in Maharashtra and Andhra Pradesh. No other state level work on NGO's health effort is undertaken. Hence, the present book is a documentation of state level study of NGOs in health care in West Bengal having considered the perspective and research gap. The reason for selecting West Bengal is its unique socio-political environment. For instance, it has history of series of movements, more than twenty seven years rule of the Left Front Government and at present more importance is being given on industrialization and work culture.

The data provided in this book have been collected and interpreted on the basis of a scientific methodology. The entire work has been carried out in five phases. In the first phase, secondary data pertaining to socio-political factors influenced the rise of NGOs in West Bengal especially after independence were gathered through literature review. In the second phase, addresses of NGOs in health care were collected based on certain criteria by using the snow ball sampling technique and a comprehensive list of 705 NGOs of West Bengal was prepared. District-wise distribution of NGOs was analysed from this list. In the third phase, questionnaires were mailed to al! the 705 NGOs and after three reminders were sent, there was a total of 216 responses. This was done to collect the necessary data in order to analyse the ideological motivations, the growth, distribution and characteristics of NGOs in health care in West Bengal. In the fourth phase, fifteen key informants were interviewed purposively to collect much more information on the influence of socio-political factors on the rise of NGOs. In the last phase, three NGOs (i.e. Southern Health Improvement Samity, CINI Moyna Rural Health Development Centre, and Rural Health Development Centre) were selected purposively based on certain criteria and studied in details. In each NGO, emphasis was given on historical background, administrative set-up, present activities, nature of programme sustainability, staff members and their job satisfaction, beneficiaries perception towards the working of NGOs, etc. to understand how far an NGO could contribute to health care.

This book is divided into eleven chapters. Chapter I is an introductory part, which begins with the emergence of welfare state, its crisis and genesis of NGOs. Ultimately, it presents a view that NGOs are prowling in the field of development and particularly in health sector. Chapter II gives an overview of relevant literature, Chapter III deals with the details of methodology and Chapter IV draws a socio-economic picture of West Bengal. The second section of the book, which includes Chapters V and VI, is devoted to understand the origin and development of NGOs in health care in West Bengal. The subsequent four Chapters (VII, VIII, IX and X) have made a portrayal on contribution of NGOs in health care in West Bengal. The last Chapter stands to make a critical analysis.

I wish to mention that this book will be worth and useful for the government, NGOs, funding agencies, academicians and researchers in designing, implementing, monitoring and evaluating health care programmes in the community. Development initiators, whether in Government or Voluntary sector, would also find answer from this book, why health programmes of NGOs should be integrated with government and private sectors. My close nexus with the beneficiaries has convinced me that people use health programmes of NGOs as stepping stone towards a better care. Therefore, my minimum expectation from writing this book would be fulfilled if development initiators who are engaged in policy formulation, research and action realize that NGOs are suitable means only for temporary, community based and preventive health services.

At the end, I would like to acknowledge the active support and cooperation of many individuals and institutions. I am thankful to Dr. Rama V. Baru, my teacher and research guide, without whose support it would not have been possible to complete the entire work. Any acknowledgement of gratitude to her in words will not suffice here. Her ideas and critical suggestions were a constant source of challenge and inspiration to give final shape of this book. I extend my deep sense of gratitude to the key informants who provided primary data and to the higher-level authorities of various Non-Governmental Organizations who replied to the mailed questionnaires. I also gratefully acknowledge the support and encouragement of three large NGOs such as Rural Health Development Center, CINI Moyna Rural Health Development Center and Southern Health Improvement Samity who have been the main source of information during the last phase of data collection. In absence of their help, this work would not have materialized. I am obliged to the librarians and their helping staff of Voluntary Health Association of India, Assam University, West Bengal Voluntary Health Association, National Library at Kolkata, Jadavpur University,

Calcutta University, Indian Institute of Management Calcutta, Indian Institute of Social Welfare and Business Management, etc. for allowing me to consult the necessary material.

I would like to place on record my sincere thanks to Mr. Manik Shah Mazumder, Mr. Ashim Das Laskar, Md. Ikbal Hussain Laskar who helped in the process of data collection, to Prof. N. Sudhakar Rao and Prof. N.B. Biswas who assisted in data analysis, to Keshab Sil and Mr. Alak Chakraborty who typed out the manuscript so neatly and gave the final shape of the same. I am indebted to Prof. Imrana Qadeer, Prof. G. Shah, Dr. K.R. Nayar, Dr. Mohan Rao and Dr. Ritu Priya for their advice and suggestions during the course of my work. With great reverence, I thank to Dr. Gopalji Mishra and Dr. B.S. Gunjal of Department of Social Work, Assam University, who took the pain to manage departmental affairs during my absence. Last but not the least, my parents, my wife Sulata and my son Teo in spite of all the taxing time pressurized me to complete this work. Thanking them would be a bit harsh. In fact, without their inspiration, this work would have never seen light of the day. I consider myself fortunate to have had such a loving family support. The strengths of this work belong to the efforts of these people while the weaknesses are mine alone.

Silchar ASOK KUMAR SARKAR
April 2004

Contents

IV. CONCLUSION

List of Tables

List of Charts

Abbreviations

ACORN	Association of Community Organizations for Reform Now
AVARD	Association of Voluntary Agencies in Rural Development
BDO	Block Development Officer
BPL	Below Poverty Line
CAARD	Report of the Committee to Review the Existing Administrative Arrangements for Rural Development
CAPART	Council for Advancement of People's Action and Rural Technology
CBR	Community Based Rehabilitation
CDPO	Child Development Project Officer
CHP	Community Health Programme
CINI	Child In Need Institute
CSP	Child Sponsorship Programme
DOT	Direct Observation Treatment
DPP	Disaster Preparedness Programme
FAIR	Foundation to Aid Industrial Recovery
FEVORD-K	Federation of Voluntary Organizations in Rural Development in
GP	Gram Panchayat
GSS	Gram Seva Sangha
ICDS	Integrated Child Development Services
ICMR	Indian Council of Medical Research
IGTH	Income Generation Through Handloom
IMF	International Monetary Fund
INHP	Integrated Nutrition and Health Programme
MC	Microscopic Centre
MCH	Mother and Child Health
MHCS	Mobile Health Care Services
MHD	Mother's Health Day

MO	Medical Officer
NACAA	National Association of Community Action Agencies
NACPC	National Advisory Committee for Public Co-operation
NAH	National Alliance to End Homelessness
NCCED	National Congress for Community Economic Development
NGOs	Non-Governmental Organisations
NIPCCD	National Institute of Public Co-operation and Child Development
PHI	Peripheral Health Institution
PRIA	Participatory Research in Asia
PU	Pre-University
RCH	Reproductive and Child Health
RHDC	Rural Health Development Center
RKLSP	Ramakrishna Mission Lokasiksha Parishad
RSP	Rural Sanitation Programme
RTI	Reproductive Tract Infections
SEVA	Society for Equitable Voluntary Action
SF	School Final
SHG	Self-Help Group
SHIS	Southern Health Improvement Samity
STD	Sexually Transmitted Disease
TC	Treatment Centre
TCP	Tuberculosis Control Programme
THR	Take Home Ration
TRYSEM	Training of Rural Youth for Self Employment
UNICEF	United Nations International Children's Emergency Fund
VLV	Village Level Volunteers
VOs	Voluntary Organizations
WB	West Bengal
WBVHA	West Bengal Voluntary Health Association
WCPMMP	Women in Cultivation, Processing and Marketing of Medicinal Plants
WEP	Women Empowerment Programme
WHO	World Health Organization

PART I

Conceptual Framework

1

Introduction

CONCEPT OF WELFARE STATE AND ITS EMERGENCE

The term 'Welfare State' evokes images of people receiving handouts from the public dole. Sometimes, it gives impression of wasteful government programmes and undeserving recipients who are content to accept public alms rather than work for their livelihood. K.V. Narayana (1991) writes, 'Welfare State' would control social and economic crisis in terms of mass unemployment, fall in production, political unrest, etc., through investment in infrastructural development, health care, education and other programmes for social integration. In fact, the "Welfare State" commits itself to ensuring, within the framework of a mixed economy, a minimum level of welfare for its citizens by enacting employment, social insurance and public assistance policies (Rudolph, 1997).

It is difficult to pinpoint when the modern welfare state first began to emerge. Otto Von Bismarck introduced workman's compensation programmes in Germany during the eighteen seventies. Sweden embarked on its path toward a social welfare system during World War I. However, in most democratic and capitalist countries, the movement toward welfare capitalism received its impetus from the hardships of the Great Depression during the nineteen thirties. In United States, Presidents like Franklin D. Roosevelt, Lyndon B. Johnson, etc. wanted to follow this path through war on poverty. The War on Poverty included few policies such as Project Head Start for educationally deprived youth, the establishment of a domestic Peace Corps for poverty zones in the inner cities and Appalachia, a retraining programme for the unskilled, a Medicare programme to guarantee health care for the elderly, and a Medicaid system to make health care more available to the poor. The United States, indeed, tended to develop its welfare state on a highly incrementalist and piecemeal basis. Conversely, most European countries embraced the concept of an integrated social welfare state that was committed to a comprehensive attack on inequality and inequities through a wide range of services that were universally available to all citizens. Perhaps the most famous blueprint of this kind was the Beveridge Plan that was developed in Great Britain in 1942 in order to combat the basic hardships of poverty, squalor, and disease in British society (Brown, 1995).

In the Western world, since the nineteen thirties, the question has not been whether a welfare state should be established but how extensive the welfare state should be and how direct the government should work in ensuring the welfare of its citizens. There was a great difference among the welfare states in the west in structuring programmes (Rudolph, 1997).

As in Western countries, India believed in the same philosophy and was declared as 'Welfare State' after independence and its constitution laid down the obligations of the state in the Directive Principles of the State Policy. Welfare of the people became the responsibility of the state. Institutionalization of social services became the hallmark of Welfare State and investments were made in a number of the state sponsored welfare programmes for the weaker and vulnerable sections of the society. The state monopolized the social service sector and was largely its sole patron (Srivastava, 1999).

The first three decades after World War II, the concept of Welfare State was implemented in many countries for postwar recovery and full employment economies. The Welfare State became concerned with relative deprivation as well as absolute poverty in their efforts to create more egalitarian societies. By the late nineteen seventies, there was a growing acceptance that the Welfare State was on the decline. For instance, in Great Britain, the contradiction of national insurance and the widening scope of means tested benefits clearly indicated that Beveridge's universalism was under considerable strain. The failures of economic management raised the question of ability of any government to secure the stable growth in the economy that seemed necessary to fund adequate health and social services. Answer, in order to save the economic illness, was rolling back of the state. In Britain, some of the policies such as the privatization of public utilities or the reduction of local government responsibilities seemed an attack on the state (Brown, 1995).

DECLINE OF WELFARE STATE AND GENESIS OF NGOs

In the beginning of the nineteen eighties, several developed and developing countries started thinking of privatization, liberalization and withdrawal of state from the social sector programmes like education, health, nutrition, etc. Because there was a movement that the state was incapable of tackling the problems of neglected and vulnerable groups of society (Bhambhri, 1987). Many Third World countries who were facing balance of payment problems, reduced their budget from social sector and started taking loan from International Monitory Fund (IMF) and World Bank (WB) for the survival of the country's economy. During the implementation of IMF and WB's programme, an understanding was developed that investment in public sector was wasteful and therefore the emphasis on Non-Governmental Organizations (NGOs) was better. It was assumed, where government failed to reach out to the marginalized sections and created gap, NGOs could bridge the same.

Since the beginning of nineteen eighties, the activities of NGOs have been growing worldwide in terms of their size and scope, their number and volume of aid. It has often been argued that this new popularity of NGOs is due to their specific characteristics such as: (a) flexible and experimental interventions due to their small size and learning process approaches; (b) their low costs and effective work at the grass roots level especially in remote areas; (c) their relationship with the beneficiaries is based on voluntarism which is the main factor allowing NGOs to achieve meaningful participation; (d) furthermore, NGOs recruit highly qualified and motivated staff on the basis of shared values and a belief in the social mission of the NGOs (Vahlhans, 1994; Baru, 1998; Rajasekhar, 2000).

In order to perform the task at the international level, NGOs have also been given importance. They are recognized as highly organized and most influential networking groups. Because, in nineteen nineties, they have helped, in the preparatory phase of almost every major U.N. Conference, such as, Conference on Environment and Development in Rio in 1992. Human Rights Conference in Vienna in 1993, the Population Conference in Cairo in 1994, Conference on Social Development in Copenhagen in 1995, Conference on Women's Development in Beijing in 1995, etc. NGO is one of the few means that manages to maintain a common identity and an agenda from one UN Conference to another. It has become customary now that every official Global Conference will be flanked by an NGO Forum (Seth, 1997).

NGOs IN INDIA

In India, Voluntary Organizations (VOs) or Non-Governmental Organizations (NGOs) have a long history. In the nineteen and early twentieth century, on the one hand, the para-state organizations, mainly of the Christian Churches, came into existence to intervene in the social and religious life of the indigenous population through improvement of health, social welfare and social reform. On the other hand, as part of anti-colonial resistance, numerous indigenous organizations emerged to accelerate social and religious reform (Sheth & Sethi, 1996). In fact, more involvement and initiatives of NGOs have been occurring in India since late nineteen seventies. For instance, The Foreign Contribution Regulation Act (1976), The CAARD Report (1985) [Report of the Committee to Review the Existing Administrative Arrangements for Rural Development], The Seventh Five Year Plan (1985-1990), etc. motivated the NGO sector for country's all round development (Garain, 1994). At present, NGOs have become very crucial in the process of decentralization of power and development (Mathew, 1999). NGOs encourage the elected representatives to strengthen panchayats financially by collecting taxes, fees, etc. from the villages and educate the poor in attending the Gram Sabha meeting to make vibrant bodies [Rajasekhar (ed), 2000].

It is evident from the above discussion, in India today, NGOs have significant role in *Development.* Now it essential to know how or at what level NGOs are associated with 'Development'.

NGOs in Development

Development, being multifarious and multi-dimensional concept, is considered as a loaded term (Apter, 1981). It is a process of advancement in totality. An integrative view of development (Chart 1A) highlights that it includes all the socio-economic, politico moral and environmental aspects (Kaur, 1997). In other words, a minimum and balanced level of social security, health, education, employment, people's participation in political process, and economic advancement manifest the true notion of development whose ultimate goal is to attain a human society imbibing the social values of dignity, moral and civic character, social justice, democracy and cultural freedom.

Chart 1A: Development—An Integrated View

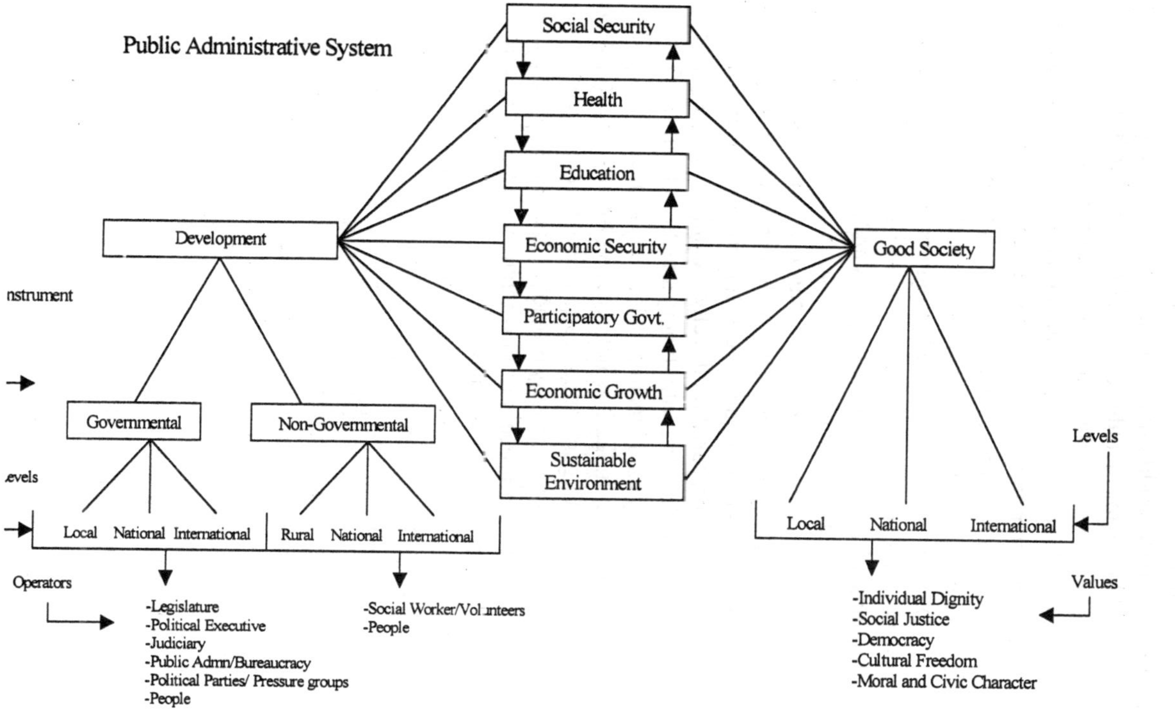

The process of this development involves different sectors in a society. According to P.D. Kulkarni (1984), there are four sectors: (a) the non-formal sector comprising of family, kith and kin and neighbourhood; (b) the market mechanism consisting of organized economy and the traditional unorganized segments of the economy; (c) the public sector includes civic and political institutions at local, state and national levels; and (d) the community sector which encompasses direct service, co-ordinating agencies and special interest groups. The community sector has the bulk of Voluntary Action.

The development process has three steps: (a) Formative—Aims and objectives of development are laid down or programmes are chalked out; (b) Distributive—To implement programmes in such a way that the services will be distributed among the people equally; (c) Sustainability—To ensure the longevity and regeneration of services.

The necessary ingredients of the successful development process in all the three steps are people's participation, commitment and dutifulness at work, economical use of resources and sharing liabilities as well as benefits on equitable basis. It is an assumption that unless a suitable ground is prepared for developmental process, any attempt to development will lead to contradictory situation (Kaur, 1997). Hence, there were so many conflicts in development process during 55 years of independence in India. It is believed, Voluntary Organizations or Non-Government Organizations can facilitate all the sectors in every step of development process by promoting the necessary ingredients.

In India, in the process of development, these NGOs play role carrying out various programmes, which are designed by their own or government, related to formal education, non-formal education, adult education, health care, social awareness, income generation training, low cost sanitation, safe drinking water, rural entrepreneurship development, computer training, agro-based training, green house, sustainable agriculture, plantation, mini saving, family counselling, legal aid for women, mahila mandal, khadi training and production, child labour, welfare for the handicapped, games and sports, aged welfare and so on (Sarkar, 2001).

NGOs in Health Care

Especially in the field of health care, NGOs have acquired a considerable importance in India since 1978 (Pattanaik, 1988). In that year, the Alma-Ala Conference, held under the joint auspices of the

WHO and the UNICEF, gave birth to a new approach in health care i.e. 'Primary Health Care Approach', which fixed a goal of 'Health For All By 2000 A.D.' That conference was proceeded by a joint study of the WHO and UNICEF for finding out alternative approaches to meet the basic health needs of the third world people. The study examined some of the isolated voluntary health projects in the third world countries like the Jamkhed in India. The conclusion drawn went strongly in favour of VOs/NGOs. At the same time, some assumptions went against the government health services i.e. the government health sector lacks infrastructural facilities, trained manpower, committed medical and para-medical personnel, and thus cannot be trusted to execute any goal oriented programme. In 1983, the National Health Policy also recognized the need for greater reliance on the voluntary and private sector for achieving the goals of 'Health For All By 2000 A.D.' (Duggal, 1988). In 1985, the Ministry of Health and Family Welfare was in full agreement with the Planning Commission on the issue of greater involvement of NGOs in the field of health care (Duggal, Gupta & Jesani, 1986). That time in a published document (Collaboration with NGOs in implementing the national strategy for health for all, GOI, New Delhi, 1985), it was categorically stated that the government had envisaged a very prominent role of VOs/NGOs in the implementation of health, family planning and 20-point programmes. In this regard, the World Development Report 1993—Investing in Health, which made a positive view regarding NGOs (The World Bank, 1993), cannot be ignored. It did influence the NGO sector of India for better provisioning of health services. National Population Policy (2000), which aims to bring down the fertility rate to replacement level by 2010 and to achieve a stable population by the year 2040, also focused on the Voluntary and Non-profit sectors for population control (Nampudakam, 2000).

We have discussed in the preceding paragraph how NGOs have been getting preference in health care in India. In fact, during last two and half decades, many NGOs have come into focus for their remarkable contribution in health care. For instance, 'Institute of Health Management Pachod' and 'Streehitakarini' in Maharashtra; 'Banwasi Sewa Ashram' in UP; 'Parivar Seva Sanstha' in Delhi; 'Society for Education Welfare and Action Rural' in Gujarat; 'Rural Unit for Health and Social Affairs' in Tamil Nadu; 'Child in Need Institute' and 'Tagore Society for Rural Development—Rangabelia Project' in West Bengal; etc. Each of these organizations is considered as model health care

NGO and has multi-dimensional activities like health awareness, clinical service, health care training, health research, etc. More or less, every state possesses this kind of NGO and also many grass roots level organizations who have limited health care activities.

NGOs in Health Care in West Bengal

The present study has been conducted to understand the NGOs in health care in West Bengal. The main reason for selecting West Bengal is its unique socio-political background, which is unlike other states. West Bengal has history of series of movements, such as, freedom movement, movement against social evils, tebhaga movement, naxalite movement, land reform of the Left Front Government, environmental movement, women's movement, etc. These movements led to form a large number of NGOs. At present, there are over 1,00,000 registered NGOs in West Bengal (as per the information of Society Registration Office, in the year 2000). According to experts, roughly over thirty per cent (i.e. over 30,000) NGOs exist only in papers and the remaining seventy per cent (i.e. 70,000) really operate in the field. Many experts are of the opinion that nearly ten per cent of these working NGOs (i.e. around 7,000 NGOs) carry out health care programmes in West Bengal. Nature of health care activity of a few NGOs can be mentioned in this regard.

Child in Need Institute (CINI), situated at South 24 Parganas District, was established in 1974. It aims at sustainable health and nutrition development for women and children. CINI has almost 350 workers who patiently listen, counsel, and provide care at the clinics, educational centres, and other outreach programmes. Workers are dedicated and ranging from semi-literate to highly qualified professional in medicine, nutrition, sociology, education and other allied fields. It initiates efforts for decentralization and community involvement with the formation and facilitation of women's groups around health issues. CINI works in close co-operation with NGOs like Voluntary Action Network India (VANI), Sishu Vikash Prachesta (SVP) and government body such as State Committee on Voluntary Action Training for NGO under Department of Health and Family Welfare, WB (CINI, 1998).

West Bengal Voluntary Health Association (WBVHA) came into being in 1974. It is a state level NGO federation that works in close association with the Government of West Bengal and other Non-Government Organizations, National and International Agencies in the field of health. More than 1,000 NGOs are connected with

WBVHA. It caters services through campaigns, policy research, press and assembly advocacy; through need based training and documentation services; through production and distribution of innovative health education materials in the form of print and audio-visuals, for a wide spectrum of users both urban and rural. WBVHA is committed to make health a reality for the distressed and under privileged people of WB on the principle of prevention, curative, promotive and rehabilitative aspects of health care (WBVHA, 1997).

Tagore Society for Rural Development—Rangabelia Project was initiated in 1975 to improve income level of the poor people to ameliorate the women status and to reduce people's health hazardous in Sundarban area of South 24 Parganas district. It is working in 9 blocks including 339 villages. It collects funds from state government, central government, foreign funding agencies, and internal sources. Its health programme is remarkable and provides service through 50 health workers frequent training programme, occasional awareness increasing camp at remote villages, mobile clinic, several sub-centres and rural hospital. Hospital is having modern treatment facility (X-ray and surgery opportunity) with medical professional and trained health manpower. Organization's preventive approach is highly appreciated. It could reduce water born disease in Sundarban area from 65 per cent in 1978 to 12 per cent in 1988 (Tagore Society for Rural Development—Rangabelia, 1995).

Ramkrishna Mission Lokasiksha Parishad (RKLSP) began its work in 1952 at Jadulal Mullick Road of North Calcutta. Later, in 1956-57, organization was shifted to its present campus Narendrapur of South 24 Parganas district. It has been working in 13 districts including 26 slums and 3,000 villages for agriculture development, health improvement, environment upgradation and income generation. Health improvement is done through environmental sanitation, family welfare and smokeless chullah programme. Environmental sanitation programme includes provision of safe drinking water; construction of low cost latrine and use of oral rehydration solution. From 1990 to 1998, RKLSP provided 2,45,167 low cost latrines, 21,535 smokeless chullahs, and 1,10,919 ORS packets. Family welfare is done through medical unit, which provides services like first aid, immunization, health check up, and medical advocacy (RKLSP, 1998).

Ananda Niketan, situated at Howrah district, was established in 1961 for social reconstruction and rural upliftment. At present, it has health, education, income generation training and savings programme.

Health programme includes health unit and sanitary mart scheme. Health unit is made of one co-ordinator and 12 health workers who provided general medical treatment to 14,000 people, advice to 300 pregnant mothers, immunization to 280 children and 275 mothers in 1997-98. Sanitary mart scheme brings awareness and provides equipments for construction of latrine to bring a massive decline of water borne disease (Ananda Niketan, 1998).

Gram Seva Sangha (GSS) began its work in 1949 under the leadership of late Sachindra Lal Kargupta and Hatthuba village of North 24 Parganas district. Mr. Kargupta was in jail for 16 years and on return from jail, he founded this organization for rural development and financial rehabilitation of the refugees from East Pakistan. Now GSS works in 520 villages through various programmes like mass education, community centre, health service and family welfare, training programme, low cost housing, family counselling centre, working women's hostel and so on. Health and family welfare programme has different wings, such as, allopathic charitable dispensary, maternity home, immunization centre and first aid booth through which respectively 504, 61, 1,547 and 1,465 people were benefited in 1997-98 (GSS, 1998).

Society for Equitable Voluntary Action (SEVA) has been working since 1985 in North 24 Parganas through village level groups or clubs. It operates in 40 villages under 4 blocks where only group or club members get benefit. It has a health unit with Homoeopathic and Allopathic intervention for mother and childcare. Popularization of indigenous systems of medicine, smokeless oven making, low cost toilet construction, etc. are some other aspects of health intervention. "Prevention is better than cure" is the basic philosophy of SEVA's all the health programmes. In 1993-94, SEVA provided health benefit to 5,775 people through Homoeo clinic and 456 people through Allopathic clinic (SEVA, 1994).

Tajmohol Gram Vikash Kendra situated at Howrah district, is working with 31 villages. It has a well known Mother and Child Care centre. It is also associated with clinics, awareness generation, immunization programme, eye operation, and blood donation camp.

Ashurali Gram Unnayan Parishad, of South 24 Parganas, established in 1975, is dedicated for exploited neglected and poor rural women. It works in 27 villages with almost 39,000 people. This organization celebrates Mother's day once in a month where discussion is initiated on child health. It runs immunization programme and clinic in six villages.

Gospel Home started working in Hoogly district in the year 1976. It covers 3 blocks including 200 villages where about 30,000 to 40,000 people are benefited both directly or indirectly through its services. It has mother and child health clinic, dental clinic and eye clinic. MCH clinic is run on every Monday and Friday for ante-natal care and post-natal care. In 1993, 13,438 children and 6,313 mothers were benefited from the MCH clinic. Dental clinic and eye clinic is respectively run on every Friday and Tuesday. In 1993, total 765 patients were benefited from dental clinic (Gospel Home, 1993).

We, from the above discussion, understand that many NGOs in West Bengal assist in health status development through rural hospital, regular health clinic, occasional health camp at remote area, awareness programme regarding prevention of disease, training of health workers, etc. Hence, initiating indepth study to understand the relative position of NGOs in providing health care vis-à-vis state in West Bengal is meaningful and realistic. In this regard, the next chapter will illuminate the relevant literature related to the research area.

REFERENCES

Ananda Niketan. 1998. *Annual Report.* Bagnan

Apter, D.E. 1981. *Introduction to Political Analysis.* Prentice Hall of India Pvt. Ltd., New Delhi, pp. 456 to 57.

Baru, R. 1998. 'Structural Adjustment and Health: Changing Role of NGOs' *Paper Presented at International Seminar on Global Governance and Social Policy.* Baltic Sea Centre: Kellokeski.

Bhambhri, C.P. 1987. 'The Modern State and Voluntary Societies.' *The Indian Journal of Public Administration.* Vol. XXXIII, No. 3, pp. 395 to 398.

Brown, J. 1995. *The British Welfare State.* Blackwell: Oxford.

Child in Need Institute (CINI). 1998. *Annual Report.* Joka.

Duggal, R. Gupta, M. Jesani, A. 1986. *NGOs in Rural Health Care.* FRCH: Mumbai.

Duggal, R. 1988. 'NGOs, Government and Private Sector in Health' *EPW.* March 26, pp. 633 to 636.

Garain, S. 1994. 'Government—NGO Interface in India: An Overview'. *The Indian Journal of Social Work.* Vol. 55(3), pp. 337 to 345.

Gospel Home. 1993. *Annual Report.* Hoogly.

Gram Seva Sangha (GSS). 1998. *Annual Report.* Habra.

Kaur, I, 1997. 'Role Perspective of NGOs in Development: Priority Areas'. *Non-Governmental Organizations in Development: Theory and Practice.* Kanishka Publishers: New Delhi, pp. 87 to 97.

Kulkarni, P.D. 1984. *Voluntary Action—The Myth and Reality.* NIPCCD: New Delhi. p. 4.

Mathew, G. 1999. 'Decentralized Institutions—Governmental and Voluntary Sector.' *'Economic and Political Weekly.'* February 27, p. 529.

Narayana, K.V. 1991. 'Political Economy of State Intervention in Health Care.' *Economic and Political Weekly.* Vol. 26(42), pp. 2427 to 2433.

Nampudakam, M. 2000. 'Views on the Population Policy.' *Health for the Millions.* January February, p. 8.

Pattanaik, S. 1988. "Voluntarism and Development—A Social Science Focus on Health." *M. Phil Dissertation.* Centre for Social Medicine and Community Health, School of Social Sciences, Jawaharlal Nehru University, New Delhi.

Ramkrishna Mission Loksiksha Parishad (RKLSP). 1998. *Annual Report.* Narendrapur.

Rajasekhar, D. 2000. "Non-Governmental Organizations (NGOs) in India: Opportunities and Challenges". *Journal of Rural Development.* Vol. 19 (2), pp. 249 to 275.

Rajasekhar, D. (ed.). 2000. *Decentralized Government and NGOs—Issues, Strategies and Ways Forward.* Concept: New Delhi.

Rudolph, J.R. 1997. "The Welfare State". *International Encyclopedia of Economics, Vol. 2.* Fitzroy Dearborn Publishers: London.

Sarkar, A. 2001. "Development Through NGOs in Barak Valley: A Critical Analysis." *Social Action.* Vol. 51, January to March, pp. 61 to 73.

Seth, P. 1997. "An Overview of Non-Governmental Agencies and Their Functions" *Non-Governmental Organizations in Development: Theory and Practice.* Kanishka Publishers: New Delhi.

Sheth, D.L. & Sethi, H. 1996. "The NGO Sector in India: Historical Context and Current Discourse." *Development Policy and Administration.* Sage: New Delhi, pp. 281 to 301.

Society for Equitable Voluntary Action (SEVA). 1994. *Annual Report.* Kolkata.

Srivastava, S.P. 1999. "Nature of Voluntary Action in India Today: A Critique." *Social Action.* January to March, pp. 1 to 14.

Tagore Society for Rural Development. 1995. *Annual Report.* Rangabelia.

The World Bank. 1993. *World Development Report 1993—Investing in Health.* Oxford University Press: Oxford.

Vahlhans, M. 1994. "The New Popularity of NGOs—Will the Enthusiasm Last." *D + C Development and Co-operation.* May-June, pp. 20-22.

West Bengal Voluntary Health Association (WBVHA). 1997. *Annual Report.* Kolkata.

2

Overview of NGOs

A Review of Relevant Literature

In this chapter efforts have been made to review thoroughly the literature pertinent to the research topic and research setting. Researcher tries here to understand the basic argument between the concepts of Voluntary Organization (VO) and Non-Governmental Organization (NGO), various types of NGOs, its rise in India and available research studies pertaining to NGOs. The main objective is to bring to fore the contradictions, plurality and trends that exist among the NGOs and to throw light on the studies carried out and the conclusions that were drawn from them. It can give an insight into the research problem and help in establishing a meaningful rationale for the present study.

VO AND NGO: A CONTRADICTION

Very often 'Voluntary Organization' and 'Non-Governmental Organization' are used as interchangeable terms. But such usage is not correct, as there is a contradiction between these terms with regard to definition.

Concept of VO

The term 'Voluntarism' is derived from the Latin word '*Voluntas*' which means 'Will'. Thus, voluntary organization may be an association to fulfil the will of its members due to material, moral or intellectual inequality in society. A number of definitions of VO have been put forth by scholars from different disciplines.

Bourdillon (1945) remarks that voluntary organization is the product of the blood, sweat and toil of a few individuals, who are known for their persistent efforts for achievement of their sincere aspirations.

Michael Banton (1968), an anthropologist, characterized it as a group organized for the pursuit of one interest or of several interests in common. Usually, it is contrasted with involuntary groups serving a greater variety of ends, such as kin groups, castes, social classes and communities.

David L. Sills (1968), a sociologist, identified it as a group of persons, organized on the basis of voluntary membership without state control, for the furtherance of some common interest of its members. Sills excluded three types of similar associations: (i) making living associations (like business firms, trade associations, labour unions, marketing and consumer co-operatives, professional associations, etc.); (ii) religious organizations; and (iii) political parties.

Smith and Freedom (1972) considered voluntary association as a structure that is formally organized, relatively permanent, secondary grouping as opposed to less structured, informal ephemeral or primary grouping. Formal organization, they said, is identified by the presence of officers, which are filled through some established procedures, scheduled meetings, qualifying criteria for membership and some formalized division and specialization of labour, although the organizations do not necessarily exhibit all these characteristics to the same degree.

According to Lord Beveridge (1979), a voluntary organization, properly speaking, is an organization, where its workers are paid or unpaid, governed by its own members without external control. Definition given by Mary Morris and Modeline Roff are also similar. The only addition is that voluntary organization should depend upon at least some voluntary resources.

Norman Johnson (1981) examined the definition of voluntary organization based on the following factors, such as: (i) Method of formation, which is voluntary on the part of a group of people; (ii) Method of government, with self-governing organization to decide on its constitution, its serving, its policy and its clients; (iii) Method of financing, with at least some of its revenues drawn from voluntary sources; and (iv) Motives with the pursuit of profit excluded.

Professor N.R. Inamdar (1987) says, a voluntary organization in development to be of durable use to the community has to nurture a strong desire and impulse for community development among its members, to be economically viable, to possess dedicated and hard working leadership and to command resources of expertise in the functions undertaken.

Harold Laski, an eminent British political scientist, defined 'Freedom of association' as a recognized legal right on the part of all persons to combine for the promotion of purposes in which they are interested (Sachdeva, 1993).

On the basis of above discussion of the concept of VO, it can be defined as "an organized group in order to promote some common interest of its members and it is voluntary, self-governing, self-financing, and non-profit in its orientation". Here, 'Voluntary' refers to spontaneous initiative of the organization for addressing social and economic inequality. This does not refer to whether workers will be paid or unpaid. On the principle the salary of the staff in voluntary organization is lower than outside as "Voluntarism" concept is attached with it. "Self-governing' indicates that the decision for the organizational constitution, policy and services is not within the domain of state control. 'Self-financing' refers at least some of its revenues drawn from voluntary sources. "Non-Profit" means the motive of the members will be the welfare of the public and profits will be used to strengthen as well as to fulfil the objectives of the organization.

Concept of NGO

Cumper (1986) describes NGOs as organizations not mainly financed by governments and not under the control of governments. It stresses on the sense of distance from the state.

Tongsawate and Tips (1988) define NGO as a non-profit, non-government, private group, at least partially formalized into an organization, that an individual joins by choice.

Duggal (1988) defines NGOs in his study. According to him, (a) NGOs are registered as public trusts or societies; (b) Programmes adopted by NGOs are welfare programmes and many a time it is government funded rural development programmes; (c) NGOs as a rule do not generate their own funds completely but rely on external financial assistance from government agencies, both national and international; (d) NGOs are private organizations, but their nature makes them somewhat different from what one gradually refers to the private sector. Thus, they are not supposed to make any profit.

According to Smith (1989), NGOs are having legal independence from government, a non-profit status and a voluntary decision making structure.

Maxine Weisgrav (1997) notes in her excellent study that NGO is a term used rather loosely to refer to any organization that is not a direct division of a national government.

D. Rajasekhar (2000) examines the term NGO that undertakes voluntary action, social action and social movements. According to him, four characteristics make the NGOs as distinct organizations. These are: voluntary formation, working towards development and amelioration of suffering, working with non-self serving aims, and relative independence. He admits that these NGOs work within the parameters of government legislations and policies formulated for them (Marthy and Rao, 1997).

In general many people feel, Non-Governmental Organizations are those, which are not government organizations. Thus, this can consider private firm, company or welfare society. It may be profit making or non-profit organization. Hence, it is better to say GOG (Group Outside Government) instead of NGO.

Actually, there is no clear definition as to what precisely constitutes an NGO, and considerable differences exist from country to country. In some countries, instead of NGO, people call it as "Private Voluntary Organization (PVO)," "Voluntary Organization" and "Charitable Organization." Although such inter-country differences are, for the purpose of setting internal government policy, not important, it is important that within a country at least a workable definition is adopted and adhered to. As working definition, in the present study, we can assume, "NGO is voluntarily formed and registered organization working towards development and amelioration of suffering with non-self serving aims and free from the state control in managing day to day affairs".

Distinction between VO and NGO

An effort is being made here to distinguish VOs from NGOs. Firstly, VOs are non-profit organizations, small in size and run outside the domain of the state control; but NGOs are a later phenomenon. There is a relationship between the state and welfare NGOs. It is a fact that NGOs are non-profit organizations but provide welfare services sometimes as a part of or on the behest of Government and sometimes outside it. Secondly, various above-mentioned definitions of voluntary organizations given by sociologists never talk about registration. Voluntary Organizations existed without any legal status before passing Societies Registration Act of 1860. But registration is must for an NGO. Actually registration becomes necessary when an organization starts accepting public grants or government money. Thirdly, in Voluntary Organization, Voluntarism exists. Volunteers initiate activities with selfless motive and many times it is done without remuneration or with a very little remuneration. But NGOs emphasises on professionalism. They use professionals from all walks of life for massive and rapid social development. Since professionals do not believe in voluntarism due to their professional ethics, NGOs are reluctant to provide voluntary service. This is proved in the history of the voluntary sector after 1976 (Foreign Contribution Regulation Act was passed). In Assam, it is found (Sarkar, 1998), there are some societies who consider themselves as voluntary organizations due to the voluntary nature of their activities and resent for being treated as NGOs. Distinction made in this paragraph is not enough. More researches need to make it clear. Many a time, these two terms (VO and NGO) are used as same meaning.

In fact, these NGOs are not involved in the same kind of activities. Very few similarities are found among them. They differ in terms of size, form, orientation, ideological affinity, resources and target groups (Vahlhans, 1994; Baru, 1998). Hence, it is important to explore various types of NGOs.

TYPES OF NGOs: A VARIATION

Various types of classification of NGOs are found in literature. V.G. Nandedkar (1987) classifies NGOs into ten categories. (i) *Individual Practice of Dharma*—This covers individual's services to the needy; (ii) *Religious Institutions*—This category includes temples/churches or similar institutions engaged in activities—development in nature; (iii) *Individual Based Philanthropic Activities*—These cover a vital sector of social and cultural life; (iv) *Social Service and Cultural Associations*—These are non-political in nature and work through the socio-cultural ethos of the system; (v) *Professional and Consultancy Associations*—They extend advice, guidance and help in their specialized fields; (vi) *Functional Associations*—These express in unambiguous terms the interests of their members and endeavours to protect the same; (vii) *Front-Line Associations*—Political parties look to these associations as recruitment grounds, e.g. Kisan Sabha, Khedut Samaj, etc.; (viii) *Action Groups*—These groups are involved in mobilization and socialization of unorganized sections of society; (ix) *Protest Groups*—These groups are like action groups, with or without political affiliation; (x) *Citizen Groups*—These associations develop secular interests with community life and encourage interaction with administration. For instance, Grahak Panchayat, Consumers Education Centre, Citizens Council, etc.

Korten (1990) classifies NGOs as per strategies of development. He states four types of NGOs i.e. Relief & Welfare Organization, Community Development Organization, Sustainable Systems Development Organization and People's Organization.

Green and Matthias (1997) have classified NGOs in the context of 'Operational area' and 'Activities.' As per operational area, NGOs are of three types, such as, Community-Based NGO, National NGO, and International NGO. Based on activities, six types of NGOs are identified. They are: service oriented NGO, research NGO, supportive NGO, NGO for policy advocacy, funding NGO and co-ordinating NGO.

According to D. Rajashekhar (2000), NGOs are of four categories, such as, Operational or Grassroots NGOs, Support NGOs, Network NGOs and Funding NGOs. *Grassroots NGOs* directly work with the oppressed sections of society. It is, again, of four types: 'Charity and Welfare NGOs' which focus on providing Charity and Welfare to the poor, 'Social Action Groups' focus on mobilizing marginalized sections around specific issues, 'Development NGOs' focus on implementation of concrete development activities, and 'Empowerment NGOs' combine development activities with issue based struggle. *Support NGOs* provide services that would strengthen the capacities of grassroots NGOs, Panchayati Raj Institutions, cooperatives and others to function more effectively. Examples of this type of NGOs are SOSVA, SEARCH, etc. *Network NGOs* are formal associations or informal groups of grassroots and/or Support NGOs, which meet periodically on particular concerns. An example to this is FEVORD–K (Federation of Voluntary Organizations in Karnataka). *Funding NGOs* are those who extend financial assistance to the grassroots NGOs, Support NGOs or people's organizations. For instance, CRY, Dorabji Tata Trust, Aga Khan Foundation, etc.

Having understood the above types of classification of NGOs, the present study has preferred to group NGOs of West Bengal into five categories i.e. religious organizations, service organizations, development organizations, research and consultancy agencies, and action groups.

In general, in India, these NGOs have been increasing in numbers by leaps and bounds over the years. They have turned out to be a cogent catalytic force in the country's development pursuits and can no longer be ignored by any quarters (Raj, 1996). A brief picture of 'Rise of NGOs in India', in this context, can give much more information on how NGOs are becoming important in this country.

RISE OF NGOs IN INDIA

It may be discussed in two phases i.e. before independence and after independence. There is plurality in terms of ideology, motivation and type of organizational form during both these periods.

Before Independence

The efforts and initiatives towards welfare and developmental activities, which originated outside the state structure and within society, came into prominence during the colonial period. The agents of these activities would be called 'Voluntary Organizations' and today we treat them as 'Non-Governmental Organizations'. With regard to rise of these organizations, three major landmarks are found before independence.

During the Early British Rule, i.e. in the eighteenth century (1707 A.D. to 1800 A.D.), the Christian Churches initiated welfare activities by establishing educational institutions, hospitals, dispensaries to serve the non-convert majorities both among the Hindus and Muslims. English educated natives, affluent businessmen, traders and members of aristocracy extended their support in this respect (Inamdar, 1987).

The second shift took place during (1801 to 1904) the Social Reform Movement. Numerous indigenous organizations devoted to social and religious reform emerged. A number of Social Reformers like R.R. Roy, K.C. Sen, M. Phule, S. Banerjee, M. Karve, etc. from different parts of the country founded organizations during the late nineteenth century. For instance, Raja Ram Mohun Roy began 'Brahmo Samaj' in 1828 to shake the belief of orthodox Hindus by opposing child marriage and propagating widow remarriage. Keshab Chandra

Sen advocated inter-caste marriage, widow remarriage and removal of the *Purdah* system. He campaigned against untouchability and founded 'The Good Will Fraternity Society' and 'The Calcutta Evening School.' Mahatma Phule established 'Satya Shodhak Samaj' in 1873 to fight against untouchability. Swami Dayananda Saraswati formed 'Arya Samaj' in 1875 to work against idol worship, child marriage and caste discrimination. The 'Indian National Congress' was established in 1885 keeping in view the objectives of National Development. Sasipada Banerjee founded 'The Home for Hindu Widow' in 1887 to reduce women sufferings and to perform a number of widow remarriages. Pandit Ramabai opened 'Sarada Sadan,' a home for Hindu Widows, in 1889 at Bombay (presently named as Mumbai). Maharishi Karve started 'The Hindu Widows Home' at Poona in 1896 for education and rehabilitation of widows. Swami Vivekananda, the disciple of Ramakrishna Parmahansa, made lasting contribution by establishing 'Ramakrishna Mission' in 1897 at Calcutta in order to provide food and famine relief; health and educational facility; etc. Behramji Malbari started 'Seva Sadan Society' in Bombay to look after destitute women and children (Lalitha, 1975).

The third trend emerged during the days of the National Movement (from 1905 to 1946). As a result of this movement, patriotism, nationalism, Swadeshi spirit, a deep faith in the power and wisdom of the common people came into existence and the same led to form a few organizations. For instance, Gokhale formed 'The Servants of India Society' in 1905. The approach of the society was secular and it sought to solve the national and social problems on a rational basis. It engaged itself in improving the condition of women, problems of untouchability, establishing cooperative enterprises and rendering relief work. Mahatma Gandhi founded the 'Harijan Sevak Sangh' and 'All India Village Industries Association' to uplift the Harijans and economically poor people. As a result of Gandhiji's effort, a number of voluntary agencies like 'All India Women's Conference,' 'Indian Adult Education Association,' 'Balken-ji-Bari,' 'Bharatiya Depressed Classes League' came into existence (Lalitha, 1975).

After Independence

As a result of exploitation, by the British imperial policies, alternative protection and state initiated welfare were necessary soon after Independence in India. The first Prime Minister of India, late Pandit

Jawaharlal Nehru, assured before the Constituent Assembly, on the eve of the country's independence, that the state would strive to eliminate poverty, ignorance, disease and inequality of opportunity (Rao, 1999). Hence, Constitution was made and Five Year Plans were started. The Plans took into consideration the available resources, prioritized different development programmes and made adequate provisions for social welfare services. The first two Plans primarily emphasized on the role of the state to provide welfare services. In the Sixth Plan there was a shift towards a more prominent role for NGOs. The rise of NGOs during different Plans can be understood from the following discussions.

During the period of the First Five Year Plan, the central government established the Central Social Welfare Board in 1953 under the Ministry of Social Welfare with the objective of providing financial assistance, coordination, training, technical guidance and consultancy to the NGOs engaged in activities for women and children. In order to reach out to the local NGOs and to release funds in time, the Central Social Welfare Board established state level Social Welfare Advisory Boards (Lalitha, 1975). During that time National Institute of Public Co-operation and Child Development (NIPCCD) was established to promote NGOs in the country. NIPCCD concentrated in the area of training voluntary workers supporting NGO activities and promoting liaison between government and NGOs (Garain, 1994). First Five Year Plan allocated four crores of rupees for the voluntary sector.

During the Third Five Year Plan NGO action was considered as an aspect of public cooperation. The National Advisory Committee for Public Cooperation (NACPC), which came into existence in 1952, had representatives during Third Plan mostly from National NGOs. As the public cooperation got institutionalized, NACPC gradually lost its credibility in the eyes of small and comparatively new NGOs (Roy, 1987).

In the Sixth Five Year Plan, NIPCCD, which came into existence during the First Plan, drastically changed its focus and had become the apex body for training functionaries and to co-ordinate, monitor, evaluate the Integrated Child Development Services Scheme of Government of India. Involvement of NIPCCD in the area of Public Cooperation and NGOs had become minimum at that time (Garian, 1994). From the middle of the Sixth Plan, there were a number of initiatives at the Government of India level to establish consultative group of voluntary agencies in each state under the chairmanship of either the Chief Secretary or the Development Commissioner. But it could not be success and the move on creating consultative committees of NGOs at the state level met a natural death (Garain, 1994).

In the Seventh Plan, for the first time, NGOs were given the freedom to plan their own schemes and follow the methodology they thought best to tackle poverty in villages they were working in (Roy, 1987). During that period (in 1986) the Council for the Advancement of People's Action and Rural Technology (CAPART) was created to seek an integrated approach to Rural Development through NGOs. CAPART was promoted as an autonomous organization under the Union Ministry of Rural Development. People and NGOs, who were engaged in rural development activities, were members of governing body and general body of CAPART (Garain, 1994). During that period, a proposal was made and linked with the Seventh Plan document to establish a council for rural voluntary agencies and code of conduct through an act of parliament. But this created a lot of debate in the NGO sector and the issue was dissolved gradually (Garain, 1994). Regarding health, in the Seventh Plan, Union Ministry of Health and Family Welfare considered following schemes for releasing funds to the Voluntary Organizations:

(i) Scheme for improvement of Medical Services for expansion/ improvement of hospitals under voluntary Organizations/ associations those are operating in rural or urban areas;
(ii) Promotion and development of Voluntary Blood Donation Programme;
(iii) Special Health Schemes for setting up of small hospitals/ dispensaries in rural areas only.

During 1989-90, grants amounting to Rs. 35.83 lakhs were granted to 27 institutions under scheme one and two above. For the third scheme, grants of Rs. 10.75 lakhs were given to four institutions (Government of India, 1990).

In the Eighth Five Year Plan, it was proposed that grants-in-aid would be given to the voluntary sector for innovative experimental schemes. In the field of health and family welfare, NGOs were expected to help in raising and promoting the small family norm by means of motivation and education of women, provision of antenatal and postnatal care, etc.

During the Ninth Plan, it has been realized that NGOs are actually complementary in nature. Both the sectors (Government and NGO) have their own strategy and strong points. Both the sectors are to work on a reciprocal basis.

Apart from the Five Year Plans, many government committees pertinent to development recognized the necessity of NGOs. The Balvantray Mehta Committee (1957), the architect of Panchayati Raj administration, emphasized the need for close cooperation and collaboration between statutory organizations and the NGOs. The Rural Urban Relationship Committee (1966) focused on the role of NGOs in mobilizing community support for local level development activities. It identified NGOs as linking organizations to keep constant and close contact with the people. The CAARD Report (1985) [Report of the Committee to Review the Existing Administrative Arrangements for Rural Development and Poverty Alleviation Programmes] had emphasized the need for the involvement of NGOs in rural development activities (Garain, 1994).

There are also a few acts and social policy those have been passed after independence and have extended avenues to the voluntary sector. For instance, the Income Tax Act 1965, the Foreign Contribution Regulation Act 1976, the National Health Policy 1983, etc. Under section 139 of the Income Tax Act 1965, every person (including societies, trusts and other legal persons) who during the previous year had an income that exceeds the maximum amount which is not chargeable to income tax is required to furnish a return of income to the income tax office before 30th June. Income, derived from property or donation or voluntary contribution, of an NGO, which is used for charitable purpose can be exempted from income tax. In order to get such benefit or exemption, NGO or charitable institution will have to get itself registered with the Commissioner of Income Tax within a period of one year from the date of its creation (Mathew, 1998). There were complaints from various quarters that some political parties, organizations and individuals were misusing the aid received from foreign countries. Hence, the Foreign Contribution Regulation Act 1976 was passed to regulate the acceptance and utilization of foreign contribution, scholarship and hospitality by certain persons and associations. This act permits voluntary organizations to receive funds from the government of a foreign country, international agencies specified by the Central Government, foreign companies, multinational corporations, trusts or societies or associations registered in a foreign country, foreign citizens, trade union in any foreign country, etc. As per this act, the necessary requirements for an NGO are: (a) it should be registered with the Central Government according to the rules; and (b) it should be agree to receive the foreign contribution only through one account in a bank specified in the application (Mathew, 1996). The National Health Policy 1983 recognized the need for greater reliance on the voluntary and private sectors for achieving the goals of 'Health For All By 2000 A.D.' Specifically it indicated: (a) the government has accepted its inability to provide adequate health care; (b) the active participation of the NGOs is most necessary for achieving goals of the health sector; and (c) 'Privatization' in the health sector will result in better provisioning of health services (Duggal, 1988).

The above mentioned discussions indicate that there is a growing popularity of NGOs in India. Now, in order to find out the research gap in NGO sector, it is worthwhile to examine the existing studies.

APPRAISAL OF PREVIOUS STUDIES

As far as published and unpublished documents are concerned, researcher has come across the following studies. These are conducted by scholars both in India and abroad. Studies on NGOs in development and especially on health are reviewed here.

Studies on NGOs in Development

Bourdillon (1945) made a survey of a small suburb of Tokyo. He found that there was a relationship between political leaders and their participation in voluntary associations. Those were associated with voluntary organizations, they took active part in politics.

Peter Rossi's (1945) study reveals voluntary association's integrative role. It evidences that government officials see voluntary associations as links between the government and the citizens.

Lalitha (1975) conducted a study on "Voluntary Work in India", which was published by NIPCCD (National Institute of Public Co-operation and Child Development), during the mid seventies. It investigated the status and role of voluntary personnel engaged in social welfare organization on an all India basis. The study covered 390 VO and 356 operational volunteers in nine cities of India, namely Delhi, Bombay, Madras, Bangalore, Ahmedabad, Hyderabad, Lucknow, Patna and Amritsar. The study examined in depth socio-economic profile of voluntary workers, nature of work they were engaged in, their motivations and aspirations connected with voluntary work, the policy and attitude of voluntary organizations towards the involvement of volunteers and difficulties encountered by voluntary agencies in matters of their recruitment, training, supervision and retention. The study made certain suggestions for increasing the effectiveness of volunteers in welfare services such as a new direction and orientation of voluntary work in view of the changed socio-economic conditions in the country, a fresh look by voluntary organizations at their policies and programmes of mobilizing volunteers to keep pace with the exigencies of the present situation, determining the role of volunteers and identifying their work areas, reviewing and redesigning methods and techniques of their recruitment, placement, supervision and development.

Robert C. Wirsing's (1977) study has proved one assumption, i.e. voluntary agencies are non-political, wrong. Their philosophy has always been extolled as "people" or "poor" oriented. In general, an idea has gained ground that these agencies serve the poor and downtrodden with rare dedication and commitment. The dirty world of "politics" never touches them, as they are beyond "politics". This view is not proven by facts. Wirsing's study of Nagpur shows clearly the close nexus between local politics and voluntary organizations.

Kapoor and Singh (1977) initiated a study on "Rural Development through NGOs" to encapsulate the history of the NGO movement in Himachal Pradesh starting from its inception till its present state. It included the governmental schemes as well as projects run by the NGOs and each NGO's structure, funding agencies, the success and failure of programmes, credibility amongst the local people, technological facilities, etc. The study admitted that NGOs could do very little in areas of massive action (with human and financial resources) required for development work. However, they were equipped to operate on a limited, demonstrative and pilot basis.

Charyulu and Natarajan (1980) conducted a case study in Cuddapah district of Andhra Pradesh. They reported that flexibility, personal touch, easy accessibility of service for the client groups, capacity to initiate the experiment with new programmes, stimulation and mobilization of resources of the community, sensitivity to field problem, self-help and self-reliance were the strong points of voluntary organizations. Voluntary organizations had terms of reference and enough resources to meet the needs of the whole man.

Tendler (1982) found that NGOs were often less successful than they thought they were reaching the poorest of the poor and instituting a participatory process. He indicated that what was termed, as 'innovation' by NGOs could be better described as replication of known techniques to previously unserved population.

Paul (1982) argues that successful projects adopt service strategies that are carefully tailored to the organization's external environment and systematically sustained by matching internal structures and processes. In other words, the emphasis is on congruence between what the project seeks to accomplish (goals and strategies), the context in which it operates (environment) and how it organizes itself to attain its goals (structures and processes). The concept of 'congruence' has many similarities with the concept of 'fit' as used by Korten (1980) to describe relationships between the organization, the programme and the beneficiaries.

Marcus Franda's (1983) study gathered information on a variety of organizations engaged in the field of rural development. Such organizations were "Social Work and Research Centre (SWRC)" at Tilonia (Rajasthan); JP's Musahri Project in North Bihar; AVARD (Association of Voluntary Agencies in Rural Development); etc. Study claimed that those voluntary initiatives were not grassroots efforts and did not represent local people's innate impulse to bring development. Interventions by outside experts, funds from the government and international agencies sustained the development efforts. Their long-term future would be uncertain and these were small "enclaves" in a vastly semi-feudal rural society.

Oakley and Dillon (1985), in a major study of NGOs in India, Bangladesh, Brazil and Ghana, point out that while NGOs were relatively successful in fostering participation of client groups, their ability to institutionalize these processes was weak. This weakness seems most marked in groups engaged in income generation activities. Collective spirit gets progressively eroded as the activity starts generating profits.

Bhatt (1988) has observed that there is a change in the profile of those who join NGOs. Earlier mostly retired persons would have been involved in relief, charity and welfare activities. Now younger people (both men and women) look towards the NGOs as a career option. The setting up of agencies like Foundation to Aid Industrial Recovery (FAIR), PRADAN, or the Institute of Rural Management at Anand, is indicative of the heightened interest of middle-class professionals in

NGOs. Equally significant is the banding together of young people locally under an NGO banner to attract funds for local/community advancement.

Garain (1993) made an effort to develop an instrument for measuring organizational effectiveness of NGO. The study was conducted in West Bengal. Having followed a systematic and exhaustive process, he identified eight dimensions and twenty-eight items. All the items had significant item-total correlation. Separate factor analysis of the items in respective dimensions was undertaken. The twenty-eight items scale yielded an interpretable structure. The instrument was consistent with the concept of Organizational Effectiveness used in the study.

Sachchidananda *et al.* (1994) have completed a study on 'Tribal Development and Voluntary Action' to review the activities of the Badlao Foundation in some districts of the 'Santhal Pargana Division' in Bihar. This organization has been working for more than ten years in the field of tribal development with assistance from the state government, central government and international donor agencies. Its main focus is on women's development, economic upgradation and supplementary service for education as well as health. The study has made an attempt to do a sympathetic assessment of the entire efforts in different fields and discover the constraints in various situations. Towards the end, a number of suggestions have been offered by the study to improve the situation and to streamline the work so that it becomes effective and fruitful.

Boyce (1994) finds, NGOs are key components of Community Based Rehabilitation (CBR). They forge relationships with other NGOs for networking purposes, and they have associations with donor organizations for funding purposes. He determines the key issues in these partnerships, their structure, dynamics and goal compatibility, in order to improve the ability of CBR NGOs to function effectively.

Kapoor (1995) carried out a research project on "Women and Welfare—A Study of Voluntary Agencies" in Punjab. The study made a historical survey of the status of women as determined or influenced, from time to time, by scriptural codes, social conventions, cultural traditions, political changes, economic and industrial development, constitutional provisions and humanistic ideas. It explored the changing nature and dimensions of voluntary action towards women welfare by understanding the working of four voluntary agencies—Association for Social Health in India, Bharatiya Grameen Mahila Samiti, Nari

Niketan, and Sewa Sadan—along with their ancillary units. The study brought out the points of strength and weakness of voluntary agencies and suggested ways so that they might be able to cope with the new challenges, in view of the changing roles and growing needs of women.

Ahlawat's (1995) study on "Women Organizations and Social Network", conducted in Haryana, was a comparative analysis of two women organizations across two different settings. It examined in detail the significant role played by social networks that operated in the functioning of the social organizations to accomplish desired goals as well as broader objectives. It also tried to focus attention upon how 'networks' would help individuals as well as organizations as a two way process of social exchange network.

A study made by the Committee for Economic Development (1995) strongly endorses that Community Groups (Non profit organizations) offer indispensable institutional and human resources, a knowledge of neighbourhoods and their problems, and the trust and participation of residents. Outside institutions (government, business) possess financial resources, technical knowledge and skills, and political power. Partnerships between these two complementary sources of strength represent the nation's best hope for revitalizing inner-city communities.

Johnson *et al.* (1996), through broad-based mail survey, studied the relationship between collaborating CBR NGOs, as well as relationship with other groups such as universities. The study focused on the effectiveness of umbrella organizations, their different characteristics, as well as the roles and responsibilities in existing linkages.

Uddin *et al.* (1996) made a study in Bangladesh, which dealt with the relationships between small NGOs, donors and government, and the NGO's abilities to effectively develop CBR. The study observed convergence and divergence of goals, differences in operational practices and personnel management and shifting from NGO "commitment" to "functionality".

Prasad's (1997) study on 'Voluntary Action and Rural Reconstruction' is an empirical endeavour to explore Gram Bharati's contribution, over 30 years, in translating the concept of Sarvodaya and Antodaya in the Gram Dan villages in selected parts of Bihar. Data for this work were collected from 90 villages under the constituency of Gram Bharati. The study finds that Gram Bharati has been doing its best in solving disputes, conflicts and violence by peaceful manner in the area. However, there is still much more needed to protect the indigenous (Adivasi) people from continued exploitation. The study suggests that the Gram Bharati can do two things for them (a) to check dispossession of adivasis by land grabbers from the plains; and (b) to restore the alienated land to the adivasis or restoring the lost land to them.

Rich *et al.* (1998) completed a study in order to develop a better understanding on relationship between Community Based Organizations (CBOs) [i.e. non-profit organizations] and City Governments who were involved to reduce poverty and revitalize neighbourhoods. A mail survey was conducted in summer 1998. The CBO mailing list was derived from the membership lists of four national associations of community based organizations: the National Alliance to End Homelessness (NAH), the National Congress for Community Economic Development (NCCED), the National Association of Community Action Agencies (NACAA), and the Association of Community Organizations for Reform Now (ACORN). A total of 2,110 survey schedules were sent to the mayors in 555 cities and to the executive directors of 1,555 CBOs located in those same cities. A total of 788 responses were received, resulting in an overall response rate of 37 per cent. The survey found, despite of many fundamental barriers, a large amount of city—CBO collaboration was occurring. The percentage of respondents reported collaborative city—CBO relationships varied across programme areas and by the type of respondent, but on balance the results indicated that a large percentage of cities and CBOs were working together regularly. The present study suggested further research to understand more the dynamics and determinants of these relationships in individual cities.

Sarkar (1998) has observed in his study that there is heterogeneity among the NGOs of Assam so far as their distribution, size, target groups, ideological philosophy, professional backgrounds, nature of services and so on are concerned. This kind of trend has serious consequences for accessibility, availability, and quality of services. The study shows, NGOs cannot be chosen, due to their non-uniformity, as means for implementation of any kind of social programmes (like health, education, etc.) since services will not reach to every one.

Seshagiri (1999) examined that neither too much nor too less importance should be given to the non-governmental activity. They are certainly significant as vital gap fillers and conduits between the governing and governed bodies. She concluded that the romances of

State-NGO inter relation and glorification of non-state intervention does not tell the true story of development. She argued, the NGO phenomenon is a reflection of organisational innovation to respond to shifting market trends and an assertion of the irreducible autonomy of individuals and communities, against an active state. But it is also a phenomenon of growing co-operation and partnership with the state.

Rao (2000) conducted a study among the NGOs involved in training the rural youth under TRYSEM. It examined that the trainees who received training from the NGOs were better employed than the others got trained in government and public institutions. NGOs took interest in arranging employment for their trainees while in government and public institutions once the training was over the trainees had to try for employment on their own. It was also found out that the facilities for training in some NGOs were much better than government and public institutions.

Manimekalai *et al.* (2000) have conducted a study in rural Tiruchirapalli to understand empowerment of women through self-help groups formed by NGOs. Study suggests: (a) a carefully drawn up training system has to address the strategic needs of rural women for survival, growth and sustainability; (b) The training system should be linked up with some kind of credit delivery mechanism whether formal or informal; (c) The group approach is the need of the hour to bring deprived women together for purpose of income generation or awareness creation; (d) The rural women would be helped to get into non-traditional activities through the provision of credit facilities and entrepreneurial skill development programmes. Researchers conclude that the government machineries neither create specific opportunities nor have specific programmes for empowerment of rural women. NGOs work effectively and efficiently to promote and encourage rural women entrepreneurs not only in traditional and feminine nature of products but also in non-traditional and non-feminine areas. NGOs should be given due importance.

The trafficking of Nepali women and girls, both within the Nepal and across the Indian border, is an ongoing human rights crisis that has received considerable interventional attention. NGOs and government agencies in the region have launched anti-trafficking interventions to raise community awareness as well as rescue women and girls from brothels, offer them counselling and care, and return them to their homes or train them in new vocational skill. To understand the different approaches of NGOs in anti-trafficking interventions, the

Asia Foundation and Horizons (2001) conducted a study. The study found significant disparity in the strategies and messages of different organisations. In the study, researchers interviewed ten Kathmandu-based NGOs, one local agency, and four key informants. Overall they found a lack of conceptual clarity and little understanding of human rights issues among many organizations. A few NGOs were confused between the trafficking with sex work and migration in search of income opportunities or a better life.

Wolleback *et al.* (2002) examined the impact of participation, in Voluntary Associations, on social capital using three dimensions—intensity (active *vs.* passive participation), scope (many *vs.* few affiliations) and type (non-political *vs.* political purpose). Those were affiliated with many associations, displayed higher levels of social capital than others. The difference between active and passive members was absent or negligible. The only cumulative effect of participation occurred when a member belonged to several associations simultaneously, preferably with different purposes. The authors demonstrated that active participation was necessary for the formation of social capital and suggested that more attention should be paid for passive and multiple affiliations with associations.

Studies on NGOs in Health

Pyle (1981) observes, under the Indian Constitution, health is not a basic human right. Yet, NGOs have used this rationale of social justice to target specific sub-population—the tribals, the Scheduled Castes, those are in slums, or those are the most poor in rural settings. NGOs have tried to achieve equity by identifying these disadvantaged and serving their needs. This rationale not only has focused NGOs efforts, but also gives them a cause for commitment.

Duggal, Gupta and Jesani (1986) conducted a study on "NGOs in Rural Health Care" at the behest of the Indian Council of Medical Research (ICMR) to gain a deeper insight into the role and functioning of the many different types of NGOs in the field of health located in Maharashtra, a state having the largest number of such agencies. That study brought out the largest variation between the aims and motivation of the various NGOs as well as their different approaches, which vary from the running of rural hospitals to community participation and conscientisation. That also brought out the change of approach of the NGOs during the past two decades from being more medical functionaries to involvement in community activities. An interesting finding of that study was that the NGOs had hitherto neglected socially and economically backward districts as compared to their better concentration in the average and highly developed districts in the state of Maharashtra. That highlighted the need to pay more attention to the deprived masses in the backward districts where infrastructure was highly underdeveloped.

American Public Health Association made an international study, which explored 180 health projects (31 in India) in the developing countries, and concluded that more detailed studies were necessary to understand the meaningfulness and feasibility of alternative low cost health projects (Duggal, Gupta and Jesani, 1986).

David Pyle's study of health projects in Maharashtra, undertaken for the Ford Foundation, had identified major factors that contributed to the success of different schemes (Duggal, Gupta, Jesani, 1986).

World Bank initiated study of 14 health, nutrition and family planning projects in India has summarized the work of these projects, highlighting the common as well as differential elements among them (Duggal, Gupta, Jesani, 1986).

Indian Institute of Management Ahmedabad (1987) conducted a comparative study among the NGO hospitals, Government hospitals and Private hospitals. It reported that, in general, the cost per hospital bed per day in the NGO sector was very less than the government and private sectors. The study suggested that NGOs might be relatively efficient providers of hospital-based care compared to others. In fact, NGOs often achieve substantial 'Cost Savings' due to lower pay scales compared to government employees and in some cases honorary physician services, both of which lead to a lower wage bill and lower overall cost. These are benefits not easily transferable to other institutions.

Baru (1987) made a study on 'Factors influencing variations in health services' in Andhra Pradesh. The study was limited in two well-developed districts (Krishna and Guntur) as well as two backward districts (Mehbubnagar and Medak). It considered public, private and voluntary sectors providing health services. With regard to voluntary sector, study explored that growth and distribution of voluntary agencies were skewed in favour of well-developed districts. The reasons for concentration of VOs in a particular area were many: (a) Well developed districts were under British rule and more number of hospitals as well as dispensaries were set up by Christian missionaries;

but backward districts were under Nizam's rule and very few hospitals were set up by missionaries; (b) In 1977, a severe cyclonic storm took place in Krishna as well as Guntur districts and hence there was a rapid growth of voluntary organizations for relief and rehabilitation work; (c) In the well-developed districts, infrastructural facilities were better for setting up VOs.

Duggal and Amin (1989) have made a study on 'Cost of Health Care'. Results indicate that the level of per capita health expenditures of NGOs is within the range of current government spending on primary health care. It is worth noting that in most cases, NGO projects function in addition to the normal government system. The similarity in average costs of NGO-provided services to those provided by government-funded primary health care suggests that these added resources are being used at least as efficiently as those in the public sector. This may reflect the unmet needs that are being met with additional NGO inputs.

The Ford Foundation has been engaged with NGO programmes in India since the 1970s. In order to systematically analyze, document and disseminate the experiences of NGOs implementing health and family planning programmes in India, it initiated a project in 1986. Under the project, twelve case studies, entitled ANUBHAV, were published. Each case study included details regarding the NGO i.e. genesis of the project and its evolution, its organizational structure, staffing pattern, funding and cost structures, the range and mode of service delivery, institutional relationships with the government and other institutions, community participation, information systems and programme impact. The lessons of these projects were shared with NGOs policy planners, researchers and donors (Pachauri, 1994). Based on these documented case studies (published in Anubhav Series) many scholars have given many interpretations. For instance, Peter Berman and Priti Dave (1994) point out that NGOs show a high degree of creativity and innovation in developing varied sources of financing to reduce dependency and enable them to sustain their programmes. Their health programmes operate as efficiently as public services and provide supplementary support rather than substitute services. They suggest further development of voluntary sector financing, which may reinforce overall health care intervention. Shanti Ghose (1994) observed that the innovation of a three-tiered structure of health services and the emphasis on comprehensive health care rather than on vertically targeted programmes were some of the factors behind the success of NGO projects. She suggested, such innovative strategies for training and programme implementation should be followed by the areas under government auspices. Rajesh Tandon (1994) studied the Anubhav Projects in order to know the nature of community participation in health. He suggested a policy framework in promoting effective community participation for better health in India. J.K. Satia (1994) noted that significant upscaling of community health programmes could take place through increased collaboration between NGOs and the government. Strengthening institutional capacity by learning from each other was the most important step in that direction.

Bhattacharjee (1996) has completed a study on "NGO Approaches to Health and Development in India: Strategies and Sustainability." He observes, in order to achieve appreciable and sustainable results, an NGO will have to make long-term commitments to the community. During its period of function, it may encounter difficulties, such as, (a) shortage of trained staff; (b) very high turnover rate of middle level staff due to low pay and uncertain future; (c) dependency on the donor agency; (d) rivalry, between the NGOs; and (e) too much interferences at the grassroots level by the political parties. Many of these problems however can be overcome if financial stability is achieved. To do so, it has to depend upon government, donors and internal resources (generated by itself). But the NGO cannot rely on the government or donor, since its activities might be controlled in the interest of the donor or the government. It would then become difficult to act as a pressure group. It will, therefore, have to generate its own funds. Such generation of funds can be done by increasing the number of pay clinics. The NGO then will become a channel to redistribute money from the rich to the poor.

The Population Foundation of India was established in 1970. It had either supported or itself commissioned around 320 projects. These projects included innovative studies, action research projects and training in family planning, maternal and child health and related areas. Many projects funded by the Foundation were not effective in the long run. Therefore, a qualitative evaluation of the action research projects was very necessary. The Population Foundation of India selected fourteen action research projects carried out by voluntary organizations during 1995-96 for the case study and qualitative evaluation. Main purpose was to assess the effectiveness of the NGOs in bringing about the desired changes in the individual and community value systems. Among the fourteen projects, three were related to infant mortality and fertility; three were pertaining to integrated health, family planning and development; four to reproductive health and family planning in urban slums; another three to reproductive health and family planning among industrial workers; and the remaining one to family planning through rural medical practitioners. Dr. Sunil Mishra (2000) brought together all the fourteen case studies (evaluation report) of action research projects in a volume and analysed the dynamics of social change, the factors that led to success and the problems. He found that NGOs could work as catalysts of change. A concern for community participation as well as a need for mass education, under an NGO, was very crucial to bringing about an attitudinal change in health behaviour.

In brief, this chapter has found, there is no doubt or confusion to understand the term VO but conflict arises for the concept of NGO. NGO is a relative term and hence always there is need to assume a working definition. The chapter has also noticed a plurality among the NGOs. They may be classified in terms of activities, philosophy or working approach, operational area and so on. Regarding rise of NGOs, it is clear that NGO is legacy of colonial system and its growth in independent India is very steady to reinforce the development process. Last part of the chapter has reviewed the existing studies on NGOs. It shows diversity among the research initiatives. Researcher finds there is no state level study in West Bengal with regard to NGOs in health care.

REFERENCES

Ahlawat, N. 1995. *Women Organizations and Social Networks.* Rawat Publications: New Delhi.

Baru, R. 1987. 'Factors Influencing Variations in Health Services—A Study of Selected Districts of Andhra Pradesh.' *M.Phil Dissertation.* Centre for Social Medicine and Community Health, Jawaharlal Nehru University, New Delhi.

Baru, R. 1998. 'Structural Adjustment and Health: Changing Role of NGOs'. *Paper Presented at International Seminar on Global Governance and Social Policy.* Baltic Sea Centre: Kellokeski.

Bhattacharjee, S. 1996. 'NGO Approaches to Health and Development in India: Strategies and Sustainability.' *M.A. Dissertation.* Prins Leopold Instituut Voor Tropische Geneeskunde: Belgiam.

Boyce, W. 1994. 'CBR NGO Relationships with Donors and the State.' *ICACBR.* Queen's University: Kingston.

Bourdillon, A.F.C. (ed.). 1945. *Voluntary Social Services: Their Place in Modern State*. Methuen: London. p. 104.

Berman, P. & Dave, P. 1994. 'Experiences in Paying for Health Care in India's Voluntary Sector.' *Reaching India's Poor—Non-Governmental Approaches to Community Health.* Sage: New Delhi.

Bhatt, A. 1988. *Development and Social Justice.* Sage: New Delhi.

Banton, M. 1968. 'Anthropological Aspects, Voluntary Associations.' *International Encyclopaedia of Social Sciences (Vol. 16).* Collier Macmillan: London, p. 358.

Beveridge, W. 1979. *Voluntary Action in a Changing World.* Bedford Square Press: London.

Committee for Economic Development (CED). 1995. *Building Inner-City Communities: A New Approach to the Nation's Urban Crisis.* Author: New York.

Charyulu, U.V.N. and Natarajan, V.K. 1980. *A Case Study of Cuddapah District.* NIRD: Hyderabad.

Cumper, G. 1986. 'The Changing Role of NGOs: No Longer the Eunuch in the Harem?' *Health Policy and Planning.* Vol. 1 (4), pp. 335-344.

Duggal, R. Gupta, M. Jesani, A. 1986. *NGOs in Rural Health Care.* FRCH: Mumbai.

Duggal, R. and Amin, S. 1989. *Cost of Health Care: A Household Survey in an Indian District.* The Foundation for Research in Community Health: Mumbai.

Duggal, R. 1988. 'NGOs, Government and Private Sector in Health.' *EPW.* March 26, pp. 633 to 636.

Franda, M. 1983. *Voluntary Associations and Local Development in India.* Young Asia Publications: New Delhi.

Ghosh, S. 1994. 'Health Delivery Strategies: Lessons from the NGO Experience.' *Reaching India's Poor—Non-Governmental Approaches to Community Health.* Sage: New Delhi.

Garain, S. 1993. 'Towards a Measure of Organizational Effectiveness for Non-Governmental Organizations.' *The Indian Journal of Social Work.* Vol. LIV, No. 2, pp. 251 to 270.

Garain, S. 1994. 'Government—NGO Interface in India: An Overview.' *The Indian Journal of Social Work.* Vol. LV, No. 3, pp. 337 to 345.

Green, A and Matthias, A. 1997. *Non-governmental Organizations and Health in Developing Countries.* Macmillan Press: London. pp. 32 to 37.

Government of India. *Annual Health Report 1989-90.* Ministry of Health & Family Welfare: New Delhi.

Indian Institute of Management Ahmedabad. 1987. *Study of Health Care Financing in India: Based on Case Studies in Maharashtra and West Bengal.* Asian Development Bank: Manila.

Inamdar, N.R. 1987. 'Role of Voluntarism in Development.' *The Indian Journal of Public Administration.* Vol. XXXIII, No. 3, pp. 421 to 422.

Johnson *et al.* 1996. 'NGOs, Health Providers, and Universities: Collaboration in CBR.' *ICACBR.* Queen's University: Kingston.

Johnson, N. 1981. *Voluntary Social Services.* Basil Blackwell & Martin: Oxford.

Kapoor, A.K. Singh, D. 1997. *Rural Development Through NGOs.* Rawat Publications: New Delhi.

Kapoor, U. 1995. *Women and Welfare—A Study of Voluntary Agencies.* Indus Publishing Company: New Delhi.

Korten, D.C. 1980. 'Community Organization and Rural Development: A Learning Process Approach.' *Public Administration Review.* Vol. 40, No. 5.

Korten, D.C. 1987. 'Third Generation NGO Strategies: A Key to People Centred Development.' *World Development.* Vol. 15, Supplement, pp. 145 to 160.

Lalitha, N. 1975. *Voluntary Works in India.* NIPCCD: New Delhi.

Manimekalai *et al.* 2000. 'Empowerment of Women Through Self-Help Groups (SHGs)' *MARGIN.* Vol. 32, No. 4, pp. 74-87.

Mathew, P.D. 1996. *Law on Foreign Contribution.* Indian Social Institute: New Delhi, pp. 1 to 4.

Mathew, P.D. 1998. *Law on the Registration of Societies.* Indian Social Institute: New Delhi, pp. 12 to 13.

Mishra, S. 2000. *Voluntary Action in Health and Population—The Dynamics of Social Transition.* Sage: New Delhi.

Nandedkar, V.G. 1987. 'Voluntary Association: A Strategy in Development.' *The Indian Journal of Public Administration.* Vol. XXXIII, No. 3, pp. 465 to 481.

Oakley, P and Dillon, B. 1985. *Strengthening People's Participation in Rural Development.* University of Reading. (Unpublished).

Prasad, A. 1997. *Voluntary Action and Rural Reconstruction.* Inter-India Publications: New Delhi.

Paul, S. 1982. *Managing Development Programmes: The Lessons of Success.* Westview Press: Boulder.

Pyle, D. 1981. 'From Project to Programme: The Study of the Scaling Up/Implementation Process of a Community Level Integrated Health, Nutrition and Population Intervention in Maharashtra (India).' *Thesis Submitted for the Degree of Ph.D.* Massachusetts Institute of Technology: Boston.

Pachauri, S. 1994. *Reaching India's Poor—Non-Governmental Approaches to Community Health.* Sage: New Delhi.

Raj, S.L. 1996. 'Editorial'. *Social Action.* January to March, p. III.

Rao, Y.V. 2000. 'TRYSEM Through NGOs.' *Kurukshetra.* Vol. 48, No. 9, pp. 22-26.

Rich *et al.* 1998. *Collaborating to Reduce Poverty: City Halls and Community Based Organizations Working Together to Revitalize Neighbourhoods.* National League of Cities: Washington.

Rajasekhar, D. 2000. 'NGOs in India: Opportunities and Challenges.' *Journal of Rural Development.* Vol. 19 (2), pp. 249 to 275.

Rao, D.N. 1999. 'Social Sector and Development Planning.' *Employment News.* Vol. XXIV, No. 1.

Roy, S. 1987. 'Voluntary Agencies in Development—The Role, Policy and Programmes.' *The Indian Journal of Public Administration.* Vol. XXXIII, No. 3, pp. 454 to 464.

Society for Particapatory Research in Asia. 1991. *Voluntary Development Organization in India.* New Delhi.

Sarkar, A. 1998. 'Characteristics of NGOs: An Exploratory Study in Assam.' *M.Phil. Dissertation.* Centre for Social Medicine and Community Health, Jawaharlal Nehru University, New Delhi (Unpublished).

Sachchidananda *et al.* 1994. *Tribal Development and Voluntary Action.* Inter-India Publications: New Delhi.

Seshagiri, S. 1999. 'Role of the Indian State and NGOs in Public Health.' *M.Phil Dissertation.* Centre for Political Studies, Jawaharlal Nehru University, New Delhi (Unpublished).

Satia, J.K. 1994. 'Upscaling Successful Innovations: Role of NGOs.' *Reaching India's Poor—Non-Governmental Approaches to Community Health.* Sage: New Delhi.

Sills, D.L.1968. *International Encyclopaedia of Social Sciences (Vol. 16).* Collier Macmillan: London.

Smith, C. and Freedman, A. 1972. *Voluntary Associations: Perspective on the Literature.* Harvard University Press: Cambridge.

Sachdeva, D.R. 1993. *Social Welfare Administration in India.* Kitab Mahal: New Delhi.

Smith, K. 1989. 'Non-Governmental Organizations in the Health Field: Collaboration, Integration and Contrasting Aims.' *Social Science and Medicine.* Vol. 29(3), pp. 395 to 402.

The Asia Foundation and Horizons. 2001. 'Assessment of Anti-Trafficking Efforts Finds Disunity Among NGOs.' *Horizon Report.* Spring 2001.

Tendler, J. 1982. *Turning Private Voluntary Organizations into Development Agencies: Questions for Evaluation.* USAID: Washington D.C.

Tandon, R. 1994. 'Where are the People? Community Participation in Health.' *Reaching India's Poor—Non-Governmental Approaches to Community Health.* Sage: New Delhi.

Tongsawate, M. and Tips, W. 1988. 'Coordination Between Government and Voluntary Organizations in Thailand's Rural Development.' *Public Administration and Development.* Vol. 8, pp. 401 to 420.

Uddin *et al.* 1996. *NGO-Donor-Government Relationships.* Voluntary Health Services Society: Bangladesh.

Vahlhans, M. 1994. 'The New Popularity of NGOs—Will the Enthusiasm Last.' *D + C Development and Cooperation.* May-June, pp. 20-22.

Wirsing, R.C. 1977. *Sociologist, Society and Free Enterprise Politics: A Study of Voluntary Associations in Urban India.* Vikash: New Delhi.

Wolleback, D & Selle, P. 2002. 'Does Participation in Voluntary Associations Contribute to Social Capital? The Impact of Intensity, Scope, and Type.' *Nonprofit and Voluntary Sector Quarterly.* Vol. 31, No. 1, pp. 32 to 61.

Wiesgrau, M. 1997. *Interpreting Development: Local Histories, Local Strategies.* University Press of America: New York.

3

Methodology

The previous chapter has given an overview on relevant literature. This chapter provides details regarding the methodology that has been adopted to carry out the present study. It encompasses rationale of the study, specific objectives, research design, sources of data, construction of tools, sampling, process of data collection, nature of analysis and so on. The actual limitations, those the study admits, are also included here. It should be noted that there is no specific methodology for research on NGOs in health care. It depends on the topic, the purpose of investigation, the data available and the experience as well as capability of the researcher. The present work is an empirical study and has shown a new methodology using a few methods together.

RATIONALE OF THE STUDY

Review of studies on NGOs, in the previous chapter, shows diversity among the research initiatives. For instance, a few are individual case studies, few are related to programme activities, few deal with the organizational structure and the remaining studies relate to the beneficiaries. These studies are largely from a management or a sociological perspective. A public health perspective, which has an interdisciplinary approach and can examine the social basis of these NGOs, their growth and distribution, their contribution, etc. is lacking in this area of research. It is also found that there are only two state level studies on NGOs in health care. Those were conducted in Maharashtra (Duggal, Gupta, Jesani, 1986) and Andhra Pradesh (Baru, 1987). No other state level work on NGO's health effort is undertaken. Hence, the present study is a state level study of NGOs in health care in West Bengal having considered the perspective and research gap mentioned above. The reason for selecting West Bengal is its unique socio-political environment. For instance, it has history of series of movements, more than twenty-five years rule of the Left Front Government and at present more importance is being given on industrialization and work culture.

Again, a few studies on NGOs express that NGOs are not reliable for social planning due to their variations. For instance the above mentioned studies conducted in Maharashtra (Duggal, Gupta & Jesani, 1986) and Andhra Pradesh (Baru, 1987) show, NGOs are skewed in favour of socio-economically developed areas in their distribution. The study of NGOs in Assam (Sarkar, 1998) shows, NGOs are varied in size, ideology, organization structure, programme and the population that they serve. These raise an important issue regarding to what extent NGOs actually serve the poorer areas and under-privileged sections. In this context, the present study tries to examine the case of West Bengal with regard to NGOs in health care.

During the last two decades, there has been a shift towards greater reliance on the market and NGOs for provision of services in the social sector. The private sector and NGOs are seen as more efficient, less bureaucratic and effective as compared to the government. With this understanding, the National Health Policy document 2001 also envisages a greater role for private sector and NGOs. The NGOs represent plurality in terms of size, services provided and inter- as well as intra-state distribution. Given these variations, the present study has decided to examine the social basis, growth, distribution and contribution of NGOs working with health care in West Bengal. Ultimate aim is to locate the relative position of NGOs in providing health care vis-à-vis the state in West Bengal.

OBJECTIVES

The specific objectives of the study are as follows:

(i) To develop an understanding of the socio-political factors influencing the rise of NGOs in West Bengal after independence and examine their role in health services.

(ii) To analyse the trends in growth and distribution of NGOs in health care in West Bengal with special focus from the early seventies.

(iii) To do an indepth study of a selected NGOs by focusing on historical background, organizational set-up, present activities, nature of programme sustainability, level of job satisfaction of the staff members and beneficiary's perception towards the working of NGOs to explore how far NGOs can contribute in health care.

RESEARCH DESIGN

There was paucity of data in the research area. It was necessary to explore different aspects and establish facts related to socio-political factors influenced the rise of NGOs in West Bengal, growth and distribution of NGOs in health care in West Bengal, these NGO's historical background, organizational set-up, programme sustainability, staff member's job satisfaction, baneficiary's perception and so on. Hence, researcher had to do literature review, experience survey and case studies of some NGOs. Literature scanning and experience survey were done to understand the socio-political factors influencing the rise of NGOs. Experience survey was made through informal interviews and mailed questionnaires. Informal interviews were conducted among the key persons and mailed questionnaires were sent to the Directors of NGOs. Case study was initiated in selected NGOs to observe and reveal various aspects pertinent to past history, programme, staff and beneficiaries. Thus, the present study has used **exploratory design.**

TYPES OF DATA REQUIRED

In order to carry out this exploratory study, the following types of data were required:

(i) For the first objective, data related to the social and political factors those led to from NGOs in WB were essential. Each factor was explored and discussed clearly. It was to examine whether there was any factor related to health.

(ii) To carry out the second objective, researcher required following data: (A) Growth of NGOs (number of organizations emerged periodically i.e. 1945 to 1950, 1951 to 1955, 1956 to 1960, 1961 to 1965, 1966 to 1970, 1971 to 1975, 1976 to 1980, 1981 to 1985, 1986 to 1990, 1991 to 1995, 1996 to

2000) in health care in West Bengal in terms of (a) operational area (urban, rural, tribal, etc.); (b) type of organization (religious organization, service organization, development organization, research and consultancy agency, action group, etc.); (c) type of service (institutionalized or community based or both); (d) nature of starting programme (awareness or service oriented or both); (e) promoter's background (medical practitioner, school teacher, retired government official, political leader, freedom fighter, activist of any movement, group of young enthusiastic friends, businessman, untrained dedicated social worker, college or university teacher, etc.); (f) year of starting health programme; (g) nature of starting health programme (awareness generation, occasional health camp, regular mobile dispensary, permanent clinic, permanent hospital and training of health workers); (h) full time separate health staff (have or do not have); and (i) health budget (nil, upto Rs. 10,000, Rs. 10,001 to 50,000, Rs. 50,001 to 1,00,000, Rs. 1,00,001 to 2,00,000, Rs. 2,00,001 to 5,00,000, Rs. 5,00,001 to 10,00,000 and above Rs. 10,00,000). (B) Distribution of NGOs (as per the area of operation i.e. Urban area, rural area, tribal area, urban and rural area, all the areas) in health care in West Bengal in terms of location, affiliation (yes or no), type of organization, type of service, total number of full time paid staff (nil, one to five, six to ten, eleven to twenty, twenty one to fifty, fifty one to eighty, eighty one to hundred, above hundred), annual budget (upto Rs. 5,00,000, Rs. 5,00,001 to 10,00,000, Rs. 10,00,001 to 25,00,000, Rs. 25,00,001 to 50,00,000, Rs. 50,00,001 to 1,00,00,000, Rs. 1,00,00,001 to 2,00,00,000, Rs. 2,00,00,001 to 4,00,00,000), promoter's background, present health programmes (awareness generation, occasional health camp, regular mobile dispensary, permanent clinic, permanent hospital, training of health workers and RCH), separate health staff, types of health staff (trained doctors, non-trained doctors, nurses, trained health workers, non-trained health workers and administrative staff), health budget, etc.

(iii) In order to fulfil the third objective, three NGOs were selected for case study. Types of required data were: NGO's

(a) historical background; (b) organizational set-up and present activities; (c) programme sustainability: programme's name, objectives, target group, various component, programme execution process, duration, area of operation, service cost, nature of infrastructure and resources required, alternative arrangement for resources after the project duration, beneficiary's needs and participation, people's organization and its link with the programme, use of volunteers, staff mobility, staff selection, staff related difficulties, innovative aspect, political intervention, integration with other programme, programme monitoring, evaluation, etc.; (d) staff member's job satisfaction: satisfaction for the facilities available at the job, satisfaction from the relationship with the boss, satisfaction for physical condition of working place, satisfaction for career advancement scheme, satisfaction for job security, etc.; (e) beneficiary's perception towards the working of NGO: health care programme of the locality, necessity of the NGO's health care programme, service cost and quality of the NGO's health care programme, NGO's health service in difficult situation, staff co-operation, beneficiary's participation, etc.

SOURCES OF DATA

Keeping in view the objectives of the study, researcher collected data from secondary as well as primary sources. First part of data requirement was collected using both the sources i.e. through literature (secondary source: Government's report, NGO's report, Books, Newspapers, reports of the State Level Society Registration Office, etc.), informal interviews (primary source), and mailed questionnaires (primary source). Second part of the data requirement was collected by means of mailed questionnaires (primary source). Same mailed questionnaire was used for first two objectives. Last part of the required data was explored using only primary source, i.e. from selected NGOs. In this connection, five separate tools were developed i.e. Information Proforma for NGOs, Interview Schedule in understanding nature of programme sustainability, Information Proforma for health care staff, Job Satisfaction Scale for full time paid health care staff and Interview Schedule for beneficiary's perception.

THE TECHNIQUES AND TOOLS

It is understood from the above paragraph that altogether one technique and six tools were used. Informal interview was the only technique used among the key persons, such as, activists, politicians, academicians, bureaucrats and NGO promoters, to know the socio-political factors influencing the rise of NGOs. There was no specific question but main thirst was to explore the roots of NGOs through a fruitful discussion.

Regarding tools, mailed questionnaire was used at first to make a survey of NGOs in health care at the state level. It carried nineteen questions, which covered NGO's origin and trends in growth as well as distribution. Director or secretary of NGO was respondent. In order to examine the reliability of this questionnaire, it was administered twice in one-month interval among the seventy NGOs of West Bengal. Ninety eight per cent of the responses were found similar between the two tests.

The remaining five tools such as two information proforma, two interview schedules and one job satisfaction scale were used during case study. Information proforma of NGO was necessary to collect the history as well as basic information (name, address, objectives, operational area, organizational structure, programmes, staffing pattern, financial aspect, monitoring and evaluation, etc.). Information proforma of health care staff was required to know various types of staff and their numbers as well as characteristics. Both the proforma were filled up with the help of Officė Superintendent or Office Incharge. Interview Schedule in understanding nature of programme sustainability encompassed total thirty three questions pertaining to programme, beneficiaries, infrastructure (organizational and local), volunteers, funding agencies, etc. Programme Coordinator or Programme Incharge was the respondent. Interview Schedule to understand the perception of beneficiaries included twenty six questions pertinent to local heath care facilities, nature and necessity of NGO's health care programme, staff cooperation, beneficiary's participation, etc. Beneficiaries under a particular group were considered as respondents for this tool. With a view to standardize these two proformas and two interview schedules, researcher selected an NGO named Seva Sangha (situated at Kanthalfully of South 24 parganas district) where he spent one week and tried out these tools. After the test, a few changes were made in various tools by putting appropriate word for the question, simplifying the complex question and correcting the question with the concerned problem.

In respect of job satisfaction scale, which was developed for full time paid health care staff, researcher had to work very extensively. It was fact that a few job satisfaction scales were available in literature for the employees of private industries, autonomous organizations, government agencies, etc., but there was no scale for the staff of NGOs specially located in West Bengal. Hence, this scale was constructed. It followed Likert's method. At the very outset, five dimensions (from where satisfaction came) were identified. Those were: (a) Facilities available at the job; (b) Relationship with the boss; (c) Physical condition of working place; (d) Career and self-improvement scheme; and (e) Job security. Hundred statements were framed and gathered with the help of experts and relevant reading giving emphasis over all the five dimensions mentioned above. The draft comprises of hundred statements was sent to few experts for cross verification of the items. After the verification, eighty statements were retained. Researcher revised this draft several times and at last the list contained seventy items, both favourable and unfavourable equal in number, under all the five dimensions. All these seventy statements were shuffled, systematically arranged and finally draft scale was developed. The score of the favourable items were decided as 5, 4, 3, 2, 1 for the responses Strongly Agree (SA), Agree (A), Undecided (U), Disagree (D) and Strongly Disagree (SD) respectively. The scores were reversed (i.e. 1, 2, 3, 4, 5) for the unfavourable items. The following Table 3.1 shows the scoring key at a glance:

Table 3.1: Scoring Key for Job Satisfaction Scale

Degree of Choice	*Scores for items*	
	Favourable	*Unfavourable*
SA	5	1
A	4	2
U	3	3
D	2	4
SD	1	5

This five-point job satisfaction scale with seventy items was tried out on a group of fifty-four employees of Seva Sangha (located at south 24 parganas district). Having collected fifty-four filled up scales from the respondents, scoring was made. The filled up scales were arranged in the ascending order on the basis of total scores obtained by the respondents. Then, one-third scales from the top as well as one-third scales from the bottom were taken and middle one-third were put aside. Thus, two scoring groups i.e. higher and lower scoring groups were formed. Then each item was taken and calculated discriminating value (D), using the percentages of correct and incorrect responses of both the groups, with the help of following formula:

$$D = \frac{P_1 - P_2}{\sqrt{\frac{P_1Q_1}{N_1} + \frac{P_2Q_2}{N_2}}}$$

Where P_1 and P_2 were percentages of staff respectively in higher and lower scoring groups who solved the item correctly; and Q_1 and Q_2 were percentages of respondents who solved the item incorrectly. N_1 and N_2 were number of staff members in higher and lower scoring groups respectively. In this regard, researcher made it clear that 'correct' answer meant reply to the positive or favourable item as 'Strongly Agree' and getting five marks against such response. Similarly, a reply to a negative, or unfavourable item as 'Strongly Disagree' was considered as 'correct' answer and five marks were awarded to such response. Thus, the researcher gave the award of five marks against each correct answer irrespective of upper and lower group.

It is known to us (Asthana, B. and Agarwal, R.N., 1995), if the value of D is 1.96 or more, then the item is discriminating. Having calculated D value of all the seventy items, through above formula, best thirty-eight items were selected whose discriminating values were more than four. These thirty-eight items were mixed up irrespective of their specific dimensions, arranged logically and gave the shape of final job satisfaction scale. The dimension-wise distribution of the items in the final scale was as follows:

Table 3.2: Dimension-wise Distribution of the Items

Dimension	*Nature of Statement*	*Serial Number of the Statement*
Facilities available at the job	Positive (+)	20, 21, 24, 30, 32, 36, 38
	Negative (-)	2, 14, 19, 34
Relationship with the boss	Positive (+)	4, 8, 9, 15
	Negative (-)	25, 31
Physical condition of working place	Positive (+)	5, 26, 37
	Negative (-)	11, 12, 16, 27
Career and self improvement scheme	Positive (+)	1, 6, 10, 17, 22
	Negative (-)	28, 33, 35
Job security	Negative (-)	3, 7, 13, 18, 23, 29

In order to determine the reliability co-efficient of this tool, split half method (Rulon) was used. The final job satisfaction scale comprises of thirty-eight items was administered once again among the thirty staff members of Seva Sangha (located at south 24 parganas). Researcher divided the scale into two equal halves by separating the odd and even items. Each halves contained nineteen items. The scores for both the halves were given separately. Each respondent had a score on first half and a score on second half. Having used these scores, reliability co-efficient was calculated by applying Rulon's formula. The process of calculation was as follows:

Table 3.3: Score Distribution of the Two Halves

Sl. No. of the Respondent	*Score of First Half (A)*	*Score of Second Half (B)*	*Difference (D) [D=A–B]*	*Total Score*
1	70	70	0	140
2	70	64	6	134
3	59	53	6	112
4	66	75	–9	141
5	66	62	4	128
6	83	75	8	158
7	59	57	2	116
8	69	71	–2	140
9	68	72	–4	140
10	59	59	0	118
11	50	62	–12	112
12	65	70	–5	135
13	78	81	–3	159
14	78	80	–2	158
15	76	83	–7	159
16	63	67	–4	130
17	46	55	–9	101
18	53	66	–13	119
19	67	69	–2	136
20	51	66	–15	117
21	51	64	–13	115
22	57	68	–11	125
23	70	72	–2	142
24	74	66	8	140
25	74	66	8	140
26	58	58	0	116
27	60	59	1	119
28	63	69	–6	132
29	65	76	–11	141
30	64	65	–1	129

r_{tt} = Reliability coefficient of the whole test
$\sigma^2 d$ = Variance of D= 45.0298
$\sigma^2 t$ = Variance of total score =235.0989

$$r_{tt} = \frac{1-\sigma^2 d}{\sigma^2 t}$$

$$= 1 - \frac{45.0298}{235.0989}$$

$$= 1 - 0.1915 = 0.8085 = 0.81$$

Thus, it was proved that the job satisfaction scale was reliable.

With regard to validity of this scale, content validity as well as face validity was ensured. Researcher took care of it while he selected the statements by undergoing statistical technique and experts opinion.

FIELD OF STUDY

The present study has covered the entire West Bengal. This state is situated in the east part of India stretching from the Himalayas in the north to the Bay of Bengal in the south. Geographically it locates between 85°50′ east longitude to 89°50′ east longitude and 21°38′ north latitude to 27°10′ north latitude. As per census 2001, West Bengal is 88,756 sq. km and having 8,02,21,171 population. Its literacy rate is 69.22 per cent and sex ratio, i.e. number of female per thousand male, is 934 (*Manorama Year Book*, 2002). Seventy per cent of West Bengal's population are engaged in agriculture. Out of total land of the state, 62.63 per cent are cultivable area and it contributes around thirty per cent of the state's income. Jute, textile, coal, steel, tea, silk, etc. are the major industries. In 1995, this state had 10,236 registered as well as functioning factories and 4,53,831 small scale industrial units (*Manorama Year Book*, 1999). Regarding health, infrastructure and manpower development are not upto mark in W.B. But, overall health status of the state is better than the national picture. For instance, in India, in 1999, birth rate, infant mortality rate and death rate were 26.1, 70 and 8.7 respectively whereas in West Bengal it was 20.7, 52 and 7.1 respectively (*Economic Survey* 2000-2001).

It should be noted that administratively West Bengal is divided into three divisions i.e. Presidency division, Burdwan division and Jalpaiguri division. Jalpaiguri division is called as North Bengal. Since this division is very far from the state capital, West Bengal government has the step-motherly attitude towards the socio-economic development of it. In order to know more regarding West Bengal, chapter IV has given the details.

PROCESS OF DATA COLLECTION

Under the study, data were collected in five phases. In the first phase, secondary data related to the socio-political factors influenced the rise of NGOs in West Bengal specially after independence were gathered through literature review. In this regard, National Library of Kolkata, Jadavpur University Library, Calcutta University Library, American Information Centre, British High Commission Library (Kolkata), Library of Indian Institute of Management Calcutta, Indian Institute of Social Welfare and Business Management Library, West Bengal Voluntary Health Association Library, etc. were visited by the researcher.

In the second phase, addresses of NGOs (registered) in health care were collected from various umbrella organizations (i.e. from Child in Need Institute, Lok Kalyan Parishad, LIONS International, Rotary International, and West Bengal Voluntary Health Association), various national or regional institutes (i.e. National Institute of Orthopaedically Handicapped, Regional Institute of Speech and Hearing Handicapped, Regional Institute of Mentally Handicapped and All India Institute of Public Health and Hygiene) and various directories of NGOs (published by Indian Institute of Management Calcutta, Family Planning Association of India, etc.). Having put all the addresses together, a comprehensive list of 705 NGOs of West Bengal was prepared.

In the third phase questionnaires were mailed to all the 705 NGOs whose addresses were collected. Having given three reminders there was a total of 216 responses, which worked out around thirty one per cent response rate. This was done to know various socio-political factors influenced the rise of NGOs and to get required data for understanding trends in growth and distribution of NGOs in health care in West Bengal. In the fourth phase, fifteen key informants (such as activists, politicians, academicians, bureaucrats and NGO promoters) were interviewed informally to know socio-political factors influenced the rise of NGOs.

At the last phase, case studies were made only in three NGOs (i.e. Southern Health Improvement Samity, CINI Moyna Rural Health Development Centre, and Rural Health Development Centre), selecting one organization from each division (i.e. Presidency division Burdwan division and Jalpaiguri division). In each NGO, researcher spent minimum twenty-five days. He collected information related to the organization, programme and staff from the campus and information pertinent to the beneficiaries from the field by forming four groups. The criteria for group formation were as under: (a) one nearby and one distant villages would be selected under each organization, (b) in each village, one male and one female group should be formed, (c) members of the group should fall within the age group of 20 to 40 years, (d) each group should contain 10 to 20 members, (e) group members (beneficiaries) should be Scheduled Caste/Scheduled Tribe/Backward Class/Minority people and fall below poverty line, and (f) members (beneficiaries) should be permanent residents for last three years in the respective villages and should get health care benefit.

SAMPLING

As per the information of Society Registration Office, in the year of 2000 in West Bengal, total numbers of registered NGOs were over 1,00,000. It was also known from the same office that nearly thirty per cent of them existed only in papers and the remaining seventy per cent really operated who would prepare annual report and audited statement of account in every year. According to experts, seven to ten per cent of the existing NGOs had health care programmes. Thus, over seven thousands NGOs would carry out health activities in West Bengal and those were considered as *Universe* of the present study.

Sampling was not required in the first phase of data collection. In the second phase, a list of 705 NGOs was developed from the Universe. Thus, sample size was 705. The unit of sample was selected by applying snowball sampling technique based on the following criteria: (a) NGO must be located within the territory of West Bengal; (b) NGO must be registered, alive and should submit annual report as well as audited statement of account regularly in the society registration office; and (c) NGO should have at least one health care programme.

During the third phase of data collection, questionnaires were mailed to all the 705 NGOs. Therefore, no specific sampling technique or criterion was used to handle questionnaires. In the fourth phase, purposive sampling technique was used to select fifteen key informants. It was done based on the following criteria: (a) Minimum qualification of the respondent should be Bachelor Degree; (b) Respondent should be either activist or politician or academician or bureaucrat or promoter of NGO; and (c) respondent must have minimum fifteen years experience in the field of NGO.

In the last phase of data collection, three NGOs were chosen purposively (purposive sampling), for case studies, based on the following criteria: (a) NGO may be in urban or semi-urban or rural area but should locate within the territory of West Bengal; (b) Only one NGO should be selected from one division (i.e. Presidency division, Burdwan division and Jalpaiguri division); (c) NGO must be registered, non-profit and welfare organization; (d) NGO should have at least twenty full time paid staff and yearly turnover of Rs. 50,00,000; (e) NGO must be having at least one full fledged health programme which has specific project proposal, budget allocation and full time paid employees. In this phase, five separate tools were used. Sampling was necessary in handling job satisfaction scale (for staff members) and interview schedule (to understand nature of programme sustainability). For job satisfaction scale, thirty staff members were selected purposively (purposive sampling) from each NGO. Efforts were made to include all types of staff (lower level, middle level and higher level) as per their availability, age, sex, marital status, educational qualification, etc. For interview schedule, four main programmes were identified purposively (purposive sampling) from each NGO based on certain criteria, such as, (a) At first, preference should be given to include health care related programme. If four health care programmes are not found, other programmes can be undertaken; (b) Each programme should have specific project proposal, budget allocation as well as full time paid employees; and, (c) Coverage of each programme should be at least three villages. No sampling technique was required to handle interview schedule for beneficiaries. Because, all the beneficiaries of each group were interviewed.

ANALYSIS OF DATA

In the present study, qualitative and quantitative both kind of analysis were done. For first objective, data were discussed qualitatively. For second objective, quantitative analysis was made. At fast available data were reorganized to develop a common framework for examining the same. The data, those were possible to code, were identified and grouped from each questionnaire. Then simple cross tabulation was done to understand the aspect mentioned in the objective.

In the third objective, data related to NGO's history and existing activities were presented having followed qualitative method. To understand the nature of programme sustainability, data were also discussed qualitatively. In this regard, programmes of each NGO were analyzed on the basis of following twelve factors:

(a) Capacity of the organization: Whether organization has—
- appropriate policy (as per constitution),
- infrastructural capacity,
- democratic decision making procedure,
- will power and united approach.

(b) Continuity in funding:
- Whether organization can arrange funds continuously to carry out the programme.
- If not, whether any alternative arrangement has been made.

(c) Need fulfilment and ensuring qualitative services:
- Whether needs are fulfilled properly.
- Whether qualitative services are ensured.

(d) Intention of the beneficiaries:
- Whether beneficiaries understand that those services are meant for them.
- Whether beneficiaries show their interest and fight judiciously to utilize this service.

(e) Nature of people's participation: Whether people participate in:
- Beneficiaries selection,
- Need identification,
- Resource contribution or collection,
- Programme planning,
- Monitoring and evaluation.

(f) Recognition of people's participation:
- Whether people's participation is recognized.

(g) Use of volunteers and continuous liaison with them:
- Scope of use of volunteers to carry out programmes.
- Continuous liaison with volunteers.

(h) Nature of staff mobility:
- How frequently staff members leave a particular programme and what reasons are found for it.

(i) Innovative component:
- Whether there is any innovative component, which helps the programme to be executed in an effective way.

(j) Local cooperation:
- Whether local people, influential persons and other organizations of the community co-operate in the programme.
- Whether problems or barriers or inconvenient issues are created by political parties or opponent groups as threat for the programme.

(k) Integrated with other programmes and multi-sectoral activities:
- Whether this programme is integrated with other programmes for its better existence.
- Whether the programme is having multi-sectoral activities. For instance, health programme can have a component of income generation since both are inter-related. If people are advised to boil water for drinking or to use soap for maintaining personal hygiene, they can not follow these instructions if they do not have money to buy fuel or soap.

(l) Regular monitoring:
- Whether various aspects of the programme i.e. staff, finance, and activities are monitored regularly.

If a programme was in favour of all the above enumerated factors, it was treated as more sustainable. If any programme was lacking one or few of the above mentioned factors, that programme was understood as comparatively less sustainable. If any one did not relate most of the factors, that indicated unsustainability of the programme.

Under the third objective, qualitative analysis was also made for the data pertinent to the perception of the beneficiaries. Information collected from each group were discussed under six separate dimensions such as (a) health care institution of the locality and their nature of services; (b) necessity of the NGO's health care programmes; (c) cost and quality of the NGO's health care services; (d) NGO's health care services at difficult situation; (e) staff cooperation; and (f) scope of beneficiary's participation. Under this objective, quantitative analysis was done only for the data related to the job satisfaction of the staff members. Simple cross tables were used to highlight profile of the staff. As per the obtained score (in the scale) of each staff, levels of satisfaction were identified on the basis of following rules:

Table 3.4: Rules to Identify Levels of Satisfaction

Level of Satisfaction	*Very Low Satisfaction (score)*	*Low Satisfaction (score)*	*Moderate Satisfaction (score)*	*High Satisfaction (score)*
Variables				
Variable-1	11-21	22-32	33-43	44 and above
Variable-2	6-11	12-17	18-23	24 and above
Variable-3	7-13	14-20	21-27	28 and above
Variable-4	8-15	16-23	24-31	32 and above
Variable-5	6-11	12-17	18-23	24 and above
Total Score	38-75	76-113	114-151	152 and above

In order to understand the association between nature of staff and level of satisfaction, chi-square (χ^2) test was used.

OPERATIONAL DEFINITIONS

NGO

It is voluntarily formed and registered organization working towards development and amelioration of suffering with non-self serving aims and free from the state control in managing day to day affairs. Study has considered those NGOs who execute at least one health care programme.

Public Health

In a narrow sense, public health refers to the health of a population, the longevity of its individual members and the extent to which they are free from disease. Alternatively, public health can be seen as a philosophy of intervention aimed at protecting and promoting the health of the population. According to Winslow, in a broader sense, "Public health is the science and art of preventing disease, prolonging life and promoting physical health and efficiency through organized community efforts for the sanitation of the environment, the control of community infections, the education of the individual in principles of personal hygiene, the organization of medical and nursing service for the early diagnosis and preventive treatment of disease, and the development of social machinery which will ensure to every individual in the community a standard of living adequate for the maintenance of health" (Baggott, 2001). It is found that state has an active role in providing public health services. Under the study, public health perspective is considered as an interdisciplinary approach which includes various aspects like health services, availability of food, nutrition, safe drinking water, sanitation, improvement of wages, education, etc. to ensure every individual in the community an adequate standard of living for the maintenance of health. Universality (reaching service to all the sections or age groups of the society), equality (services are accessible and available to all the people irrespective of caste or class) and comprehensiveness (includes all sorts of services like preventive, curative, promotive, rehabilitative, etc.) are the three main principles of this perspective.

Health Care

It is defined as "Multitude of services regarded to individuals, families or communities by the agents of the health services or professions, for the purpose of promoting, maintaining, monitoring or restoring health." Such services might be staffed, organized, administered and financed in every imaginable way, but they all have one thing in common: people are being 'Served', that is, diagnosed, helped, cured, educated and rehabilitated by health personnel (Park, 1995). In the present study, health care refers to NGO's service or intervention those are provided by the health personnel in order to promote, maintain and restore health.

Social Basis of NGO

According to *Webster's New World Dictionary* (1991), the word 'Basis' refers to the base or foundation or chief supporting factor of anything. It may be the fundamental principle or theory, as of a system of knowledge. As per the *Cambridge International Dictionary of English* (1997), 'Basis' means the most important facts, ideas, etc. from which something is developed. A basis is also a way or method of doing something. Under the study, 'Social Basis of NGO' refers to the important facts or social phenomena or ideas from which NGOs are developed in West Bengal. Social basis of NGO basically indicates to various socio-political factors those lead to promote NGOs.

Socio-Political Factor

The term 'Social' refers to attribute which is related to people and community or which is influenced by people's common problems, life styles, customs, welfare and reforms or which is pertaining to society. It does not talk about only one or individual; it encompasses more than one. The word 'Political' indicates to the matter, which is related, to state or government or public affairs in general (rights or liberties). It may be something related to conflict or rivalry between two or more parties. It can also imply to the people interested in or active in politics. Under the study, *Socio-Political Factors* refer to the aspects like people's common problems, customs, welfare, reforms and state affairs or public affairs those have influenced the rise of NGOs in West Bengal.

Rise

As per *The Oxford Dictionary for International Business* (1998), 'Rise' means to appear or to be visible above the horizon. It may be getting up from lying, sitting, kneeling or from bed. Sometimes, 'Rise' indicates increase in amount, degree, quantity, price, etc. It may also refer origin or begin or spring up. Under the study, the word 'Rise' is used to understand the increase of NGOs in numbers or quantity.

Growth and Distribution

The term 'Growth' is generally used to indicate changes of a quantitative nature, such as change in weight, height, number, etc. (Dandekar, 1995). It may be increase in economic activity or profitability. It is sometimes abnormal or diseased formation in the body (e.g. a tumer or cancer). The word 'Distribution' is meant to understand an instance of giving some items among several people (e.g. prize distribution, form distribution, etc.). It may be positioning or location of items, features, etc. within an area. Thus, the words 'Growth' and 'Distribution' are used in the study to understand trends of NGO's increase in numbers and its positioning or location within the West Bengal State.

Programme

Under the study, the programme of an NGO refers to activities having specific project proposal, programme staff and budget allocation.

Sustainability

It refers ability to bear something without breaking or falling. It is also considered as ability to keep somebody or something alive or in existence. Present study uses the word 'Sustainability' to know nature of programme continuation i.e. whether one programme will exist for long time (more sustainable) or for short time (less sustainable) or will be stopped (unsustainable) when project duration will be over or organization will withdraw its programme from the operational area.

Job Satisfaction

According to Herbert Simon (1966), 'Satisfying' means picking a course of action that is satisfactory or good enough under the circumstances. Koontz H. and Weihrich H. (1990) feel, 'Satisfaction' refers to the contentment experienced when a want is satisfied. 'Job satisfaction' is a result of employees' perception of how well their job provides those things that are viewed as important (Luthans, 1998). Locke (1976) gives a comprehensive definition of job satisfaction as 'a pleasurable or positive emotional state resulting from the appraisal of one's job or job experience'. Smith, Kendall and Hulin (1969) have suggested five factors those influence job satisfaction. These are: (a) *The work itself* i.e. the extent to which the job provides the individual with interesting tasks, opportunities for learning and the chance to accept responsibility; (b) *Pay* which as equal as in other organizations; (c) *Promotion opportunities* i.e. the chances for advancement in the organization; (d) *Supervision*—the abilities of the supervisor to provide technical assistance as well as behavioural support; and (e) *Coworkers*—Whether fellow workers are technically proficient and socially supportive. In the present study, job satisfaction refers to the emotional responses and several related attitudes of the staff members under an NGO as a result of job situation or job experience.

Perception

According to the *Encyclopedia Americana* (1992), the core meaning of perception is immediate awareness. To perceive something is to become directly or immediately aware of it. For example, by means of our senses, we perceive, or become aware of, the objects, events, and persons in our environment. As per the *New Encyclopedia Britannica* (2002), perception is the process whereby sensory stimulation is translated into organized or meaningful experience. Mc Grow-Hill

Encyclopedia of Science and Technology (1987) defines perception as the subjective experiences of objects or events that ordinarily result from stimulation of the receptor organs of the body. According to A.F. Witting, perception would be the set of mental experiences arising when the Brain processes sensory data (Ray, 2000). Under the study, perception refers to the way of seeing or awareness of beneficiaries towards the working of NGO.

Contribution

Under the study, contribution refers to NGO's activities or support or help towards development in general and health care in particular.

LIMITATIONS OF THE STUDY

(i) This study is limited only in West Bengal. As roots of NGOs are influenced by the socio-political factors of the state, entire findings of the study may not be applicable in case of other state.

(ii) In the second phase of data collection, when a list of NGOs in health care was compiled, few umbrella organizations and directories of NGOs were consulted. It was not possible to collect all the addresses (over seven thousands) of NGOs in health care in West Bengal.

(iii) At the last phase of the study, case studies (of three NGOs) have been done. It is important to note that outcome of case study may not be generalized everywhere in West Bengal.

So far we have understood the methodology of the study. Now the following chapter will try to give an overview of West Bengal and its milieu.

REFERENCES

Asthana, B. Agarwal, R.N. 1995. *Measurement and Evaluation in Psychology and Education.* Vinod Pustak Mandir: Agra.

Baru, R. 1987. 'Factors Influencing Variations in Health Services—A Study of Selected Districts of Andhra Pradesh.' *M.Phil Dissertation.* Centre for Social Medicine and Community Health, School of Social Sciences, Jawaharlal Nehru University, New Delhi.

Baggott, R. 2001. *Public Health: Policy and Politics.* Macmillan Press Ltd: London.

Duggal, R. Gupta, M. Jesani, A. 1986. *NGOs in Rural Health Care.* FRCH: Mumbai.

Dandekar, W.N. 1995. *Psychological Foundations of Education.* Macmillan: Chennai, p. 55.

Encyclopedia Britannica Inc. 2002. *The New Encyclopedia Britannica,* Vol. 9. Chicago.

Government of India. 2001. *Economic Survey 2000-2001.* Ministry of Finance: New Delhi.

Grolier Incorporated. 1992. *The Encyclopedia Americana,* Vol. 21. USA.

Koontz, H. & Weihrich, H. 1990. *Essentials of Management.* McGrow-Hill Publishing Company: New York.

Locke, E.A. 1976. 'The Nature and Cause of Job Satisfaction', in M.D. Dunnettee (ed.), *Handbook of Industrial and Organisational Psychology.* Rand McNally: Chicago, p. 1300.

Luthans, F. 1998. *Organisational Behaviour.* Irwin-McGrow-Hill: New York, p. 144.

Malayala Manorama, 1999, *Manorama Year Book 1999.* Kottayam.

Malayala Manorama, 2002, *Manorama Year Book 2002 (Bengali Version).* Kottayam.

McGrow-Hill Book Company. 1987. *McGrow-Hill Encyclopedia of Science and Technology,* Vol. 13. London.

Neufeldt, V (ed). 1991. *Webster's New World Dictionary.* Webster's New World: New York.

Park, K. 1995. *Preventive and Social Medicine.* Banarsidas Bhanot: Jabalpur.

Procter, P., (ed). 1997. *Cambridge International Dictionary of English.* Cambridge University Press: London.

Ray, S. 2000. *Educational Psychology.* Soma Book Agency: Kolkata

Sarkar, A. 1998. 'Characteristics of NGOs: An Exploratory Study in Assam'. *M.Phil Dissertation.* Centre for Social Medicine and Community Health, School of Social Sciences, Jawaharlal Nehru University, New Delhi. (Unpublished).

Simon, H. 1966. *Organizations.* John Wiley & Sons: New York.

Smith, P.C. Kendall, L.M. and Hulin, C.L. 1969. *The Measurement of Satisfaction in Work and Retirement.* Rand McNally: Chicago.

The Market House Book Ltd. 1998. *The Oxford Dictionary for International Business.* Oxford University Press: New York.

4

West Bengal and its Milieu

Series of annals place a high impression regarding the Bengal. For instance, the people of this region were adapted in seafaring and crossed the seven seas of the world for the purpose of trade and commerce. From the very dawn of history, the Bengalis were noted for their spirit of independence. They resisted the intrusion of Vedic culture into Bengal for long. They evolved their own schools of art and architecture. Their *Viharas* or Universities drew students from far and wide. Their evangelist sons went to establish cultural colonies in Central Asia, China and Indonesia. Apart from that, Bengal is also popular for the contribution of Ramakrishna and Rabindranath, Renaissance of the Nineteenth Century, art and literature of the Twentieth Century and its fight against British Imperialism (Sur, 1992). Since the present study is initiated in West Bengal, this chapter attempts to give a brief history and socio economic development of the same state.

HISTORICAL BACKGROUND

The old Bengal is known as Gauda or Vanga in ancient Sanskrit literature. At the time of Aryan penetration into the East, Vanga had a well-settled civilization and culture. During the third century B.C, Bengal was considered as a part of the Mauryan Empire and from the fourth to the sixth century A.D., it came under the Gupta dynasty. Till 800 A.D., the Palas ruled Bengal. They were very powerful and enlarged their territories into the nearby countries of Bihar, Orissa and Assam. As a result of power, they developed diplomatic relations with Sri Vijaya, the Indonesian King.

In the eleventh century, Bengal was ruled by the Senas whose capital was located at Nadia. In the beginning of the thirteenth century, Boktiar

Khalji occupied Nadia and started Muslim rule for first time in Bengal. After the death of Aurangzeb, the last of the great Mughals, Bengal became independent under its Muslim governors. Siraj Daula, the last independent Muslim ruler of Bengal, lost at the battle of Plassey in 1757 and a sort of British control was realized in Bengal society. Britishers took over the administration of Bengal in 1764 after the battle of Buxar.

When Bengal was formed as a province, under the British rule, it included present Bihar, Orissa and expanded upto Agra. Agra was detached from Bengal in 1861 but Assam was attached to it, which was constituted as a separate province again in 1874.

Lord Curzon divided Bengal, in 1905, into two provinces. Assam and East Bengal with its capital at Dacca was carved out of old Bengal. The remaining part along with Bihar and some parts of Orissa formed Bengal. Many people opposed this partition as an attempt at disintegrating Bengal. When India was free from British rule in 1947, Bengal was divided between India and Pakistan. Pakistan's share was called as East Pakistan and India's share was named as West Bengal. Under the state Reorganization Act, some parts of Bihar were transferred to Bengal. Now this state is divided into eighteen districts (*Manorama Year Book,* 1999).

GEOGRAPHICAL CHARACTERISTICS

Location

West Bengal covers a part of India in the east stretching from the Himalayas in the north to the Bay of Bengal in the South. It is bounded on the north by Sikkim and Bhutan, on the east by Assam and Bangladesh, on the south by Bay of Bengal and on the west by Orissa, Bihar and Nepal (*Manorama Year Book*, 1999).

Physiography

West Bengal has two natural divisions. One, the Himalayan north, which comprises of three hill districts such as Darjeeling, Jalpaiguri and Cooch Behar. Two, the alluvial plain, the handiwork of many big rivers that is in the southern part of the state. Temperature fluctuates here between 8°C to 40°C throughout the whole year. Rainfall varies from 1,006 mm to 2,933 mm (*Manorama Year Book*, 1999).

Rivers

The main rivers of this state are Ganga, Hoogly, Mayurakshi, Ajoy, Damodar, Mahananda, Tista, Torsa, Jaldhaka, Kansabati, Subarnarekha,

MAP OF WEST BENGAL

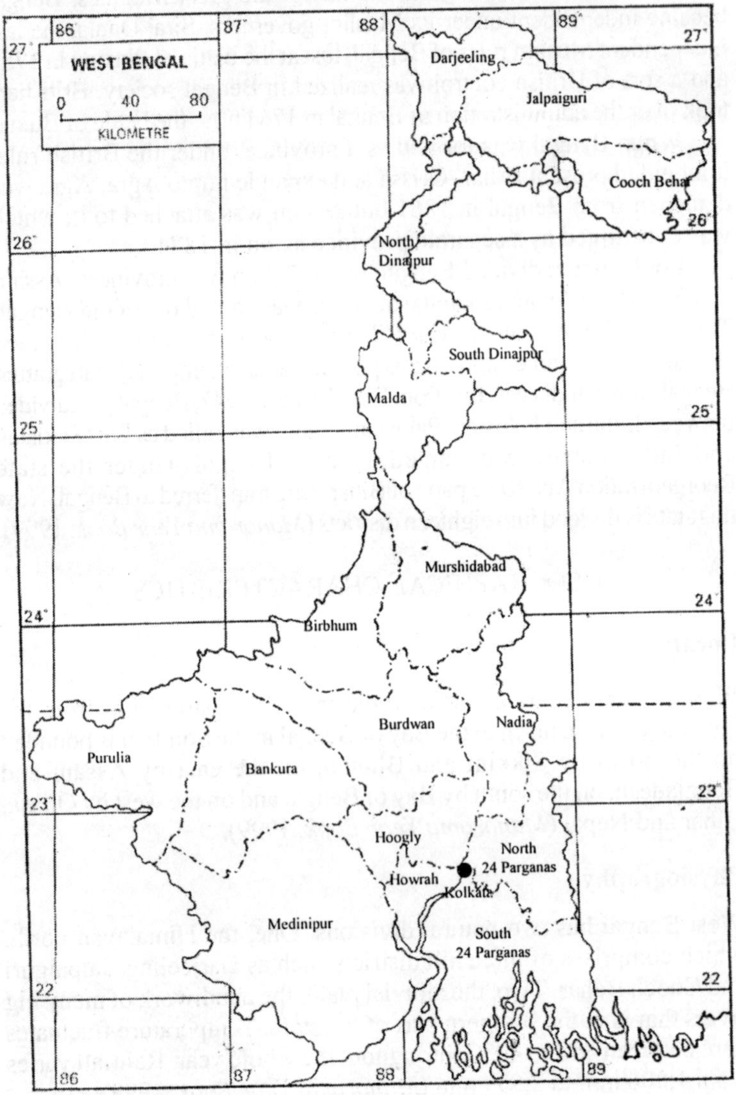

Rupnarayan, Darakeshar, Kalindi, Kaljani, Raydak, Sankosh, etc. Apart from these, there are also a few small rivers, such as Vidyadhari, Piali, Matla, Icchamati, Punarbhaba, Atrai, Kulik, Tangan, Machi, Balasan,

Rangit, Jalangi, Churni, Shilai, Kumari, Tarafeni, Bramhani, Kopai, Haldi, Saraswati, Behula, Kunti, Mundashari, Kana, etc.

Actual Forest Area

In 1993, actual forest area of West Bengal was 8,186 sq. km, which increased to 8,349 sq. km in 1997. At the all India level this situation was different. Actual forest area of 6,40,107 sq. km in 1993 decreased to 6,33,397 sq. km. in 1997 (TERI, 1996; TERI, 2001).

DEMOGRAPHIC CHARACTERISTICS

Population

As per primary calculation of the census 2001, total population of West Bengal is 8,02,21,171, out of which 4,14,87,694 are male and 3,87,33,477 are female. Table 4.1 gives the details regarding population of various districts in 1991 and 2001.

Table 4.1: Population of West Bengal

Sl. No.	*District*	*Population 1991*	*Percentage (%)*	*Population 2001*	*Percentage (%)*
1.	Medinipur	83,31,912	12.24	96,38,473	12.02
2.	North 24 Parganas	72,81,881	10.70	89,30,295	11.13
3.	Burdwan	60,50,605	8.89	69,19,698	8.63
4.	South 24 Parganas	57,15,030	8.39	69,09,015	8.61
5.	Murshidabad	47,40,149	6.96	58,63,717	7.31
6.	Hoogly	43,55,230	6.40	50,40,047	6.28
7.	Nadia	38,52,097	5.66	46,03,756	5.74
8.	Kolkata	43,99,819	6.46	45,80,544	5.71
9.	Howrah	37,29,644	5.48	42,74,010	5.33
10.	Jalpaiguri	28,00,543	4.11	34,03,204	4.24
11.	Malda	26,37,032	3.87	32,90,160	4.10
12.	Bankura	28,05,065	4.12	31,91,822	3.98
13.	Birbhum	25,55,664	3.75	30,12,546	3.76
14.	Purulia	22,24,577	3.27	25,35,233	3.16
15.	Coochbehar	21,71,145	3.19	24,78,280	3.09
16.	Uttar Dinajpur	18,97,045	2.79	24,41,824	3.04
17.	Darjeeling	12,99,919	1.91	16,05,900	2.00
18.	Dakshin Dinajpur	12,30,608	1.81	15,02,647	1.87
	Total	6,80,77,965	100.00	8,02,21,171	100.00

Source: *Manorama Year Book* 2002 (Bengali Version)

Population Density

West Bengal occupies sixth place, in India, for population density. Delhi, Chandigarh, Pondicherry, Lakshadweep, Daman and Diu are ahead of this state. Table 4.2 has drawn a picture of population density in various districts of West Bengal. Kolkata, Howrah and North 24 Parganas respectively stand first, second and third. It also shows that population density in West Bengal, as per census 2001, is 904 per sq. km. In 1991, this density was 767 per sq. km. During last ten years, 137 people have increased in each sq. km.

Table 4.2: Population Density

Sl. No	*District*	*Area (Sq. km)*	*Density (per sq. km)*	
			2001	*1991*
1.	Kolkata	185	24,760	23,783
2.	Howrah	1,467	2,913	2,542
3.	North 24 parganas	4,094	2,181	1,779
4.	Hoogly	3,149	1,601	1,383
5.	Nadia	3,927	1,172	981
6.	Murshidabad	5,324	1,101	890
7.	Burdwan	7,024	985	861
8.	Malda	3,733	881	706
9.	Uttar Dinajpur	3,180	778	604
10.	Coochbehar	3,387	732	641
11.	South 24 Pgs	9,960	694	574
12.	Medinipur	14,081	685	592
13.	Dakshin Dinajpur	2,183	677	555
14.	Birbhum	4,545	663	562
15.	Jalpaiguri	6,227	547	450
16.	Darjeeling	3,149	510	413
17.	Bankura	6,882	464	408
18.	Purulia	6,259	405	355
	West Bengal	88,756	904	767

Source: (i) *Manorama Year Book* 2002. (ii) Government of India. *India 2001—A Reference Annual*. Ministry of Information and Broadcasting: New Delhi.

Sex Ratio

As per the Census Report 2001, sex ratio, i.e. number of female per 1,000 male, of West Bengal is 934. In 1981 and 1991, it was 911 and 917 respectively. During last twenty years, the situation had improved considerably. Now West Bengal has achieved seventeenth place, with regard to sex ratio, which was twenty-third in 1991 among all the states and union territories.

Table 4.3: Sex Ratio (Number of female per 1,000 male)

Particulars	*1981*	*1991*	*2001*
India	935	927	933
West Bengal	911	917	934

Source: *Manorama Year Book* 2002. (Bengali Version).
Ali, A. and Sisodia, P., 1995.

SC, ST and Urban People

Table 4.4 illuminates the percentage of SC, ST and Urban people against the total population of each district. It is found that more than half of the people of Coochbehar and more than one-third of the people of South 24 Parganas as well as Jalpaiguri are SC. Kolkata has the lowest number of SC people. With regard to ST people, Jalpaiguri and Purulia have more contribution whereas Kolkata, Howrah and Cooch Behar have very few. Kolkata is a metropolitan city. Apart from it, respectively North 24 Parganas, Howrah and Burdwan stand first, second and third so far as urban-based population is concerned.

Table 4.4: Percentage of SC, ST and Urban People (Within the total population of district)

Sl. No.	*District*	*SC (%)*	*ST (%)*	*Urban (%)*
1.	North 24 Parganas	21.49	2.33	51.23
2.	South 24 Parganas	34.45	1.23	13.30
3.	Uttar Dinajpur	28.97	5.41	13.13
4.	Dakshin Dinajpur	29.10	16.92	13.67
5.	Kolkata	6.45	0.20	100.00
6.	Coochbehar	51.76	0.61	7.81
7.	Jalpaiguri	36.99	21.04	16.36
8.	Darjeeling	16.15	13.78	30.47
9.	Nadia	29.01	2.35	22.63
10.	Purulia	19.35	19.23	9.44
11.	Burdwan	27.44	6.21	35.09
12.	Bankura	31.37	10.34	8.29
13.	Birbhum	30.68	6.95	8.98
14.	Malda	18.12	6.50	7.07
15.	Murshidabad	13.40	1.30	10.43
16.	Midnapore	16.34	8.28	9.85
17.	Howrah	15.79	0.27	49.58
18.	Hoogly	24.12	4.05	31.19

Source: *Manorama Year Book* 2002. (Bengali Version).

SOCIAL CHARACTERISTICS

Employment

As per the data available till March 2000, in West Bengal, total 22.65 lakhs people are employed in organized sector. Out of them, 14.54 lakhs have government service. According to seventy-one State Employment Centres, sixty Block Level Employment Information Centres and four University Employment Information Centres, till October 1999, total registered unemployed were 55.85 lakhs. In 1998, it was little bit more i.e. 56.49 lakhs (*Manorama Year Book* 2002). It should be noted that these data cannot give correct information pertinent to unemployed persons. It informs only those who seek employment in organized sector. During 1999-2000, total production has increased in various fields like agriculture, pisciculture, forestry, trade and industry and those have generated employment for many more people. In order to increase employment rate in unorganized sector, various programmes such as Jawahar Gram Samridhi Yojana, Swarnjayanti Gram Swarozgar Yojana, Prime Minister Rojgar Yojana, Small Scale Entrepreneurs Programme, Special Employment Programme for Urban and Semi Urban Areas, etc. are in operation.

Education

There are eleven Universities in West Bengal. These include Calcutta University, Jadavpur University, Rabindra Bharati University, Vidyasagar University, Burdwan University, North Bengal University, Kalyani University, Visva-Bharati (Central University), Calcutta University of Animals and Fisheries, Bidhan Chandra Agricultural University and Netaji Subhas Open University. There is also a Deemed University i.e. Bengal Engineering College. Table 4.5 brings to our notice the number of various recognized educational institutions of West Bengal during 1997-98. Government of this state has decided to update the course curriculum of various Universities. Microbiology and Information technology are being added with the syllabus of various courses.

Apart from the Universities and Colleges, there are 2,383 lower Madrasha as well as lower Madhyamik schools and 9,501 high Madrasha, Secondary and Higher Secondary Schools.

With regard to *universal primary education,* West Bengal requires a total of 58,261 primary schools. At present total of 52,385 schools are existing. State Government is developing Child Education Centre for those who do not get opportunity of formal education at the age of five to nine years. These centres are in operation under Gram Panchayat with the advise of Village Education Committee. Women having age of above forty years are appointed as teachers. Till November 2000, 7,920 Child Education Centres have already been established with 14,851 teachers.

Table 4.5: Number of Recognized Educational Institutions (1997-98)

				Degree Colleges									
State/Country	*Universities*	*Deemed Universities*	*Institutions of National Importance*	*Science, Arts & Commerce Colleges*	*Oriental Learning Colleges*	*Agricultural Colleges*	*Law Colleges*	*Medical Colleges*	*Veterinary Colleges*	*Teachers Training Colleges*	*Engineering & Technical Colleges*	*Other Colleges*	*Total*
W.B.	11	1	2	333	1	2	6	24	–	28	13	12	433
India	178	43	11	–	761	90	333	798	46	618	486	371	10,910

Source: Government of India. Statistical Abstract India 1999. Ministry of Statistics and Programme Implementation: New Delhi.

As far as number of *students* are concerned, during 2000-01, there were a total of 1,00,54,191 students in class I to class V. For class VI to XII, total students were 17,49,367 including 11,35,597 male and 6,13,770 female.

Regarding *literacy* rate, census data show, it has increased in West Bengal during last ten years. In 2001, percentage of literacy is 69.22 whereas in 1991 the same was 57.70. Though literacy rate has been escalated, the performance of West Bengal among all the states and union territories has not been improved much. As per literacy, this state has now secured eighteenth place which was nineteenth in 1991. Table 4.6 highlights literacy rate in various districts of West Bengal.

Kolkata, North 24 Parganas. and Howrah respectively stand first, second and third. Purulia, Murshidabad, Malda and Uttar Dinajpur are lagging behind in this respect.

Table 4.6: District-wise Literacy Rate

Sl. No	*District*	*1991*		*2001*	
		Population	*Literacy Rate (%)*	*Population*	*Literacy Rate (%)*
1.	Kolkata	43,99,819	77.61	45,80,544	81.31
2.	North 24 Parganas	72,81,881	66.81	89,30,295	78.49
3.	Howrah	37,29,644	67.62	42,74,010	77.64
4.	Hoogly	43,55,230	66.78	50,40,047	75.59
5.	Medinipur	83,31,912	69.32	96,38,473	75.17
6.	Darjeeling	12,99,919	57.95	16,05,900	72.87
7.	Burdwan	60,50,605	61.88	69,19,698	71.00
8.	South 24 Parganas	57,15,030	55.10	69,09,015	70.16
9.	Coochbehar	21,71,145	45.78	24,78,280	67.21
10.	Nadia	38,52,097	52.53	46,03,756	66.55
11.	Dakshin Dinajpur	12,30,608	46.40	15,02,647	64.46
12.	Bankura	28,05,065	52.04	31,91,822	63.84
13.	Jalpaiguri	28,00,543	45.09	34,03,204	63.62
14.	Birbhum	25,55,664	48.56	30,12,546	62.16
15.	Purulia	22,24,577	43.29	25,35,233	56.14
16.	Murshidabad	47,40,149	38.28	58,63,717	55.05
17.	Malda	26,37,032	35.62	32,90,160	50.71
18.	Uttar Dinajpur	18,97,045	34.58	24,41,824	48.63
	WEST BENGAL	6,80,77,965	57.70	8,02,21,171	69.22

Source: *Manorama Year Book* 2002. (Bengali Version).

Health Status

Table 4.7 indicates, during 1983 to 1999, birth rate, infant mortality rate and death rate have gradually come down in West Bengal as well as India. Health status of West Bengal is far better than the all India situation.

The cumulative value of the age specific fertility rate of the end of the child bearing ages gives a measure of fertility known as *Total Fertility Rate (TFR)* which indicates the average number of children expected to be born per women during her entire span of reproductive period assuming that the age specific fertility rate to which she is exposed to continue, to be the same and also there is no mortality.

Table 4.7: Birth Rate, Infant Mortality Rate and Death Rate

Year	*Birth Rate*		*Infant Mortality Rate*		*Death Rate*	
	West Bengal	*India*	*West Bengal*	*India*	*West Bengal*	*India*
1983	32.0	33.7	84	105	10.3	11.9
1988	28.4	31.5	69	94	8.4	11
1993	25.7	28.7	58	74	7.4	9.3
1998	21.3	26.4	53	72	7.5	9.0
1999	20.7	26.1	52	70	7.1	8.7

Source: Ali, A. and Sisodia, P. 1995; *Economic Survey* 1999-2000; *Economic Survey* 2000-2001; *Manorama Year Book* 2002.

Table 4.8 highlights, during 1996-1998, TFR was 2.29 in WB. It was comparatively lower than many states like U.P. (3.99), Rajasthan (3.78), Bihar (3.48), M.P. (3.31), Haryana (2.88), Gujarat (2.71), Maharashtra (2.52), Orissa (2.46) and Assam (2.31) [Bose, 2000].

Table 4.8: Total Fertility Rate (TFR) during 1996-98 (15 to 49 years)

State	*Urban*	*Rural*	*Total*
West Bengal	1.69	2.49	2.29

Source: Bose, A., 2000.

Health Services

At present, including government and private sectors, there are 414 *hospitals* and 1,268 *health centres* (covering rural areas) in West Bengal. Among these institutions, respectively 58,065 and 12,319 bed facilities are available. Apart from these, 8,126 *sub-centres* are in operation. Regarding distribution of services for Out-Patients and In-Patients (Table 4.9), private sector has limited role in West Bengal as compared to India.

With regard to *health care personnel,* Table 4.10 and Table 4.11 give clear picture. It is required to mention that growth rate for registered medical practitioners have gradually come down in both West Bengal as well as India during 1991 to 1998. But, in this respect, West Bengal is lagging behind as compared to the all India situation.

Table 4.9: Percentage Distribution of Services for Out-Patients and In-Patients over Sources of Treatment in WB and India

Nature of Patients	*State*	*Public Hospital & Dispensary*	*Primary Health Centre*	*Private Hospital*	*Charitable Institution*	*Nursing Home*	*Others*	*All*
Out-Patients	WB	20.26	0.58	1.95	2.03	0.34	74.84	100
	India	24.35	1.19	16.18	0.81	1.15	56.32	100
In-Patients	WB	72.64	1.26	10.06	2.45	13.48	0.11	100
	India	59.51	0.75	29.55	1.91	7.04	1.24	100

Source: Baru, R., 1998.

Table 4.10: Number of doctors possessing recognized medical qualifications and registered with State Medical Council

State / *Year*	*West Bengal (No. of doctors)*	*Growth rate (%)*	*India (No. of Doctors)*	*Growth Rate (%)*
1991	41,722	–	3,93,640	–
1992	42,723	2.34	4,09,742	3.92
1993	43,612	2.03	4,26,469	3.92
1994	44,294	1.53	4,42,643	3.65
1995	45,123	1.83	4,59,676	3.70
1996	45,794	1.47	4,77,326	3.69
1997	46,591	1.71	4,95,164	3.60
1998	47,358	1.62	5,07,313	2.39

Source: Government of India. *Statistical Abstract India 1999*. Ministry of Statistics and Programme Implementation: New Delhi.

Table 4.11: Number of registered nursing personnel (1997)

State	*Nurses & Mid Wives*	*Health Visitors*	*ANM*
West Bengal	34,701	2,983	36,094
All India	6,07,396	24,824	3,01,691

Source: Government of India. *Statistical Abstract India 1999*. Ministry of Statistics and Programme Implementation: New Delhi.

ECONOMIC CHARACTERISTICS

Agriculture

Agriculture plays an important role in the economy of West Bengal. Out of the total land of the state, 19.19 per cent are outside the agriculture, 13.72 per cent are forest area, 62.63 per cent are cultivable area and 4.46 per cent have infertile soil. Rice, wheat, potato, pulses, oilseeds, jute, vegetables, flowers, etc. are the main agricultural products of this state. Table 4.12 gives details regarding cultivated area and production of various agricultural products.

Table 4.12: Agricultural Products and their Production in West Bengal

Agricultural Products	*Cultivated Area (Lakh hectares)*		*Production (Lakh tonnes)*	
	1998-99	*1999-2000*	*1998-99*	*1999-2000*
Rice	59.04	61.50	133.17	137.59
Wheat	3.67	3.64	7.78	8.51
Pulses	2.04	2.14	1.26	1.42
Potato	3.18	3.16	66.92	78.82
Oilseeds	4.93	5.02	3.79	4.06
Jute	6.12	6.13	73.74 (Lakh bales)	75.94 (Lakh bales)
Vegetables	–	–	98	99.32
Flower	–	–	0.63	0.64
Fruits	–	–	15.36	18.16
Milk	–	–	–	34.65
Fish	–	–	–	10.45
Meat	–	–	–	4.36

Source: *Manorama Year Book* 2002.

During the last twenty years, lots of improvements have taken place in agricultural sector. Till September 2000, under the Land Reform system, 4.26 lakh hectares of lands have been distributed among 25.44 lakh people. Among these people, 9.39 lakh are scheduled castes and 5.02 lakh are scheduled tribes. Under the Operation Barga system, names of 14.95 lakh sharecroppers have been registered. For construction of houses, till September 1999, 7,244.95 hectares of lands have been allocated among the landless farmers. Apart from these, various facilities such as irrigation, loan, high yielding seeds, fertilizers and insecticides have been extended to improve agricultural production.

Industry

In 1994, West Bengal government declared New Industrial Policy. As per the policy, foreign investment as well as technology was invited in the state. Since Central Government in 1991, declared the abolition of license system under its industrial policy, total 2,474 proposals came for establishment of industry in WB during 1991 to 2000. In 1999, total 94 industrial projects were implemented where total 1,848.13 crores of rupees had been invested (*Manorama Year Book*, 2002). On 1st January 2001, West Bengal government declared to extend support for setting up new industry. It wanted to provide grants and electricity in cheap rate. As per this declaration, districts were divided into B and C categories. North and South 24 Parganas, Howrah, Hoogly, Burdwan and Nadia were under B category and Kolkata as well as other districts came under C category. It was decided that 15 per cent of the total investments would be provided as grants to the new industries under B category and 25 per cent to the industries under the districts of C category. It was also assumed that grants would be sanctioned up to Rs. 2,50,00,000 to each industry and relaxation with regard to electricity will be given maximum for five years from the date of starting production. Table 4.13 gives an idea of production in various industries of West Bengal.

Table 4.13: Production in various Industries of West Bengal

Industries	*Production*	
	1998	*1999*
Jute	15.51 (Lakh tonnes)	13.48 (Lakh tonnes)
Textile	223.59 (Lakh metres)	25.37 (Lakh metres)
Coal	165.40 (Lakh tonnes)	170.00 (Lakh tonnes)
Steel	11.88 (Lakh tonnes)	12.85 (Lakh tonnes)
Tea	19.79 (Cr. Kg)	18.02 (Cr. Kg)
Silk	870 (Metric tonnes)	1,173 (Metric tonnes)

Source: *Manorama Year Book*, 2002.

Energy

With regard to energy resources, West Bengal is self-sufficient as compared to all India situations. Table 4.14, 4.15, 4.16 and 4.17 bring to our notice the various energy resources available in this state. It is found that Coal resource is gradually decreasing in West Bengal. This may be as a result of continuous domestic and industrial use. In case of power generation, this state had capacity (installed) of 3,282.9 MW in 1993, which increased to 4,372.91 MW in 2000. During five years, power generation capacity increased 24.9 per cent in West Bengal whereas it was 26.07 per cent at the all India level. It is reported, quite a good percentage of power is wasted during distribution and transmission through electricity boards. In West Bengal, this wastage was 23.7 per cent, 20.7 per cent and 19 per cent respectively on 31.3.1993, 31.3.1996 and 31.3.2000. Data show, in 1994-95, people have made 81,151 family type biogas plants, which has come down to 76,713 in 1996-97. It has also been noticed that energy is being used for pumsets or tube wells. In 1993, number of energized pump sets or tube wells were 94,710 in West Bengal, which increased to 1,07,238 in 1999.

Table 4.14: Coal Resource (Million tonnes)

State	*1995*				*2000*			
	Indicated	*Proved*	*Inferred*	*Total*	*Indicated*	*Proved*	*Inferred*	*Total*
W.B	11,438	11,271	4,010	26,718	10,894	10,779	4,236	25,909
India	89,754	68,598	41,677	2,00,029	89,501	82,396	39,697	2,11,594

Source: TERI, 1996; TERI, 2001.

Table 4.15: Installed Capacities of Power (MW)

State	*Hydro*		*Steam*		*Diesel & Wind*		*Gas*		*Nuclear*	
	1993	*2000*	*1993*	*2000*	*1993*	*2000*	*1993*	*2000*	*1993*	*2000*
West Bengal	46.5	164.01	3146.4	4086.4	0.0	22.50	90.0	100.0	0.0	0.0
All India	19575.3	23816.01	46596.5	59900.8	224.6	1881.09	3928.0	9558.9	2005.0	2680

Source: TERI, 1996; TERI, 2001.

Table 4.16: Family Type Biogas Plants in WB (Number of insertions)

1994–95	*1996–97*
81,151	76,713

Source: TERI, 1996; TERI, 2001.

Table 4.17: Potential Availability of Agriculture Based Biomass (MT) on 31.03.1994

State	*Rice Husk*	*Wheat Straw*	*Maize Cobs*	*Bajra Straw*	*Sugar Cane Bagasse*	*Coconut*			*Jute Sticks*
						Shell	*Fibre*	*Pith*	
West Bengal	5.7	0.8	0.1	–	0.2	0.0	0.1	0.1	1.4

Source: TERI, 2001.

Financial Assistance

We come across, from the Table 4.18, regarding various financial institutions those have sanctioned and disbursed assistance in West Bengal during 1995 to 2000. It is found that AFCI, ICICI and IDBI respectively stand as first, second and third every year in case of extending financial support. IVCF and TFCI have very limited role in lending money.

SOCIO-ECONOMIC STATUS OF THE DISTRICTS IN WB

An effort has been made through Table 4.19 to develop a tentative idea on socio-economic status of various districts of West Bengal. It is found that six districts such as North 24 Parganas, South 24 Parganas, Kolkata, Burdwan, Howrah and Hoogly are developed districts; three districts such as Midnapore, Nadia and Jalpaiguri are mediocre and the remaining districts are socio-economically backward.

In a nutshell, West Bengal ranks fairly high in terms of sex ratio, literacy rate and health status indicators. Primarily it is an agricultural state. It is unique in that the Communist Party led government has initiated land reform movement. There has been redistribution of land among poorer sections of society. As far as industrial development is concerned, it lags behind other states and unemployment levels are quite significant. There is growth of health services and manpower in the public sector. Regarding the health services in private sector, growth rate is very low unlike some other states.

Table 4.18: Per Capita Assistance Sanctioned (S) and Disbursed (D) in West Bengal (During 1995-2000)

Financial Institutions	*1995-96*		*1996-97*		*1997-98*		*1998-99*		*1999-2000*	
	S	*D*	*S*	*D*	*S*	*D*	*S*	*D*	*S*	*D*
AFI	321.1	151.7	279.1	174.1	442.7	317.3	459.7	414.2	496.7	427.9
IDBI	56.5	42.2	71.0	43.9	125.8	107.2	66.6	87.6	119.6	81.1
IFCI	56.0	22.3	22.8	32.0	20.9	9.0	7.5	17.5	9.7	12.6
ICICI	88.1	35.7	104.5	45.1	193.5	116.4	280.8	191.4	248.2	224.1
SIDBI	19.7	16.9	21.0	19.2	32.1	24.3	38.5	27.0	28.2	23.7
IIBI	11.3	10.6	17.3	7.1	29.8	16.7	24.3	27.5	41.3	24.2
IVCF	–	–	0.3	–	–	0.3	–	–	–	–
TFCI	1.3	0.4	1.9	0.6	–	0.7	–	0.6	–	0.1
LICI	34.0	5.5	18.4	12.2	21.1	19.2	15.8	18.7	25.8	39.3
GICI	4.6	5.3	12.4	4.8	2.3	9.0	1.7	12.2	7.1	8.8
SFCs	9.3	6.5	8.1	6.8	13.6	9.6	9.6	7.9	10.3	7.1
SIDCs	5.0	4.4	7.0	5.7	9.9	7.2	29.3	29.3	6.6	6.6

Source: Industrial Development Bank of India. Report on Development Banking in India—1999-2000. Mumbai.

AFI = All Financial Institutions.
IDBI = Industrial Development Bank of India.
IFCI = Industrial Finance Corporation of India Ltd.
ICICI = Industrial Credit and Investment Corporation of India Ltd.
SIDBI = Small Industries Development Bank of India.
IIBI = Industrial Investment Bank of India Ltd.
IVCF = IFCI Venture Capital Funds Ltd.
TFCI = Tourism Finance Corporation of India.
LICI = Life Insurance Corporation of India.
GICI = General Insurance Corporation of India.
SFCs = State Financial Corporations.
SIDCs = State Industrial Development Corporations.

Table 4.19: Socio-Economic Status of the Districts

Districts	*Net Agricultural Land (%)*	*Number of Regd. Industry*	*Number of Small Scale Industry*	*Number of Health Care Institutions and Bed Capacity*		*Number of Family Planning Centre*	*Number of Banks and Cooperatives*		*Socio-Economic Status*
				Institutions	*Bed Capacity*		*Banks*	*Coop.*	
North 24 Parganas	70.08	5332 (N&S)	36729	717	4254	47	370	485	Developed
South 24 Parganas	39.93	–	14907	842	2410	33	234	493	Developed
Dinajpur (N)	82.41	61(N&S)	5813	298	701	11	81	198	Backward
Dinajpur (S)	85.53	–	701	196	580	10	62	207	Backward
Kolkata	–	951	29793	77	18899	48	969	–	Developed
Cooch Behar	74.76	28	3580	362	1552	14	110	238	Backward
Jalpaiguri	51.86	423	12362	439	2477	18	136	183	Mediocre
Darjeeling	43.53	247	7174	227	2702	16	105	100	Backward
Nadia	77.02	166	13155	456	5140	20	181	360	Mediocre
Purulia	55.15	65	7817	472	2441	23	112	245	Backward
Burdwan	66.77	711	25801	838	6665	41	369	612	Developed
Bankura	48.30	133	10581	607	2976	24	166	421	Backward
Birbhum	75.06	138	7838	481	2197	22	174	279	Backward
Malda	77.23	33	6402	427	1249	16	143	229	Backward
Murshidabad	76.68	22	14903	743	2937	30	220	490	Backward
Midnapore	64.10	208	28069	1495	4836	62	478	1796	Mediocre
Howrah	59.37	2386	28653	428	3422	26	217	210	Developed
Hoogly	71.31	512	15221	689	3738	26	248	510	Developed

Source: *Manorama Year Book* 2001.

REFERENCES

Ali, A. and Sisodia, P. 1995. 'Health Profile of India: An Overview'. *Health For The Millions.* Vol. 21, Souvenir No. October, pp. 47 to 53.

Baru, R. 1998. *Private Health Care in India: Social Characteristics and Trends.* Sage: New Delhi, pp. 74 to 80.

Bose, A. 2000. 'The National Population Policy and After'. *Health for the Millions.* Vol. 26, No. 4, pp. 17 to 19.

Government of India. *Statisical Abstract India 1999.* Ministry of Statistics and Programme Implementation: New Delhi.

Government of India. *India 2001—A Reference Annual.* Ministry of Information and Broadcasting: New Delhi.

Government of India. *Economic Survey 1999-2000.* Ministry of Finance: New Delhi.

Government of India. *Economic Survey 2000-2001.* Ministry of Finance: New Delhi.

Industrial Development Bank of India. *Report on Development Banking in India—1999-2000.* Mumbai.

Malayala Manorama. *Manorama Year Book 1999.* Kottayam.

Malayala Manorama. *Manorama Year Book 2002 (Bengali Version).* Kottayam.

Sur, A.K. 1992. *History and Culture of Bengal.* Best Books: Kolkata.

Tata Energy Research Institute (TERI). *TERI Energy Data Directory and Year Book 1995–1996.* New Delhi.

Tata Energy Research Institute (TERI). *TERI Energy Data Directory and Year Book 2000–2001.* New Delhi.

PART II

Emergence and Development of NGOs in Health Care in West Bengal

5

Socio-Political Factors influencing the Rise of NGOs in West Bengal

In the context of social, economic and political crisis, NGOs have always been appearing as change agents since British regime. When colonial exploitation was on the peak and imperialism was the policy for development, welfare activities for impecunious and stymied people were embarked on by non-profit organizations that were extraneous of the British Government. During last hundred years, these non-profit agencies have increased by leaps and bounds and spread out in the form of social organizations, cultural organizations, sports organizations and so on. They are formed either as development agents of the community or as a result of specialized technical knowledge or induced by the government. In the post-independence era, freedom fighters, philanthropists, trained social workers, sociologists, anthropologists, development experts, planners, architects, etc. have contributed to promote NGOs (Kapoor *et al.*, 1997). In fact, unique socio-political forces of the state influenced rise of NGOs (Sarkar, 1998).

The socio-political forces of West Bengal are very unique. It is proved by the Renaissance of the Nineteenth Century, annals of series of movements of the Twentieth Century, more than 25 years rule of the Left Front Government and so on. These conspicuous socio-political traits of West Bengal, as usual, have caused NGO's emergence. Therefore, the present chapter makes an effort to understand how the socio-political factors are influencing the rise of NGOs in West Bengal.

It is indeed impossible to spell the date of inception of NGO in West Bengal, but the initiatives pertaining to NGO development have been reinforced in Bengal in the wake of freedom. Hence, attention is paid in this chapter to understand the socio political factors influencing the rise of

NGOs after independence. The chapter, in the last part, also examines whether these factors have any contribution in case of health care.

SOCIO-POLITICAL FACTORS INFLUENCING THE RISE OF NGOs IN WEST BENGAL AFTER INDEPENDENCE

There are several diverse socio-political factors. These are as follows:

1. The Christian Missionaries

In the last quarter of Eighteenth Century, the Serampore of West Bengal was the headquarters of the Missionaries delegated from the Europe, for the purpose of converting the natives of Hindustan to the Christian religion (Basu, 1985). Their main target was fulfilled for first time in the year 1800, when a Bengali carpenter of the Serampore named Krishna Paul became Christian. Till 1817, Missionaries motivated almost 700 people in and around Serampore and converted them into Christian. Along with the conversion of religion, they started charitable work and fight against social evils. In different parts of Bengal, they founded orphanages, opened hospitals, started schools, literacy centres, vocational training institutes, etc. (Basu, 1985). In fact, that was the starting of voluntary action on the part of the Missionaries in Bengal. In 1937, number of hospitals and dispensaries led by Missionaries were respectively twelve and fifteen in Bengal. In 1947, these numbers came down to nine and six. A major reason for closing down hospitals and dispensaries could be due to the financial crunch faced by these institutions because of cutbacks in funding from foreign churches. There may have also been problems in administration and availability of manpower, especially after the Foreign Missionaries handed over institutions to Indian Missionaries (Baru, 1999). However, after independence, many Christian Missionaries have promoted Voluntary Organizations to serve the vulnerable people by means of improvement in education, health care, nutrition, income generation, etc. in urban slums, remote villages and hill areas. For instance, Cathedral Relief Service (1974), Palli Unnayan Samiti Baruipur (1978), St. Joseph's Rehabilitation Centre and Relief Services (1985), etc. They receive financial support from the foreign churches.

2. Movement against Casteism

In West Bengal, movement against Casteism gives very less evidence in promoting NGOs but it is an important landmark and should not be ignored in this regard. After independence, role of this movement to form caste organizations in Bengal cannot be discussed in isolation. It has a close nexus with the pre-independence era and movement of other parts of the country.

From 1870s, many organized societies initiated caste movement in different regions of India. For instance, Satya Shodhak Samaj (1873) in Maharashtra and Arya Samaj (1875) in Northern India started raising voice against the oppressions of lower castes. The Non-Brahmin movement in southern provinces also became prominent. The Conversion of Mahars, a low caste in Maharashtra, into Buddhism under the leadership of Ambedkar in the 1940s was another way of addressing the caste oppression (PRIA, 1999).

Before independence, all India trend of this movement led to form a couple of NGOs in West Bengal to fight against untouchability and caste discrimination. Some of them were Humanity Association (1924), Harijan Sevak Sangh, Bengal (1932), Harijan Kalyan Sangha (1946), etc. After independence, those organizations and some more newly emerged societies like West Bengal SC/ST council (1970), Harijan Nav Jubak League (1970), Vivekananda Adivasi Kalyan Samity (1971), Adarsha Harijan Jubak Sangha (1973), etc. continued Harijan Welfare. In West Bengal, these organizations are of two types due to ideological difference i.e. Gandhian group and non-Gandhian group. Gandhian group never followed inter-caste marriage or taking food with higher caste people but non-Gandhian group did the same. After 1947, Bengal made various landmarks in history. Tebhaga movement, Naxalite Movement, Land Reform Movement of Left Front Government, etc. were the evidences. Poor, exploited and lower caste people were always the centre of attention in every movement. Again, the present Government is supported by these working class people and has been continuing for more than 25 years. Hence, Casteism problem in West Bengal is not as visible as in other parts of the country. Thus, number of NGOs, emerged after independence to fight against casteism, are very less in West Bengal.

3. Scouts and Guides Movement

The term 'Scouts' in the Military is used for the party of soldiers who go into the enemy territory to find out antagonists whereabouts and report back to their own army officers for attack or defense. Robert Stephenson Smyth Baden Powell used the term 'Scouts' for boys who could be given training in small groups under responsible leaders for games, journeys and competitions. He applied the word 'Guides' for girls to attempt the same objective. In fact, Baden Powell was the father of Scouts and Guides Movement which was introduced in 1907. Main purpose was to counteract, if possible, the physical, moral and spiritual degradation of boys as well as girls and to train them to be more efficient and characterful citizens. The movement had National, International and Universal Character. It was National as it worked through National Organization; it was International as it recognized the National Barrier in the comradeship of the Scouts and Guides; it was Universal as it insisted upon Universal fraternity between all Scouts and Guides of every Nation, Class or Creed. Baden Powell rightly pointed out that there was not enough scope for boys and girls training and, therefore, focus should be given on character building and general intelligence, skill of handicraft, services for others and for the state physical development and health knowledge, etc. (Singh, 1993).

In the above paragraph we have tried to understand the Scouts and Guides Movement. We do not know anything about Baden Powell. In fact, he was born in 22nd February 1857 in London. From the paternal side, he was the descendant of a Minister on the one hand and an adventurous as well as loyal colonist of the world on the other. From the maternal side he belonged to the mobile and loyal men of the British Navy and the North American Army. He lost father at the age of three years. His eldest brother Warrington became the leader of the Patrol of four brothers. All the brothers used to go for hiking, camping, tramping, canoeing and sailing round the coast of Great Britain and even across the North Sea to Norway. He was an all-rounder but not an outstanding sportsman. Though he was not good in mathematics or French or Greek, he was an enthusiastic. He was learner of 'How to do things'. In 1876, he joined in Army and at the age of 26 became a captain by his hard work. In the army Polo Horseback, Pig sticking, Shooting, Scouting and Acting in the Theatricals were his favourite hobbies. He initiated Scouts and Guides movement in 1907 in England. January 8, 1941 was his last day on the earth (Singh, 1993).

Now we need to find out the nature and extent of Scouts and Guides Movement in West Bengal, which directly as well as indirectly led to the formation of NGOs. The first scouting camp (i.e. The First Gilwell Wood Badge Course) of India was held in Calcutta at Tolly Gunj from 3rd to 12th February 1922. Sir Alfred Pickford, Dy. Camp Chief acted as the Scoutmaster and Mr. I.S. Wilson, Dy. Camp Chief as Asstt.

Scoutmaster. The second scouting camp was also held again at Tolly Gunj, Calcutta, from 19th to 30th January 1923 by J.S. Wilson as Scoutmaster. The Bharat Scouts and Guides—West Bengal, was established in 1924 to organize many camps to train the youth. On November 7, 1950 the Bharat Scouts and Guides formed its headquarters at Delhi. Thereafter, activities of the Bharat Scouts and Guides, West Bengal have increased. It extended programmes to almost all the districts of West Bengal. It inspired young people to be involved in relief work during natural calamities; social service projects like patient's libraries in hospitals; voluntary service on various occasions like free eye-operation camps, flag days for several humanitarian causes, Red Cross hospital sweeping, crowd control in religious gatherings; Scouting and Guiding in refugee homes, tea gardens, slums and industrial area, etc. (Mishra, 1982). These sort of activities influenced the youth to form club related organizations in their own locality with a purpose of service to humankind.

4. LIONS Movement

'The International Association of Lions Clubs' began on June 7, 1917 as the dream of Chicago insurance man Melvin Jones. Its slogan was 'Liberty, Intelligence, Our Nation's Safety (LIONS).' Various business and professional leaders participated in this association to promote civic life, education, health and international amity. Association became "International" with the formation of the Windsor, Ontario and Canada Lions Club in 1920. Clubs were later organized in China, Mexico, and Cuba. At present, there are 187 countries with the membership of 1.5 million people under this association. Helen Keller, the great international crusader against Blindness, attended two International Lions Conventions and appealed to the association to work for 'Sight Conservation'. From that period, Lions Clubs International is involved in Blindness Control Programme. 'Lions Sight First Programme' was introduced at the '1990 International Convention'.

This LIONS movement has influenced the NGO sector of West Bengal. Especially after eighty's decade, the well-known business families like Agarwal, Khaitan, Surana, Mehta, Jain, Jaiswal, etc were interested by the message of Lions Clubs International and promoted a good number of NGOs. Right at this moment, there are over 120 Lions Clubs who are working in different corners of West Bengal. More than 80 of these clubs are situated in the Calcutta since promoters live there. Lions Clubs of West Bengal run programmes like free homoeopathic dispensaries, free health check up camp at school, free eye operation camps, adult literacy centre, vocational training centre, civic welfare (e.g. tube well sunk), relief work during flood, etc. Though a wide range of activities are covered by them, majority of these clubs mainly pay attention towards prevention and control of blindness at the community level with active participation of the masses. In West Bengal, Lions Clubs have become more relevant and significant to achieve the goal of VISION BY 2010 AD, which will enable the community to lead a socially and economically productive life. They conduct eye screening camps at the community to find out defective eyes and thereafter, if operation is required, patients are referred either to the own eye hospital or treated at the community level having organized eye operation camp. These clubs come across the problems like cataract, refractive errors, aphakic blindness, glaucoma, corneal opacity and trachoma as the major causes of blindness (Choudhury, 2000). Cataract contributes more towards eye problems and hence awareness camps are initiated by Lions Clubs in schools as well as in community level as preventive measures. Having realized these gigantic roles and appreciation of the common people, numbers of Lions Clubs are increasing in West Bengal.

5. Gandhian Movement

M.K. Gandhi was a revolutionist and reformist in Indian society. His ideas pertaining to reconstruction of society were manifested through social struggle. His movement, during 1920s and 1930s, aimed at the welfare of all human beings and the creation of a stateless and classless society by means of 'Swaraj' and 'Sarvodaya'. In this regard, Gandhi initiated various programmes like Khadi and Village Industries, abolition of untouchability, village sanitation, basic education, tribal and labour welfare, women welfare, etc. The movement wanted to make village communities self-reliant, self-sufficient and free so that they would stand up for their own rights. Gandhiji made his movement strong with the formation of 'Shanti Senas' (Peace Brigades) in cities and towns to promote communal harmony in 1938. The individuals, who had interest, joined these groups as volunteers. It was the most systematic attempt towards development of moral and spiritual values among the people (Dayal, 1986). Another important aspect i.e. Bhoodan, initiated by Vinoba Bhave in 1951, reinforced this Gandhian

Movement after Gandhiji's death. The object of Bhoodan was to effect a voluntary transformation in the distribution of land in rural India according to the principle of equality (Radhakrishna, 1987). It used neither 'force' nor 'blackmail', but simple logic to share with one another in order to coexist.

The above mentioned nature of Movement promoted NGO sector in Bengal. 'West Bengal Sarvodaya Mondal' and 'Gandhi Seva Sangha' were established in Kolkata in 1948 and 1951 respectively in order to bring change in society as per Gandhiji's dream. Gandhi Vichar Parishad (GVP) was formed in Bankura District, 175 Km. from Calcutta, in the year 1956, when Vinoba Bhave visited the place to propagate Gandhiji's message. Late Prof. Sudarshan Singh, Shri D.N. Banerjee (a Judiciary Officer), Prof. S.N. Chakraborty, Prof. Rathindra Mohan Choudhury, Shri Sambhunath Chakraborty (Freedom Fighter) contributed to run GVP at the preliminary stage. Initially, they organized seminars, conferences and meetings to spread the social, economic and political ideas of Mahatma Gandhi. After 1968, having understood the concept of Gram Swaraj of Gandhiji, GVP formed village level committees and with their help community activities were initiated to make the villagers self-reliant. During the violent days of Naxalite movement in Bengal, GVP engaged in mobilizing peace force. Like GVP, innumerable NGOs have been developed in West Bengal with a view to serve the community as a result of Gandhian movement specially in the 1960s and 1970s. Some of the popular organizations among them are Gandhi Peace Foundation (1960), Sarvodaya Karm Mandir (1961), Sarvodaya Siksha Niketan (1961), Gandhi Memorial Committee (1971), etc. Till the end of 1970s, in West Bengal, Gandhian organizations more or less would initiate agriculture and animal husbandry, irrigation, adult education, extension service, appropriate technology, removal of untouchability, sanitation, medical care, skill formation and relief oriented activities. Since 1980s, when state policies were made favourable to non-profit sector, environmental NGOs have been emerging in West Bengal with Gandhian philosophy. They use the concept of non-violent action to control depletion of natural resources. Thus, Gandhiji's idea is still active in developing new NGOs in West Bengal.

6. Women's Movement

This movement was initiated formally in 1920s when the All India Women's Congress (AIWC) came into existence, the first women's organization at the national level, to fight for status and rights of women as well as to extend support for freedom movement (Karat, 1997). Its formation coincided with Mahatma Gandhi's call to the nation. Gandhiji too emphasized on women's empowerment. After independence, the failure of the state to eradicate gender inequalities gave impetus to this movement. Self Employed Women's Association (SEWA)—a trade union of women vendors, established in 1972, raised voice for first time in independent India to address issues like gender discrimination at the work place, unequal wages and the domestic labour (PRIA, 1999). The first report on Status of Indian Women was produced by Government in 1975 on the occasion of International Year of Women. This report too helped the Indian women's movement to seek support from the International Women's Movement. The social oppression of women in the form of dowry, rape and bride burning have galvanized the women's movement again in the late 1970s and early 1980s (PRIA, 1999). In fact, after 1947, women's multiple struggles—in national development, in politics, in their own families and lives—have shaped the Indian Women's Movement (Karat, 1997).

In West Bengal, root of this movement is older than the all India scenario. Raja Ram Mohun Roy fought for abolition of child marriage, removal of *sati* practice, widow remarriage and women education through 'Brahmo Samaj' in 1828 (Lalitha, 1975) Ishwar Chandra Vidyasagar started campaign in favour of widow remarriage and women education in 1850s. Keshab Chandra Sen too advocated for better women status. In fact, R.R. Roy, Vidyasagar, K.C. Sen played the role of advocacy and active involvement of the women was very limited. During 1905 to 1946, as a result of women's movement at the national level, women's movement in West Bengal became very strong with women's active participation. This situation led to the formation of huge numbers of NGOs in Bengal in order to uplift the social and economic status of women. Some of these organizations are West Bengal Council for Women (1919), Saroj Nalini Dutta Memorial Association (1925), Mahila Silpa Vidyalaya (1940), Umasashi Nari Silpa Siksha Mandir (1940), Serampore Mahila Silpasram (1942), Nari Seva Sangha (1944), Vivekananda Nari Karma Mandir (1945), Sandhani Mahila Samity (1945), etc. In the preceding paragraph, it is mentioned that women's movement intensified at the national level in 1970s and 1980s as a result of state inability, to maintain gender equality and to control domestic violence. The same flow of the nation-wide women's struggle did affect the Bengal. Various bourgeois liberals, left women, autonomous groups as well as NGOs in West Bengal became interested to address women issues at that time. Therefore, after independence, in 1970s and 1980s, again many women's organizations emerged in Bengal to fight against crime involving women and to bring women empowerment. Some of these organizations are Nari Kalyan Kendra (1970), Rajarhat Mohila Samity (1970), Bapujinagar Mohila Samity (1971), Sri Ma Mahila Mangal Samity (1976), Santipur Nari Silpa Udyog (1976), Mohila Silpa and Siksha Samity (1977), Nari Kalyan Samiti (1977), Gramin Mohila Kalyan Samity (1978), Kaichar Mohila Kalyan Samity (1979), Nari Colony Sishu Mahila Kalyan Samity (1980), Tarkeswar Mohila Samity (1980), Kalyani Mohila Samity (1980), Mathur Mahila Samity (1982), Kalaghata Mahila Mandal Samity (1982), Kalidaha Mahila Mandal (1982), etc.

7. Tebhaga Movement

The Tebhaga movement (1946–47 and 1948–49) was a major peasant upheaval in Bengal in the twentieth century. The main objective of this movement was to establish the rights of the Borgadars on two-thirds of the total agricultural produce (Bandyopadhyay 2001). In the villages of North Bengal the Borgadars were known as Adhiyars. Small landowners used to live in the villages, but the big Jotedars lived in towns and were involved in money-lending as well as other commercial activities. These urban Jotedars were totally different from the rural Adhiyars. Most of the lands in the rural areas were under the direct control of the urban Jotedars and the Adhiyars were sharecroppers who cultivated these lands. The entire crop cultivated by the Adhiyars used to be taken away by the Jotedars. The Adhiyars received a small share of the yield, most of which had to be again handed over to the landlord for the payment of interest on the loans they had taken in the kind during the pre-harvesting season. The land owners/Jotedars always exploited the helplessness of Adhiyars. Even the bodyguards of Jotedars used to sexually exploit the womenfolk of Adhiyar families. The Rajbanshi Adhiyars tried to set themselves free from such type of exploitation of the Jotedars by organizing the Tebhaga movement. Small farmers, landless labourers, petty artisans, factory workers and the urban middle class extended their support in order to reinforce this movement. In fact, this was one of the few struggles in the land of West Bengal where different oppressed people's voices can be heard.

This movement led to form many voluntary groups, in the late 1940s, as Kisan Sabha, Depressed Classes League, Small and Marginal Farmers Club, etc. in Jalpaiguri, Malda, Midnapore, 24 Parganas and Mymensingh districts. These groups could be treated as NGOs. Their common slogans were "Tebhaga Chai" (We want two-thirds share) and "Nij Khamare Dhan Tolo" (stock the paddy on your own threshing floor and not, as earlier, at the joteder's house). These organizations fought for: no eviction, two-thirds share, right to stock harvested crop in the Bargadar's farmyard, and reduction in the exorbitant interest rates on advance and elimination of all illegal exactions. But these organizations could not run the movement in the same way they dreamt of. It was derailed not because of people's failure but because of Communist Party's strategic retreat or hobnobbing with Congress/Muslim League. Later on, these farmers and depressed classes organizations added fuel during Naxalite Movement and Operation Barga (which was a showpiece land reform package of the Left Front Government of West Bengal).

8. Freedom Fighters

In West Bengal, several freedom fighters have promoted many NGOs during 1950s, 1960s and 1970s in order to combat sufferings of the poor people. They were involved in freedom movement to make the Indian people free from British control and suffered imprisonment for a long period. After independence, when it was impossible for the country to address the wide range of social problems, having considered the woeful condition in remote villages (i.e. poverty, illiteracy, ill health, pressure of refugees from East Pakistan, etc.), these freedom fighters promoted social organization. Their social, humanitarian and philanthropic ideas helped to organize people and to extend services at the community level. Few examples can be cited in this regard. Late Sachindra Lal Kargupta promoted Gram Seva Sangha (1949); Sri Sambhunath Chakraborty helped to promote Gandhi Vichar Parishad (1956); Late Pannalal Dasgupta helped to promote Tagore Society for Rural Development (1969), Institute for Motivating Self-Employment (1973), Rural Development Consortium (1974), Kirtipur Agradut Samiti (1976), etc.

9. Naxalite Movement

In the late 1960s, social oppression was more in West Bengal and its political atmosphere had a burning phase. About 60 per cent of the rural households were either landless or owned less than 2.5 acres each. Since the big peasants manipulated the laws to hoard the foodgrains and sell them at a higher price, the food shortage aggravated malnutrition and starvation among the rural poor. The poor peasants were least protected by the laws and subjected to pay exorbitant rent in the form of crops produced to the big landlords. The agricultural labourer's wages were very low and insufficient. As a result, people used to borrow money from the village moneylenders at a high interest rate in the lean season when they failed to find work elsewhere. The expected non-payment led many of the poor people to work as bonded labourers for the rest of their lives.

The Naxalite movement sprang up first in West Bengal to address the above mentioned social issues pertaining to poor peasantry. It began in a small village named Naxalbari in the Darjeeling and quickly spread to 24 Parganas, Midnapore as well as Birbhum districts of West Bengal. The movement was led primarily by the youths who wanted to make an exploitation free, classless society, by means of violent action. Student's hostels and university campuses were the breeding centres of Naxals. There were full time cadres among the students and they used to go to spread Naxal ideology in rural areas during holidays. Police attack at hostels, clubs and residences during night time to arrest young stars was a common phenomenon. Most of the parents and housewives of the activists would be under great tension and many of them had fate to carry loving one's dead body from the police station (Sengupta 1997). The ideological orientation of the Naxalite movement mounted a vociferous attack against the state and problematised the very basis of relationship between the democratic state and its citizenry. Since the movement took a more militant turn, it was forcefully suppressed by the state (PRIA, 1999).

The State Government banned the Naxalite movement and issued order to arrest leaders who were directly involved in violent action. Activists absconded in the remotest rural areas of West Bengal where police would not reach. Few of them left the state and went to other Bengali speaking areas like Silchar (Assam) and Agartala (Tripura); few reached Bihar, Andhra Pradesh and Kerala to add extra fuel in the on going movement of those areas. Activists did hide in big cities like Delhi, Bombay, Madras, etc. to earn their livelihood. Since Naxals had an ethical orientation and they developed a strong resentment against government rules and government services, these activists preferred to find jobs in the NGO sector. Many of the Naxal leaders who escaped in rural areas of West Bengal, promoted people's organizations (NGOs) with a dream to rebuild the society. The promoters of the organizations did not disclose their identity and initiated activities like income generation training, health care unit, farmers co-operative, adult and non-formal education, interest free loan, etc. At the same time, occasionally those organizations provided leadership to intensive mass movements, mass mobilizations, meetings, processions, etc. against the social, political and economic oppressions in rural areas (Institute for Motivating Self-Employment, 1981).

10. Devastating Flood

West Bengal covers a part of India in the east stretching from the Himalayas in the north to the Bay of Bengal in the south. Many big rivers like Ganga, Bhagirathi, Mayurakshi, Damodar, Ajoy, Tista, Torsa, etc. flow through it. Again, the Bhagirathi, called Hoogly in its lower reaches and is itself a branch of the Ganga, provides Kolkata its link with the sea (*Manorama Year Book*, 1999). Therefore, flood is not an exceptional issue here. After independence, devastating floods have occurred time to time in West Bengal. 1959, 1978 and 1980 are the years when major floods have occurred. The flood situation, which causes havoc and demands relief, directly or indirectly led to the forming of many NGOs. There are basically four distinct ways, as we find in West Bengal, who are responsible for the promotion of NGOs during post-flood work.

Firstly, a group of like-minded enthusiastic people congregate to mitigate the sufferings of the flood victims. They start emergency relief work removing the people to the safe place; distributing medicine, food, halogen tablet, cloth and blanket, polythene paper, cooking utensils, etc.; making necessary arrangement to reduce the further loss of lives and properties. Relief giving necessitates close contact with local panchayats, block development offices, outside voluntary as well as religious organization, etc. to mobilize external resources. To expedite this process of post-flood activities in a sustainable manner and to bring a long lasting socio-economic change in the flood affected villages, sometimes these enthusiastic people get interested to form NGOs. For instance, 'Village Welfare Society' situated at Kolkata.

Secondly, sometimes workers, on behalf of other NGO, come to the flood affected area and make relief-giving camps on an emergency basis. This camp focuses on medical care and runs mobile health care unit. After three to six months, when mother organization would like to terminate the camp, local people oppose it and demand their service continuously. Then, with the on going medical care programme, mother NGO initiates economic programmes side by side in the flood affected villages. Having understood the dedication and gigantic role of this NGO, local people ask for its permanent existence. As people donate land, new branch of the mother NGO is set up. After a couple of years, when new branch auspicates multifarious programmes, separate legal identity is made to manage its whole affairs. Thus, a new NGO emerges. For instance, CINI Moyna Rural Health Development Centre situated at Midnapore.

Thirdly, during flood, when external resources in the form of cash and kind reach to the local NGO, staff members may follow unfair means at the time of relief distribution. Workers who are honest, dedicated and have good ideological orientation cannot tolerate such type of malpractices. They feel embarrassed and compel to leave the organization. However, zeal of social work persists among them and thus they promote new NGO to cherish their dream. Ashurali Vivekanananda Smriti Sangha situated at south 24 Parganas district is an example of his kind of NGO.

Fourth, flood brings many outsiders like religious workers, foreigners, NGO workers, government employees, etc. to the affected area for relief work. Unique nature of dedication and enthusiasm for voluntary service, which are expressed through their activities, bring drastic change to the local people's mind. Local people understand the importance of voluntary work and feel to promote NGO. An example can be cited in this regard. During the flood of 1978, Brother Gaston Dayanand (from Switzerland) came to Howrah district for relief work. He was moving by boat to rescue people as well as to distribute food, water, cloth and medicine. Mr. M.A. Wohab was impressed by his work and met him to know the mechanisms of charitable work under the banner of an organization. Later on, he (M.A. Wohab) promoted an NGO i.e. Southern Health Improvement Samity (SHIS).

11. Environmental Movement

Conflicts over land, water and forests are not new in India. The previous contentions over land would revolve around the question of inequalities germane to productive relations. The contemporary environmental movement does not discard these questions but address injustices with regard to development, ecological degradation and survival of nature dependent people (PRIA, 1999). Guha (1994) says: "In contemporary India, conflicts over nature, ... raise important questions about distributive justice and economic efficiency." This environmental movement pays attention to conflicts arising from a wider range of issues such as commercial use of forests, mechanized fishing, loss of livelihood of poor people, displacement caused by dams, mines, industries, etc. The movement also criticizes the top down, centralized and bureaucratic developmental planning that leads to environmental loss. The Chipko Movement (in UP) and Narmada Bachao Andolan (involving the states of MP, Gujarat, Maharashtra and Rajasthan) are two well-known movements which stand out the poor people's voice and occupy some important portion in the entire spectrum of environmental movement in India.

In West Bengal, environmental movement raises a gamut of interrelated questions on economy, ecology, society and politics. This movement has gained momentum since 1980s as a result of emergence of the new definition of development, i.e. Sustainable Development, at the international level. 'Sustainable Development' emphasizes that development should be environmentally non-degrading, preferable enriching, economically viable, technologically appropriate, equitable and culturally acceptable (World Commission on Environment and Development, 1987). Since 1980s, several NGOs have been promoted in West Bengal only to reinforce the environmental movement. Environmental education through camp, seminars and workshops; controlling deforestation; afforestation; promoting biogas; sustainable food preservation; sustainable agriculture; pollution control; save the wetlands; wildlife conservation; protecting river embankment in the Gangetic islands; etc. are the concern for these NGOs. Friends of the Trees Calcutta (1980), Alipurduar Nature Club (1981), Conservation of Nature and Ecology Cell (1986), Punisole Environment and Rural Development Samity (1997), Save the Environment, etc. can be cited as examples of environmental NGOs.

12. Concern to Reduce Poverty through Economic Upliftment

The systematic treatment of India as a poor country is more than a century old. The leading personalities such as Dadabhai Naoroji, R.C. Dutt, M.G. Ranade, G. Subramania Iyer, G.K. Gokhale and Gandhiji pointed out that poverty in India was a result of British exploitation through trade and transfer (Kurien, 1987). Therefore, after independence, poverty alleviation has been an important issue before the nation. Governments after governments and five year plans after plans have been promising to alleviate poverty, but the target date for removal of poverty has been shifting and one does not know how many more years would be needed for removing poverty altogether (Prasad, 2000). Few studies (Ravallion & Dall, 1996; Sen, 1996) on the long term trends of poverty in India indicate that the period from 1970 to 1990 is characterized by a reduction of both urban and rural poverty, since National HI* falls from 53 per cent to 37 per cent. The incidence of poverty has declined from 54.9 per cent in 1973-74 to 36 per cent in 1993-94 (Sivasubramanian, 1999). In fact, reduction in poverty during 1970s and 1980s was the result of activities of the state in various forms (Franco, 1999). One of these activities was to give recognition and importance to the NGOs. They would work at the grassroots level and impart income generation training to the poor, treat credit as a resource to fight poverty (Thakur, 1995) and extend this facility, emphasize empowerment of the poor women and thereby form self-help groups, etc.

The same policy of the Government of India, i.e. preferring NGOs for poverty reduction, has also been observed in West Bengal. Therefore, during 1980s in West Bengal, while existing NGOs were taking up anti-poverty programmes, uncounted new NGOs have emerged only with a view to ameliorate the economic conditions of the poor by means of various programmes such as income generation training, micro credit, self-help group formation, etc. Agradut Pally Unnayan Samity (1984), Darabari Srikrishna Seva Sangha (1987), etc. are the examples of this kind of NGOs.

13. Youth Force

After independence, in West Bengal, various interests of youths and ideologies of renowned religious leaders, social reformers as well as freedom fighters time to time have brought the youngsters together, organized themselves and led to form many Clubs or NGOs with a view to serve the poor, destitute and exploited community people. These common causes for emergence of youth organizations can be discussed in details.

---

* HI refers to Head Count Ratio or Index. It is defined as the percentage of population living in households with average or mean consumption expenditure below a specified level.

Youth's Interests: At the tender age, people get interested towards sports, games, gymnastic, cultural activities, etc. Very often, they meet to exercise body building, football, cricket, kabbadi and so on; to organize various tournaments; and to celebrate some puja (Kali, Saraswati, etc.), Rabindra Jayanti (Rabindranath Tagore's birthday), Republic Day (26th January), Independence Day (15th August), etc. In order to maintain youths interest pertaining to indoor as well as outdoor games and to perform well in celebrating programmes, contribution is collected from the group members, local people and sometimes from outside the village. But entire money is not used for the scheduled programmes. Some funds remain. During natural calamities like floods, droughts, failure of crops, youth members try their level best to help people from their previous accumulated extra funds. Thus, voluntarism starts to help the helpless. When youth members come under one umbrella and think of helping people to get rid of social crisis, lack of funds create problems. Collecting huge amount of money becomes difficult due to lack of seal, pad, registration, etc. Thus, the question of registration of the organized youth society comes into focus and they get the same registered. This is how numbers of NGOs, as youth organization, have emerged in West Bengal. They continue various social development activities along with their original programmes i.e. sports, games, gymnastics and so on. Mass Welfare Society, Saraswati Samity, Ratulia Palli Bikash Kendra etc. are the examples of this kind of NGO.

Ideologies: Culture of Bengal is very rich for the contribution of Rabindranath Tagore, Swami Vivekananda, Raja Ram Mohun Roy, Ishwar Chandra Vidyasagar, Netaji Subhash Chandra Bose and so on. Especially, ideals of Vivekananda and Netaji have influenced the youths to a greater extent than any other section of the society of West Bengal. 'Service to man as worship to God', 'Let the poor and distressed Indians be our deity', 'Let us start work, now and at once', 'Let the giver kneel down and give thanks, let the receiver stand up and permit'—these words preached by Swami Vivekananda have inspired many youths to promote organization to fight against ignorance, illiteracy, untouchability and ill health. Ideal of Netaji too has encouraged the youngsters to come forward in order to raise voice for inequalities and exploitations in rural areas. This has also led to develop youth organizations. Vivekananda Swasthya Seva Kendra, Atma Shakti Sangha, Pallishri Sangha, Swamiji Netaji Ideal Youth Society, Patdaha Netaji Sangha, etc. are the examples of this kind of NGOs who stand for an ideology. Apart from the youth's interests and influence of ideologies, few of the youth organizations have been developed by the help of Nehru Yuvak Kendra (NYK).

14. Social Problems of Handicapped

As a result of disability, when a person experiences certain disadvantages in life and is unable to discharge the functions as well as obligations in the society, he is termed as 'handicap' (Park, 1995). Persons affected by polio, muscular dystrophy, contracture, arthritis, cretinism, epilepsy, mental retardation, cerebral palsy, deafness, blindness, lathyrism and so on problems are treated as handicapped (Werner 1996). They are categorized as orthopaedically handicapped, mentally handicapped, visually handicapped, speech and hearing handicapped, etc. There are different roots of the organizations working with disabled in West Bengal. Firstly, many disabled persons have promoted quite a few NGOs after experiencing difficulties in their personal life. In day-to-day affairs, they have found helplessness everywhere, starting from the family to social environment. Exploitation and deprivation of the parents and relatives; neglected attitude of the friends in public places like schools, colleges, restaurants, social functions; indifferent attitude of the politicians; and bureaucratic policy of the government (which does not make the service easily accessible) have given impetus to start this kind of organization in order to help the handicapped. For instance, Bankura Zilla Saririk Pratibandhi Kalyan Samity, Adarsha Protibandhi Samity, etc. Secondly, persons having specialized knowledge and curiosity (e.g. Child specialists interested towards mentally retarded children), training and working exposure (attended some training programme and thereafter worked with handicapped) have felt to promote NGO for treatment and rehabilitation of handicapped considering the lack of service in and around the district. They have a purpose to make it reputed service organization in the whole state. Indian Institute of Cerebral Palsy (1974), Alokendu Bodh Niketan Residential (1978), etc. are the examples of this kind of NGOs. Thirdly, physically handicapped find very minor scope for job opportunities. Employers neither feel them competent nor feel capable to carry out responsibility. Their disabilities make them dependent upon others. This deprives them to exercise basic rights and increases psychological stress. Many NGOs (e.g. Nadia—Murshidabad Pratibandhi Samaj Kalyan Union Samity, Nadia Zilla

Pratibandhi Kalyan Samity, etc.) have been promoted by dedicated people with a view to run income generation programme, vocational training centre, etc. for handicapped in order to make them independent, tension free and to run smooth life finding a life partner. Fourth, many government institutes like National Institutes of Orthopaedically Handicapped, Regional Institute of Mentally Handicapped, Regional Institute of Speech and Hearing Handicapped, etc. are situated at Kolkata. Their contribution in making the technical facilities available, trained manpower generation and awareness creation for handicapped welfare have developed favourable conditions in West Bengal to promote new NGO as well as to start work in this field for the existing grassroots level NGOs.

15. Health Care Motive

Voluntary initiatives in order to reduce squalor, illness and death are not new in the history of Bengal. This motive has given rise to many health care NGOs. Of course, these motives are of different types. Firstly, in order to enrich general health care facilities, by means of free medicines, surgery facilities and low cost treatment, for poor and marginalized sections in rural as well as in urban slum areas, a considerable number of NGOs have emerged. Secondly, 'Blood' cannot be manufactured in industries. It has to be donated regularly by generous compassionate people to save lives. Again, 'Eyes' cannot be produced in factories. It requires awareness for eye donation, collection of posthumous eyes and systematic preservation of the same. Having understood the importance of blood as well as human organs collection and utility for their preservation, a few NGOs have emerged completely based upon voluntary initiatives. Association of Voluntary Blood Donors—West Bengal (1980), International Eye Bank Calcutta (1980), West Bengal Voluntary Blood Donors Forum (1989), etc. are examples of this kind of NGOs. Thirdly, Leprosy and Tuberculosis are stigmatized communicable diseases. In past, persons with these diseases would have been thrown out of the community or treated with cruelty. Having taken into account the dismayed conditions of these patients, to reduce incidence and prevalence of these diseases, and to implement National Disease Control Programmes (i.e. TB and Leprosy) a scanty number of NGOs have been developed. For instance, Mahakuma Kustha Nibarani Samity (1974), Greater Calcutta Leprosy Treatment and Health Education Scheme (1975), Jhargram Leprosy Project (1977), etc. Fourthly, a deep social concern, for truck drivers, helpers and migrant workers to improve their sexual health; for alcoholics, drug addicts and their family members who are searching inner peace; has led to develop a few NGOs (e.g. St. Joseph's Centre, Bharukha Public Welfare Trust, etc). Ultimate purpose is to make the victims alive, active, responsible and useful in the existing society. Fifthly, apart from the voluntary initiatives, professionalism has also contributed in this regard. Few NGOs, associated with highly qualified professionals, have been developed to extend training and consultancy service (pertaining to health) to the grassroots organizations.

16. Other Factors

The major socio-political factors influencing the rise of NGOs in West Bengal have been illuminated above. There are also a few factors, those can never be ignored, contribute or contributed in increasing a scanty number of NGOs. For instance, to run an NGO, finance is one of the most important factors and, therefore, good connection with sources of funds, ruling party and the bureaucracy is very much needed to sanction a project proposal. Government officials, political leaders, etc. know this procedure of obtaining funds because of their working experience. Hence, after retirement, government officials or political leaders get organizations registered to pass their time through welfare activities.

Again, in order to cater relief, rehabilitation and settlement for East Pakistani refugees after 'Independence' as well as for Bangladeshi refugees after 'Bangladesh War of Liberation', a couple of NGOs have emerged. For instance, Madhyamgram Kalyan Samity (1952), Cathedral Relief Service (1974), etc.

The ethnic flare up of the early 1990s in the state of Manipur created tribal death and destruction. The fallout was beyond description between 1991 and 1995. More than 700 people were killed, 6000 houses were burnt and 11,000 families were homeless. Many wives lost their husbands and hundreds of children became orphan. The destitution of the holocaust even landed up in West Bengal, Bihar, Delhi, etc. To work with these helpless migrated tribals with a view to provide emotional and economic rehabilitation, several Tribal Welfare agencies emerged in 1990s in West Bengal. For instance, Tribal Welfare Society (1994).

Few Rotarians to improve health, literacy and awareness in

backward areas; some teachers to promote science awareness among the students; and several doctors to provide ambulance service on an emergency have also promoted quite a few NGOs in West Bengal.

ROLE OF SOCIO-POLITICAL FACTORS IN INITIATING HEALTH CARE ACTIVITIES IN NGOs

The term 'Health Care' refers to services, provided by any institution (may be government organization or private institution or NGO), to alleviate pain and suffering caused by a variety of diseases. Under the study, it indicates to NGO's service or intervention, those are provided by the health personnel, in order to promote, maintain and restore health. This part examines how far the above mentioned socio-political factors have contributed to initiating health care activities.

Christian Missionary Organizations initiated health care programme as an aspect under wide range of services towards vulnerable section of society. They would offer free treatment facilities and run health prevention programme at the community level. In the activities of 'Bharat Scouts and Guides—West Bengal', health care was a small component. It would provide curative services like medical treatment during natural disaster, free eye operation facility at the village level camp, etc and preventive services such as maintaining cleanliness in hospital campus, giving awareness on personal health and hygiene to the youths and so on. LIONS movement intended to promote civic life, education, health and international amity. Health care was also one of their major concerns. Health care, under LIONS movement, mostly insisted on 'Sight Conservation' and 'Blindness Control by 2010'. Gandhian NGOs wanted to make the village communities self-sufficient and exploitation free. Improving environmental sanitation and creating health awareness were a part of overall village development work. Women organizations fought against dowry, rape, bride burning and wanted to gain social as well as economic empowerment of woman. Improving Mother and Child health was an ingredient of their entire activities in order to increase social empowerment. NGOs led by freedom fighters aimed to address problems like poverty, illiteracy, illness, refugee's pressure, etc. Health care was extended by these organizations under an independent programme. NGOs, promoted by Naxal leaders, wanted to rebuild the society through income generation training, health care unit, farmers co-operative, adult and non-formal education, interest free loan, etc.

Health care was only one of the inputs in their initiative. NGOs, whose origins were closely connected with devastating flood or some other natural disasters, had health care unit or community level health programme within the wide range of activities since their initial days. Environmental NGOs were concerned mainly in preventive aspects of health. For instance, they were involved in controlling pollution, creating sanitation awareness, making smokeless oven to reduce women health hazards, etc. Youth organizations emerged to serve the poor, destitute and exploited community people by means of removal of ignorance, illiteracy, untouchability, ill health and so on. Setting up free treatment centres, creating awareness on personal hygiene, improving sanitation system in the locality, etc were various components of health care programme under youth organizations. NGOs offering service to the handicapped had two types of activities i.e. treatment and rehabilitation. All NGOs would not provide treatment facilities but had rehabilitation services (Physical rehabilitation, economic rehabilitation, social rehabilitation, etc.). None but health care NGOs were exceptional. Their all the programmes contributed, either through curative or preventive or promotive approach, in order to improve health status. Some of the NGOs, which emerged as a result of Tebhaga movement, movement against casteism and concern to reduce poverty, did not have any health care aspect at the time of starting.

Extensive discussion in the preceding paragraph show, health care is a fraction of wide range of services under almost every root. Except 'Health Care Motive', no other root is entirely meant for health services or health development. Again, those NGOs initiated health care programme as a part of their overall work, many of them preferred to provide preventive, community based and temporary health services. Permanent institutionalized treatment facilities were found in very limited number of NGOs.

In brief, the chapter has divulged the socio-political factors influencing the rise of NGOs in West Bengal. These factors include Christian Missionaries, Movement Against Casteism, Scouts and Guides Movement, LIONS Movement, Gandhian Movement, Women's Movement, Tebhaga Movement, Humanitarian Attitude of Freedom Fighters, Naxalite Movement, Devastating Flood, Environmental Movement, Concern to Reduce Poverty, Youth Force, Social Problems of Handicapped, Health Care Motive, Welfare Tendency of Retired Officials and Politicians, Refugee Welfare Tendency, Minority Issue and so on. It is true that one particular factor is responsible to develop an

NGO, but sometimes a few factors have synchronized to shape an NGO. The Chapter also declares the role of these factors in health care. Except Tebhaga Movement, Movement Against Casteism and Concern to Reduce Poverty, all other socio-political factors contributed in initiating health care activities. Health care programme is found as a part of entire activities under most of the NGOs.

REFERENCES

Baru, R. 1999. 'Missionaries in Medical Care'. *Economic and Political Weekly*. February 27, pp. 521 to 524.

Basu, S. 1985. *History of Renaissance of Bengal (Bengali Version)*. Pustak Biponi: Kolkata.

Bandyopadhyay, D. 2001. 'Tebhaga Movement in Bengal: A Retrospect.' *Economic and Political Weekly*. October 13, pp. 3901-3907.

Choudhury, B.L. (Ed.). 2000. *Communication Strategy of NGOs for Rural Development*. Assam University: Silchar, p. 25.

Dayal, P. 1986. *Gandhian Approach to Social Work*. Gujarat Vidyapith: Ahmedabad, p. 141.

Franco, F. 1999. 'Poverty Reduction: Challenges and Opportunities'. *Social Action*. Vol. 49, No. 4, p. 355.

Guha, R. and Gadgil, M. 1994. 'Ecological Conflicts and the Environmental Movement in India.' *Development and Change*. Vol. 25.

Institute of Motivating Self-Employment (IMSE). 1981. 'IMSE—A New Type of Social Movement'. *News Bulletin*. Vol. 1, No. 1.

Kapoor, A.K. Singh, D. 1997. *Rural Development Through NGOs*. Rawat Publications: New Delhi, p. 5.

Karat, B. 1997. 'Years of Independence and the Multiple Struggles of Women.' *Frontline*. October 3.

Kurien, C.T. 1987. 'Poverty'. *Encyclopedia of Social Work in India*. Vol. II, p. 297.

Lalitha, N. 1975. *Voluntary Work in India*. National Institute of Public Co-operation and Child Development: New Delhi, p. 2.

Mishra, M.S. 1982. *Directory of Organisations in Rural Development*, Vol. I, Indian Institute of Management: Calcutta, p. 33.

Monorama Year Book. 1999. Malayala Manorama: Trivandrum, p. 672.

Mathias, E. and Raj, S.L. 1998. *People's Power and Panchayati Raj—Theory and Practice*. India Social Institute: New Delhi, p. vii.

Park, K. 1995. *Park's Text Book of Preventive and Social Medicine*. Banarsidas Bhanot Publishers: Jabalpur, p. 37.

PRIA, 1999. *Civil Society and Governance—An Overview of Issues and Trends in India*. Participatory Research in Asia: New Delhi, pp. 5-15.

Prasad, K. 2000. 'Poverty Alleviation: Shift in Paradigms' *Kurukshetra*. Vol. 49, No. 1, p. 11.

Ravallion, M. and Datt, G. 1996. 'India's Checkered History in Fight Against Poverty. Are There Lessons for the Future?' *Economic and Political Weekly*. Vol. XXXI; No. 35, 36, 37; pp. 2479-85.

Radhakrishna. 1987. 'Sarvodaya Movement in India.' *Encyclopedia of Social Work in India*. Vol. III, p. 6.

Sarkar, A. 1998. *Characteristics of NGOs: An Exploratory Study in Assam,* M.Phil Dissertation. Centre for Social Medicine and Community Health, School of Social Sciences, Jawaharlal Nehru University, New Delhi, p. 66.

Sengupta, A. 1997. *High Tide and Low Tide in Seventies and Eighties* (Joer Bhatay Shat Sottor). Pearl Publishers: Calcutta, p. 225.

Sen, A. 1996. 'Economic Reforms, Employment and Povety: Trends and Options'. *Economic and Political Weekly*, Vol. XXXI; No. 35, 36, 37; pp. 2459-77.

Sivasubramanian, M.N. 1999. 'Credit Based Poverty Alleviation Programme: Innovative Approach.' *Kurukshetra*. Vol. 48, No. 2, p. 38.

Singh, R.D.E. 1993. *The Story of B.P.* The Bharat Scouts & Guides: New Delhi. pp. 1, 2, 5, 6, 94, 101, 102.

Thakur, S.G. 1995. 'Women, Poverty and Empowerment.' *The Administrator*. Vol. XL, No. 4, p. 127.

Werner, D. 1996. *Disabled Village Children*. Voluntary Health Association of India: New Delhi.

World Commission on Environment and Development. 1987. *Our Common Future*. Oxford University Press: New Delhi, pp. 1-4.

6

Growth and Distribution of NGOs in Health Care in West Bengal

Development is contingent on various aspects such as social and economic security of the people, social status of women, female literacy, adoption of new technology, work participation of women, the internalization of investments to generate resources and so on. Better health, income, information, education, communication, gender justice, etc. can improve these aspects and thereby lead to development. These preconditions of development cannot be superimposed. They have to be built on the expectations, aspirations and motivation of the people. Therefore, people's own organizations i.e. NGOs are emerging gradually and participating actively in the process of social and economic transformation. The earlier chapter traces how the influence of socio-political forces has resulted in the growth of NGOs in West Bengal after independence. Since health is a necessary ingredient of a state's overall development and the present study intends to focus on NGOs in health care, detail description on when these organizations have grown and where they are located in West Bengal is important for development in general and health improvement in particular. It may guide the policy makers and bureaucrats for better health planning in this state. The present chapter, hence, provides a clear picture on trends in growth and distribution of NGOs in health care in West Bengal.

The Methodology Chapter has given the justification and details of the methods used in the present study. In the second phase of data collection, addresses of NGOs in health care of West Bengal were collected from various National Institutes, Umbrella Organizations, Directories of NGOs, etc. Having put all the addresses together, a comprehensive list of 705 NGOs was prepared. In the third phase, questionnaires were mailed to all these NGOs of which 216 NGOs replied. The data have been presented in this chapter as per the responses received from the mailed questionnaires.

TRENDS IN GROWTH OF NGOs IN HEALTH CARE

Out of 216 NGOs, 12 NGOs did not reply the year of registration. Therefore, only 204 NGOs have been considered in few cases under this part. Growth of NGOs in health care has been depicted year-wise under the following heads.

1. Operational Area

Table 6.1 shows the growth of NGOs in different areas of West Bengal during last hundred years. In urban area, during 1950s (i.e. from 1951 to 1960), 1960s (i.e. from 1961 to 1970), 1970s (i.e. from 1971 to

Table 6.1: Operational Area (No. of NGOs located in each area)

Year of Registration	*Area*					*Total*
	Urban Area	*Rural Area*	*Tribal Area*	*Urban & Rural Areas*	*Urban, Rural & Tribal Areas*	
Before 1901					1 2.4%	1 49%
1921-1940				2 5.2%	2 4.8%	4 1.96%
1941-1950	3 12.5%			2 5.2%	3 7.3%	8 3.92%
1951-1960	2 8.4%	5 6.8%	1 3.7%	1 2.6%	1 2.4%	10 4.90%
1961-1970	4 16.7%	7 9.6%	4 14.8%	3 7.7%		18 8.82%
1971-1980	8 33.3%	25 34.2%	6 22.2%	9 23.1%	12 29.3%	60 29.41%
1981-1990	3 12.5%	30 41.1%	11 40.7%	14 35.9%	16 39.1%	74 36.28%
1991-2000	4 16.7%	6 8.2%	5 18.5%	8 20.5%	6 14.6%	29 14.22%
Total	**24** **100%**	**73** **100%**	**27** **100%**	**39** **100%**	**41** **100%**	**204** **100%**

Source: Responses received from the mailed questionnaires.

1980), 1980s (i.e. from 1981 to 1990), and 1990s (i.e. from 1991 to 2000) 8.4 per cent, 16.7 per cent, 33.3 per cent, 12.5 per cent and 16.7 per cent respectively NGOs were registered. Thus, registration ratio of urban NGOs during these five decades was 8.4 : 16.7 : 33.3 : 12.5 : 16.7. Similarly, in rural area this ratio was 6.8 : 9.6 : 34.2 : 41.1 : 8.2 and in tribal area it was 3.7 : 14.8 : 22.2 : 40.7 : 18.5. It is proved here, growth rate for NGOs of urban area has been very high during 1970s and the same for rural area as well as tribal area has been very high during 1980s. In the entire West Bengal, maximum percentage (36.3%) of NGOs was registered during 1980s. It is found that 65.69 per cent of the total NGOs (204) under the study have been registered during 1971 to 1990. The table also indicates that there is fall in the registration of NGOs after 1990 in West Bengal. In this regard, Chart 6A shows the trend in a better way.

Chart 6A: Growth of NGOs as per Operational Area

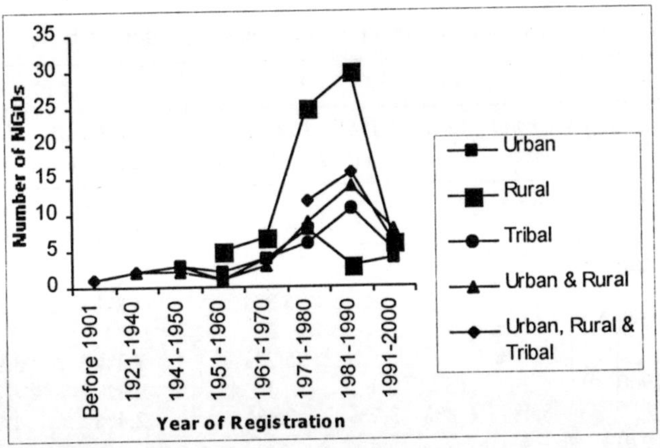

2. Types of Organization

In West Bengal, NGOs have been categorized as (a) religious organizations; (b) service organizations; (c) development organizations; (d) research and consultancy agencies; and (e) action groups. Some of the organizations are combination of these categories. Religious organizations assume service to human being is service to God; service organizations are basically philanthropic organizations work through social cultural ethos of the people; development organizations are involved in the progress of human beings through self sufficiency and

Table 6.2: Types of Organization (in numbers)

Year of Regist.	*Organization*										*Total*
	A	*B*	*BC*	*BCD*	*BCE*	*C*	*CD*	*CE*	*D*	*E*	
Before 1901		1									1
		1.8%									.49%
1921-40	1	1				2					4
	20.0%	1.8%				2.2%					1.96%
1941-50		5	1		1	1					8
		9%	4.8%		20%	1.1%					3.92%
1951-60	1	3	1		1	3		1			10
	20.0%	5.4%	4.8%		20%	3.2%		20%			4.90%
1961-70		5	4		1	8					18
		9%	19.1%		20%	8.6%					8.82%
1971-80	2	15	8	4		27	2	1	1		60
	40.0%	26.8%	38.1%	57.2%		28.7%	50%	20%	33.3%		29.41%
1981-90	1	14	6	1	2	41	2	2	2	3	74
	20.0%	25%	28.6%	14.3%	40%	43.6%	50%	40%	66.7%	75%	36.28%
1991-2000		12	1	2		12		1		1	29
		21.4%	4.8%	28.6%		12.8%		20%		25%	14.22%
Total	5	56	21	7	5	94	4	5	3	4	204
	100%	100%	100%	100%	100%	100%	100%	100%	100%	100%	100%

Source: Ibid.

sustaining the same; research and consultancy agencies carry out research activities and extend advice, guidance as well as help in their specialized fields; and action groups are involved in mobilization and socialization of unorganized sections of society. As per Table 6.2, service organizations (B) and development organizations (C) are found more in numbers in West Bengal. Under the study, during 1950s, 1960s, 1970s, 1980s and 1990s respectively 5.4 per cent, 9 per cent, 26.8 per cent, 25 per cent and 21.4 per cent service organizations (B) emerged. Similarly, for development organizations (C), these percentages were respectively 3.2 per cent, 8.6 per cent, 28.7 per cent, 43.6 per cent and 12.8 per cent. It is understood, growth rate of service organizations (B) has been very high in 1970s and the same for development organizations (C) has been very high during 1980s.

3. Types of Services

NGOs under the study, fulfilled the needs of the beneficiaries by means of either only institutionalized service or only community based service

Table 6.3: Types of Services in NGOs

Year of Registration	*Service (in number of NGOs)*				*Total*
	Institutionalized	*Community Based*	*Institutionalized & Community Based*	*Occasional Camp*	
Before 1901			1 .92%		1 .49%
1921-1940		1 1.19%	3 2.78%		4 1.96%
1941-1950	1 9.09%	3 3.57%	4 3.70%		8 3.92%
1951-1960	1 9.09%	2 2.38%	7 6.48%		10 4.90%
1961-1970	1 9.09%	4 4.76%	13 12.04%		18 8.82%
1971-1980	4 36.36%	23 27.38%	32 29.63%	1 100%	60 29.41%
1981-1990	1 9.09%	38 45.24%	35 32.41%		74 36.28%
1991-2000	3 27.28%	13 15.48%	13 12.04%		29 14.22%
Total	**11 100%**	**84 100%**	**108 100%**	**1 100%**	**204 100%**

Source: Ibid.

or both institutionalized as well as community based service or only occasional camp at the community level. Table 6.3 highlights, during 1950s, 1960s, 1970s, 1980s and 1990s, respectively 9.09 per cent, 9.09 per cent, 36.36 per cent, 9.09 per cent and 27.28 per cent NGOs emerged to provide institutionalized service. Growth of these NGOs was very high during 1970s. Similarly, growth of the NGOs provided community based service has been high during 1980s. So, it could be assumed that there was a shift from institutionalized approach to community based approach from 1970s to 1980s. NGOs who provided both types of services had a steady growth till the decade of 1980s and thereafter a fall was found. Regarding types of service, Chart 6B shows the trend in better way.

Chart 6B: Growth of NGOs as per Types of Services

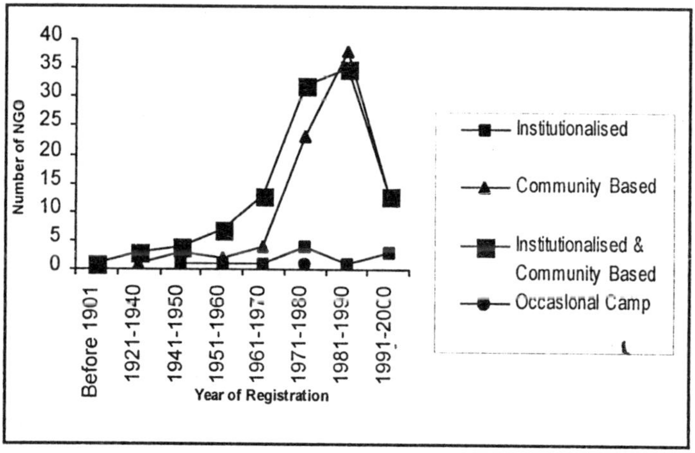

4. Nature of Starting Programme

The present study points out, NGOs, at the time of starting, had either only awareness programme or only service-oriented programme or both. Table 6.4 describes, during 1971 to 1990, growth of NGOs is very high. During this period, 64.15 per cent NGOs emerged with only awareness programme, 39.13 per cent NGOs emerged with only service oriented programme and 71.09 per cent emerged with both kinds of services. So, it is evident that awareness programme received maximum focus and importance during 1970s and 1980s. The trend pertaining to nature of starting programme is better understood pertaining to nature of starting programme is better understood from the Chart 6C.

Table 6.4: Nature of Starting Programme

Year of Registration	*Nature (in number of NGOs)*			*Total*
	Awareness	*Service Oriented*	*Both*	
Before 1901			1 0.78%	1 .49%
1921-1940	1 1.89%		3 2.34%	4 1.96%
1941-1950		4 17.39%	4 3.13%	8 3.92%
1951-1960	3 5.66%	3 13.04%	4 3.13%	10 4.90%
1961-1970	4 7.55%	2 8.70%	12 9.38%	18 8.82%
1971-1980	12 22.64%	5 21.74%	43 33.59%	60 29.41%
1981-1990	22 41.51%	4 17.39%	48 37.50%	74 36.28%
1991-2000	11 20.75%	5 21.74%	13 10.15%	29 14.22%
Total	53 100%	23 100%	128 100%	204 100%

Source: Ibid

Chart 6C: Growth of NGOs as per Nature of Starting Programme

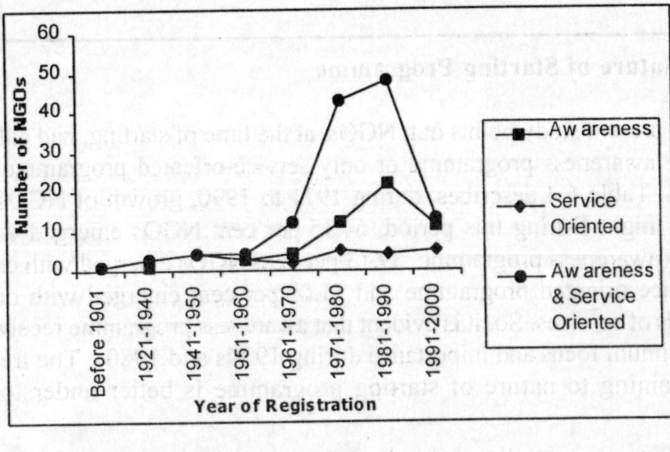

5. Promoter's Background

Article 19 (1) (C) of the Constitution of India lays down that all citizens shall have the right to form associations or unions. Hence, every one can take initiative to develop an NGO. In the present study, medical practitioners, school teachers, retired government officials, political leaders, freedom fighters, activists of any movement, group of young enthusiastic friends, businessmen, untrained dedicated social workers, college or university teachers and others were found as promoters of NGOs. Table 6.5 shows, those NGOs were led by freedom fighters, 50 per cent of that emerged during 1950s and 1960s. Similarly, those NGOs were led by activists of various movements, a high percentage (47.06%) of that came into existence during 1970s. The same table states, under the study, 60 per cent of the total medical practitioners, 48.65 per cent of the school teachers and 50 per cent of the retired government officials promoted NGOs during 1980s. It is also understood from the table that 60 per cent of the political leaders, 50 per cent of the total youth groups, 83.33 per cent of the total businessmen and 57.9 per cent of the untrained dedicated social workers promoted NGOs between 1981 to 2000. On the basis of above discussion, we can say, after independence, growth of NGOs is reinforced by freedom fighters in 1950s and 1960s, by activists of various movements in 1970s, by professionals as well as common people in 1980s, and by common people (i.e. political leaders, youth, businessmen, dedicated untrained social workers, etc.) in 1990s.

6. Year of Starting Health Programme

Responses with regard to the year of starting health programme were received from all the 216 NGOs. These NGOs have various approaches such as religious approach (A), service oriented approach (B), development approach (C), research and consultancy approach (D), social action approach (E) and multiple approaches (i.e. combination of few approaches). Concepts of these approaches have already been discussed earlier. It is observed from the Table 6.6 that 50 per cent of the total NGOs stated their health programme after 1985 (i.e. during 1986-2000). The same table also traces, respectively 44.8 per cent and 54.9 per cent of the B and C types of organizations followed the same trend. It is evident here that growth of health care programmes is found more in C type (i.e. development) organizations after 1985.

Table 6.5: Backgrounds of Promoters

Year of Registration	*Promoters (in number of NGOs)*											*Total*
	Medical Practitioner	*School Teacher*	*Retd. Govt. Official*	*Political Leader*	*Freedom Fighter*	*Activist of any Movement*	*Group of Young Friends*	*Business man*	*Untrained Dedicated Social Worker*	*College or University Teacher*	*Others*	
Before 1901											1 5%	1 .49%
1921-1940		1 2.70%	1 6.25%			1 5.88%			1 2.63%			4 1.96%
1941-1950	1 4.0%			1 10%	3 16.67%	.	1 8.33%		1 2.63%		1 5%	8 3.92%
1951-1960	1 4.0%	1 2.70%	1 6.25%		5 27.78%	2 11.77%						10 4.90%
1961-1970	1 4.0%	2 5.41%	1 6.25%	2 20%	4 22.22%		3 25%	1 16.67%	3 7.89%		1 5%	18 8.82%
1971-1980	6 24.0%	13 35.13%	4 25%	1 10%	3 16.67%	8 47.06%	2 16.67%		11 28.95%	2 40%	10 50%	60 29.41%
1981-1990	15 60.0%	18 48.65%	8 50%	3 30%	1 5.55%	5 29.41%	5 41.67%	3 50%	10 26.32%	3 60%	3 15%	74 36.28%
1991-2000	1 4.0%	2 5.41%	1 6.25%	3 30%	2 11.11%	1 5.88%	1 8.33%	2 33.33%	12 31.58%		4 20%	29 14.22%
Total	25 100%	37 100%	16 100%	10 100%	18 100%	17 100%	12 100%	6 100%	38 100%	5 100%	20 100%	204 100%

Source: Ibid.

Table 6.6: Year of Starting Health Programme (in number of NGOs)

Type of Organi-zation	*Year*							*Total*
	Before 1971	*1971-1975*	*1976-1980*	*1981-1985*	*1986-1990*	*1991-1995*	*1996-2000*	
A	2	2			1		1	6
	33.3%	33.3%			16.7%		16.7%	100.0%
B	14	3	10	5	12	1	13	58
	24.1%	5.2%	17.2%	8.6%	20.7%	1.7%	22.4%	100.0%
BC	3	1	5	6	5		1	21
	14.3%	4.8%	23.8%	28.6%	23.8%		4.8%	100.0%
BCD	1		2		1	3		7
	14.3%		28.6%		14.3%	42.9%		100.0%
BCE	2		1		1		1	5
	40.0%		20.0%		20.0%		20.0%	100.0%
C	10	7	9	20	17	16	23	102
	9.8%	6.9%	8.8%	19.6%	16.7%	15.7%	22.5%	100.0%
CD	1		1				2	4
	25.0%		25.0%				50.0%	100.0%
CE	1			1	1	2	1	6
	16.7%			16.7%	16.7%	33.3%	16.7%	100.0%
D					3			3
					100.0%			100.0%
E				1		2	1	4
				25.0%		50.0%	25.0%	100.0%
Total	34	13	28	33	41	24	43	216
	15.7%	6.0%	13.0%	15.3%	19.0%	11.1%	19.9%	100.0%

Source: Ibid.

7. Nature of Starting Health Programme

Those health programmes were started for first time in NGOs under the study, they were of various kinds such as awareness generation (A), occasional health camp (B), regular mobile dispensary (C), permanent clinic (D), permanent hospital (E) and training of health workers (F). Many of the NGOs had more than one of these programmes (e.g. AB, ABCDF, ABCD, ABD, ABDF, ABF, ADF, AC, AD, AE, AF). Table 6.7 provides a clear picture that most of the starting health programmes were related to only awareness generation (A) or only occasional health camp (B) or only training of health workers (F) or combination of these programmes (e.g. AB, AF, ABF). Again, most of the NGOs started these few programmes during 1986 to 2000.

Therefore, it can be said that preventive and developmental approaches dominated over the health programmes in late 1980s and 1990s.

Table 6.7: Nature of Starting Health Programme (in number of NGOs)

Nature of Starting Health Programme	*Year of starting health Programme*							*Total*
	Before 1971	*1971–75*	*1976–80*	*1981–85*	*1986–90*	*1991–95*	*1996–2000*	
A	5	1	4	3	12	7	7	39
	12.8%	2.6%	10.3%	7.7%	30.8%	17.9%	17.9%	100.0%
AB	4	1	2	3	9	6	10	35
	11.4%	2.9%	5.7%	8.6%	25.7%	17.1%	28.6%	100.0%
ABCD	1	1		1	2		2	7
	14.3%	14.3%		14.3%	28.6%		28.6%	100.0%
ABCDF	3		1	1	1			6
	50.0%		16.7%	16.7%	16.7%			100.0%
ABD			3	1	1	1	1	7
			42.9%	14.3%	14.3%	14.3%	14.3%	100.0%
ABDF	1		6	5	3		1	16
	6.3%		37.5%	31.3%	18.8%		6.3%	100.0%
ABF	3	3	2	3	6	3	6	26
	11.5%	11.5%	7.7%	11.5%	23.1%	11.5%	23.1%	100.0%
AC			3	2				5
			60.0%	40.0%				100.0%
AD	1			2			2	5
	20.0%			40.0%			40.0%	100.0%
ADF				2	3	1		6
				33.3%	50.0%	16.7%		100.0%
AE	4	1		1			1	7
	57.1%	14.3%		14.3%			14.3%	100.0%
AF			2	2	2	4	1	11
			18.2%	18.2%	18.2%	36.4%	9.1%	100.0%
B	1	1	3	3	1	1	10	20
	5.0%	5.0%	15.0%	15.0%	5.0%	5.0%	50.0%	100.0%
C	3						1	4
	75.0%						25.0%	100.0%
D	7	4	2	4	1		1	19
	36.8%	21.1%	10.5%	21.1%	5.3%		5.3%	100.0%
E	1	1				1		3
	33.3%	33.3%				33.3%		100.0%
Total	34	13	28	33	41	24	43	216
	15.7%	6.0%	13.0%	15.3%	19.0%	11.1%	19.9%	100.0%

Source: Ibid.

8. Full Time Separate Health Staff

Table 6.8 explains, under the study, 66.7 per cent of the total NGOs have full time separate health staff and 33.3 per cent do not have the

Table 6.8: Full Time Separate Health Staff (in number of NGOs)

Year of Starting Health Programme	*Separate Health Staff*		*Total*
	Do not have	*Have*	
Before 1971	11 (32.3%) (15.3)	23 (67.7%) (16.0)	34 (100.0%) (15.7)
1971–1975	2 (15.3%) (2.8)	11 (84.7%) (7.6)	13 (100.0%) (6.0)
1976–1980	8 (28.5%) (11.1)	20 (71.5%) (13.9)	28 (100.0%) (13.0)
1981–1985	6 (18.2%) (8.3)	27 (81.8%) (18.8)	33 (100.0%) (15.3)
1986–1990	13 (31.7%) (18.1)	28 (68.3%) (19.4)	41 (100.0%) (19.0)
1991–1995	9 (37.5%) (12.5)	15 (62.5%) (10.4)	24 (100.0%) (11.1)
1996–2000	23 (53.5%) (31.9)	20 (46.5%) (13.9)	43 (100.0%) (19.9)
Total	72 (33.3%) (100.0%)	144 (66.7%) (100.0)	216 (100.0%) (100%)

Source: Ibid.

Chart 6D: Growth of NGOs as per Full Time Separate Health Staff

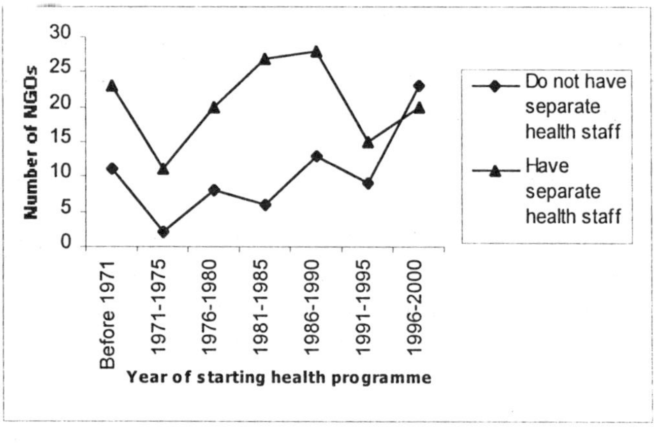

same. Again, those NGOs do not have full time separate health staff, a major portion (i.e. 31.9%) of them started health programme during 1996-2000. In the same period, those NGOs started health programme, 53.5 per cent of them did not have separate health staff. So, it can be assumed from the table that there was a growing tendency for not having full time separate health staff during late 1990s. NGOs managed to run their programmes either by general staff or by part timer. Chart 6D also shows the trend in this regard.

9. Health Budget

Table 6.9 looks into the health budget of the NGOs under study for the financial year 2000-01. Health work and health budget is nil for 0.9 per cent of the total NGOs and 3.7 per cent have health work but do not have any separate health expenditure. Rest of the NGOs have been classified into seven categories based on health budget such as up to Rs. 10,000, Rs. 10,001 to 50,000, Rs. 50,001 to Rs. 1,00,000, Rs. 1,00,001 to Rs. 2,00,000, Rs. 2,00,001 to 5,00,000, Rs. 5,00,001 to Rs. 10,00,000 and above Rs. 10,00,000. Table 6.9 describes that 70.8 per cent of the total NGOs have health budget up to Rs. 2,00,000. None but 12.1 per cent of the NGOs have a good amount of health budget (i.e. above 10,00,000). It means only a few NGOs have wide range of health activities. Again, those NGOs have health budget up to Rs. 10,000, Rs. 10,001 to 50,000, Rs. 50,001 to 1,00,000 and Rs. 1,00,001 to 2,00,000, respectively 58 per cent, 66.1 per cent, 46.8 per cent and 60.7 per cent of them started health programmes after 1985 (i.e. during 1986 to 2000). Therefore, it can be argued that NGOs who initiated health programmes after 1985 majority of them have very limited health activities.

TRENDS IN DISTRIBUTION OF NGOs IN HEALTH CARE

In this part, distribution of NGOs in health care has been understood as per the district and area of operation. In order to know district-wise distribution, all the 705 NGOs of the comprehensive list have been considered. Distribution on the basis of area of operation has been discussed taking into account 216 NGOs who replied to the mailed questionnaire.

Table 6.9: Health Budget of 2000–2001 (in number of NGOs)

Year of Starting Health Programme	*Health Budget*									*Total*
	No Health Work and Health Budget	*Health Work without Budget*	*Upto Rs. 10000*	*Rs. 10001 to 50000*	*Rs. 50001 to 100000*	*Rs. 100001 to 200000*	*Rs. 200001 to 500000*	*Rs. 500001 to 1000000*	*Above Rs. 1000000*	
Before 1971		3 37.5%	10 20.0%	7 12.5%	3 15.8%	3 10.7%	3 15.0%	2 28.6%	3 11.5%	34 15.7%
1971–1975			5 10.0%	1 1.8%	1 5.3%		1 5.0%	1 14.3%	4 15.4%	13 6.0%
1976–1980		3 37.5%	3 6.0%	2 3.6%	4 21.1%	4 14.3%	3 15.0%	1 14.3%	8 30.8%	28 13.0%
1981–1985	1 50%		3 6.0%	9 16.1%	4 21.1%	4 14.3%	5 25.0%	3 42.9%	4 15.4%	33 15.3%
1986–1990		1 12.5%	6 12.0%	14 25.0%	3 15.8%	6 21.4%	5 25.0%		6 23.1%	41 19.0%
1991–1995	1 50%		8 16.0%	7 12.5%	2 10.5%	4 14.3%	1 5.0%		1 3.8%	24 11.1%
1996–2000		1 12.5%	15 30.0%	16 28.6%	2 10.5%	7 25.0%	2 10.0%			43 19.9%
Total	2 (.9) 100%	8 (3.7) 100%	50 (23.1) 100%	56 (25.9) 100%	19 (8.8) 100%	28 (13) 100%	20 (9.3) 100%	7 (3.2) 100%	26 (12.1) 100%	216 (100) 100%

Source: Ibid.

(A) District-wise Distribution of NGOs

Table 6.10 shows distribution of NGOs in health care in various districts of West Bengal. Kolkata, 24 Parganas (South and North) and Midnapore respectively stand as first, second and third in terms of number of NGOs. Under the study, no NGO is found in Cooch Behar. It is found 72.19 per cent of the total NGOs are centralized in Kolkata and its adjacent area (i.e. Howrah, 24 Parganas and Hoogly). This may be because: (a) this region is socio-economically developed and near to capital of the state; (b) it is very old and historically important area of Bengal; and (c) most of the movements were led from this place.

Table 6.10: District-wise Distribution of NGOs

Sl. No.	*Division/District*	*No. of NGOs*	*Percentage (%)*	*Socio-economic Status of the Area*
A	**Presidency Division**			
1.	Kolkata	272	38.58	Developed
2.	24 Parganas (S & N)	148	20.99	Developed
3.	Howrah	51	7.23	Developed
4.	Nadia	24	3.40	Medium
5.	Murshidabad	13	1.84	Backward
B.	**Burdwan Division**			
1.	Midnapore	81	11.49	Medium
2.	Hoogly	38	5.39	Developed
3.	Burdwan	26	3.69	Developed
4.	Bankura	17	2.41	Backward
5.	Birbhum	06	0.86	Backward
6.	Purulia	05	0.71	Backward
C.	**Jalpaiguri Division**			
1.	Malda	08	1.13	Backward
2.	Jalpaiguri	06	0.86	Medium
3.	Darjeeling	05	0.71	Backward
4.	Dinajpur (S & N)	05	0.71	Backward
5.	Cooch Behar	00	0.00	Backward
	Total	705	100.00	

Source: List of NGOs compiled from the lists provided by various umbrella organizations (mentioned in the methodology chapter) of Kolkata.

(B) Distribution of NGOs as per the Area of Operation

It has been discussed under the following heads:

1. *Area of Operation*

Table 6.11 throws light on how many NGOs work in which area. It indicates, maximum number of NGOs (i.e. 35.6%) operate only in rural area. Respectively 11.1 per cent and 13 per cent of the NGOs work only in urban area and only in tribal area. It is also found, 19.0 per cent NGOs work both in rural as well as urban area and only 21.3 per cent NGOs run programmes in all the three areas (i.e. urban, rural and tribal). It can be summarized that except 11.1 per cent NGOs all other NGOs under the study have rural based activity. In this connection, Chart 6E gives a better understanding.

Table 6.11: Area of Operation of NGOs

Area	*Frequency*	*Percentage (%)*
Urban Area	24	11.1
Rural Area	77	35.6
Tribal Area	28	13.0
Urban and Rural Area	41	19.0
Urban, Rural and Tribal Area	46	21.3
Total	216	100.0

Source: Responses received from the mailed questionnaires.

Chart 6E: Distribution of NGOs as per Area of Operation

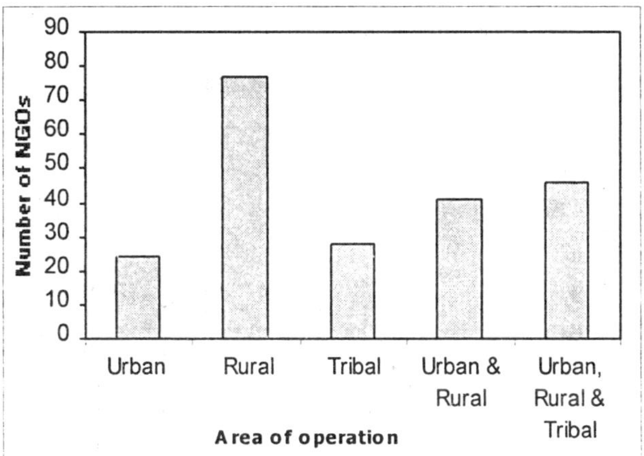

2. *Affiliation*

In this regard, Table 6.12 highlights two important aspects. One, most of the NGOs (i.e. 65.7%) work independently. They are not affiliated

Table 6.12: Affiliated to Federations (No. of NGOs)

Operational Area	*Affiliation*		*Total*
	No	*Yes*	
Urban Area	16	8	24
	66.7%	33.3%	100.0%
	11.3%	10.8%	11.1%
Rural Area	55	22	77
	71.4%	28.6%	100.0%
	38.7%	29.7%	35.6%
Tribal Area	20	8	28
	71.4%	28.6%	100.0%
	14.1%	10.8%	13.0%
Urban & Rural Area	22	19	41
	53.7%	46.3%	100.0%
	15.5%	25.7%	19.0%
Urban, Rural and Tribal Area	29	17	46
	63%	37.0%	100.0%
	20.4%	23.0%	21.3%
Total	**142**	**74**	**216**
	65.7%	**34.3%**	**100.0%**
	100.0%	**100.0%**	**100.0%**

Source: Ibid.

Chart 6F: Distribution of NGOs as per the Affiliation

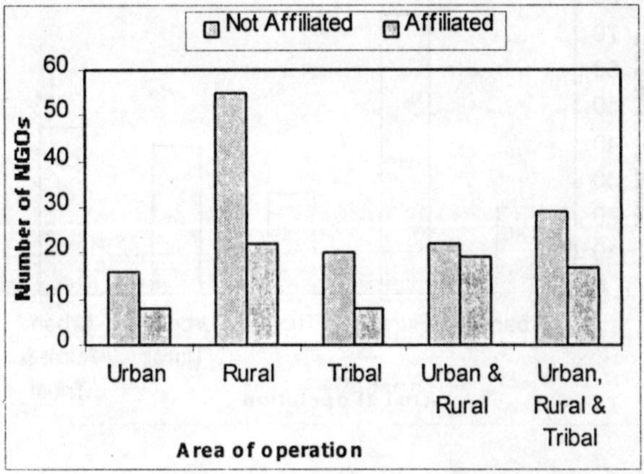

to any federation. Two, under the study, those NGOs work only in urban area, 33.3 per cent of them have affiliation; who work only in rural area and only in tribal area, respectively 28.6 per cent and 28.6 per cent of them have affiliation. It works out that NGOs operating only in urban area have more tendencies to be affiliated to any federation. Chart 6F gives graphical representation to understand the trend in this regard.

3. *Types of Organization*

Various types of organizations (e.g. A, B, BC, BCD, BCE, C, CD, CE, D, E) have already been mentioned while discussed the growth of NGOs. Table 6.13 points out, more than one-fourth (i.e. 26.9%) of the NGOs under study are service organizations (B) and 29.3 per cent of them operate only in urban area. Again, almost half (i.e. 47.2%) of the total NGOs are development organizations (C) and 52 per cent of these organizations operate only in rural area. Other types of organizations, mentioned in the table, are not found in significant numbers. It is observed that those NGOs are working only in urban area, 70.8 per cent of them are service organizations (B). NGOs who operate respectively only in rural area and only in tribal area, 68.8 per cent and 64.3 per cent of them are development organizations (C). It is also understood that those NGOs have both urban as well as rural based activity, respectively 48.8 per cent and 31.7 per cent of them are service (B) and development (C) organizations. Similarly, those NGOs run programme in all the areas, 34.8 per cent and 28.3 per cent of them are respectively treated as service (B) and development (C) organizations. From the above discussions, we can come to a consensus that most of the service organizations operate in urban area and development organizations work in rural area.

4. *Types of Service*

Services provided by the NGOs are of various types such as only institutionalized, only community based on regular basis, both institutionalized as well as community based and only occasional camp at the community level. Table 6.14 comes across with few important aspects regarding 'services'. Firstly, only 6 per cent of the total NGOs have institutionalized services. These services are visible more (46.2%) among the NGOs who work only in rural area. Secondly, 41.7 per cent

Table 6.13: Types of Organization (in Numbers)

Operational Area	*Organization*										*Total*
	A	*B*	*BC*	*BCD*	*BCE*	*C*	*CD*	*CE*	*D*	*E*	
Urban Area		17 70.8% 29.3%	2 8.3% 9.5%			5 20.8% 4.9%					24 100.0% 11.1%
Rural Area	2 2.6% 33.3%	5 6.5% 8.6%	11 14.3% 52.4%		2 2.6% 40%	53 68.8% 52.0%	1 1.3% 25.0%	1 1.3% 16.7%	1 1.3% 33.3%	1 1.3% 25.0%	77 100.0% 35.6%
Tribal Area	1 3.6% 16.7%		4 14.3% 19.0%			18 64.3% 17.6%	2 7.1% 50.0%	2 7.1% 33.3%	1 3.6% 33.3%		28 100.0% 13.0%
Urban & Rural Area	1 2.4% 16.7%	20 48.8% 34.5%	3 7.3% 14.3%	2 4.9% 28.6%		13 31.7% 12.7%			1 2.4% 33.3%	1 2.4% 25.0%	41 100.0% 19.0%
Urban, Rural & Tribal Area	2 4.3% 33.3%	16 34.8% 27.6%	1 2.2% 4.8%	5 10.9% 71.4%	3 6.5% 60%	13 28.3% 12.7%	1 2.2% 25.0%	3 6.5% 50.0%		2 4.3% 50.0%	46 100.0% 21.3%
Total	**6 2.8% 100%**	**58 26.9% 100%**	**21 9.7% 100%**	**7 3.2% 100%**	**5 2.3% 100%**	**102 47.2% 100%**	**4 1.9% 100%**	**6 2.8% 100%**	**3 1.4% 100%**	**4 1.9% 100%**	**216 100% 100%**

Source: Ibid.

of the total NGOs under the study provide only community based services. Among these NGOs, maximum numbers (i.e. 37.8%) run programmes only in rural area. Thirdly, more than half (51.9%) of the NGOs have both institutionalized as well as community based services. Almost one-third (33%) of them operate only in rural area. Fourth, those NGOs work only in rural area, many of them i.e. 48.1 per cent cater both institutionalized as well as community based services. Fifth, fifty per cent of the NGOs, work only in tribal area, carry out community based services. Sixth, respectively 51.2 per cent and 67.4 per cent of the NGOs function in 'Urban as well as Rural area' and 'Urban, Rural and Tribal Area' have both institutionalized and community based services. Having summarized the above discussion, we can say institutionalized services or community-based services or both are likely to be found more among the NGOs having rural based programme. Trend in distribution of NGOs as per the types of service can be understood in a better way from the Chart 6G.

Table 6.14: Types of Service (in number of NGOs)

Operational Area	*Service*				*Total*
	Institu-tionalized	*Community Based*	*Institutionalized & Community Based*	*Occasional Camp*	
Urban Area	2 8.3% 15.4%	12 50.0% 13.3%	10 41.7% 8.9%		24 100.0% 11.1%
Rural Area	6 7.8% 46.2%	34 44.2% 37.8%	37 48.1% 33.0%		77 100.0% 35.6%
Tribal Area	1 3.6% 7.7%	14 50.0% 15.6%	13 46.4% 11.6%		28 100.0% 13.0%
Urban & Rural Area	3 7.3% 23.1%	16 39.0% 17.8%	21 51.2% 18.8%	1 2.4% 100.0%	41 100.0% 19.0%
Urban, Rural & Tribal Area	1 2.2% 7.7%	14 30.4% 15.6%	31 67.4% 27.7%		46 100.0% 21.3%
Total	**13** **6.0%** **100.0%**	**90** **41.7%** **100.0%**	**112** **51.9%** **100.0%**	**1** **.5%** **100.0%**	**216** **100.0%** **100.0%**

Source: Ibid.

Chart 6G: Distribution of NGOs as per the Type of Service

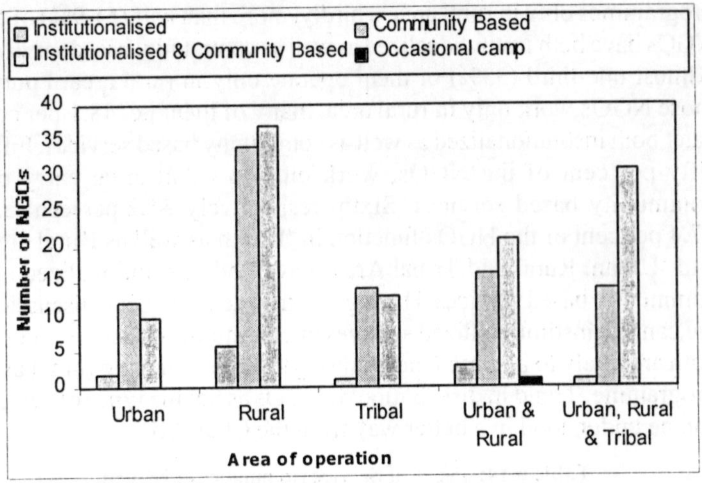

5. *Total Number of Full Time Paid Staff*

Out of 216 NGOs, 199 (i.e. 92.1%) NGOs replied with regard to total number of staff. Table 6.15 indicates, almost one-fourth (i.e. 24.1%) of the total NGOs (replied) have no full time paid staff and 35.4 per cent of these organizations work only in rural area. They manage day-to-day affairs through part time workers. 19 per cent, 13 per cent, 16 per cent, 14.6 per cent and 5.5 per cent of the NGOs have staff members between 1-5, 6-10, 11-20, 21-50 and 51-80 respectively. Those NGOs have moderate number of staff (i.e. 21 to 50), 31 per cent of them function only in rural area. Only 7 per cent of the NGOs have a good number of working staff (i.e. above 100). Many of these organizations (35.7%) are situated only in rural area. Again, table shows that NGOs who operate only in urban area, 30.4 per cent do not have full time paid staff and 26 per cent have staff members between 11 to 20. Those NGOs work only in rural area, 22.1 per cent do not have full time staff and 41 per cent have staff members between 1-10. Those NGOs carry out development activities only in tribal area, 12.5 per cent do not have full time paid staff, 51 per cent have below 21, and 25 per cent have staff member between 21 to 50. NGOs who run programmes in both urban as well as rural area, 41.7 per cent do not have staff and 36.8 per cent have below 21 staff. Those NGOs function in 'Urban,

Table 6.15: Total Number of Staff

Operational Area	*Number of Staff (in number of NGOs)*								*Total*
	0	*1–5*	*6–10*	*11–20*	*21–50*	*51–80*	*81–100*	*Above 100*	
Urban Area	7	2	2	6	3	1		2	23
	30.4%	8.7%	8.7%	26%	13.0%	4.3%		8.7%	100.0%
	14.6%	5.3%	7.7%	19%	10.3%	9.1%		14.3%	11.6%
Rural Area	17	18	14	12	9	2		5	77
	22.1%	23%	18%	16%	11.7%	2.6%		6.5%	100.0%
	35.4%	47%	54%	38%	31.0%	18.2%		35.7%	38.7%
Tribal Area	3	6	3	3	6	1		2	24
	12.5%	25%	13%	13%	25.0%	4.2%		8.3%	100.0%
	6.3%	16%	12%	9.4%	20.7%	9.1%		14.3%	12.1%
Urban & Rural Area	15	6	1	6	2	4	1	1	36
	41.7%	17%	2.8%	17%	5.6%	11.1%	2.8%	2.8%	100.0%
	31.3%	16%	3.8%	19%	6.9%	36.4%	100%	7.1%	18.1%
Urban, Rural & Tribal Area	6	6	6	5	9	3		4	39
	15.4%	15%	15%	13%	23.1%	7.7%		10.3%	100.0%
	12.5%	16%	23%	16%	31.0%	27.3%		28.6%	19.6%
Total	**48**	**38**	**26**	**32**	**29**	**11**	**1**	**14**	**199**
	24.1%	**19%**	**13%**	**16%**	**14.6%**	**5.5%**	**.5%**	**7.0%**	**100.0%**
	100%	**100%**	**100%**	**100%**	**100%**	**100%**	**100%**	**100.0%**	**100.0%**

Source: Ibid.

Rural and Tribal area', maximum of them (i.e. 23.1%) have staff members between 21 to 50. On the basis of above articulations, we can develop an understanding that rural area dominates in every aspect. Maximum numbers of NGOs under each category, such as, who do not have full time paid staff, who have less number of staff and who have a good number of staff, are found only in rural area.

6. *Annual Budget*

In the present study of 216 NGOs, only 182 (i.e. 84.3%) organizations answered regarding the financial position. Table 6.16 provides a clear picture in this connection for the year 2000-01. It shows, 58.2 per cent of the total NGOs (replied) have annual budget of below Rs. 5,00,000. 8.8 per cent, 11.5 per cent, 8.8 per cent and 6.6 per cent of the organizations have annual budget between Rs. 5,00,001–Rs. 10,00,000, Rs. 10,00,001–Rs. 25,00,000, Rs. 25,00,001–Rs. 50,00,000 and Rs. 50,00,001–Rs. 1,00,00,000 respectively. Again, NGOs who, operate only in urban area, only in rural area and only in tribal area, 61.1 per cent, 61.4 per cent and 58.3 per cent respectively of them have annual budget of below Rs. 5,00,000. Those NGOs carry out programmes in 'Urban as well as Rural area' and in 'Urban, Rural and Tribal area', 61.8 per cent and 47.2 per cent respectively of them have annual budget of below Rs. 5,00,000. The aforesaid informations reveal that most of the NGOs, whether urban based or rural based or tribal based, have very less amount of annual budget and thereby they work only at the grassroots level with limited coverage.

7. *Promoter's Background*

It is already mentioned (while discussed the growth of NGOs) that medical practitioner, school teacher, retired government official, political leader, freedom fighter, activist of any movement, group of young enthusiastic friends, businessmen, untrained dedicated social workers, college or university teachers, and others are the promoters of NGOs under the study. Table 6.17 clearly brings out the fact that almost half (i.e. 49.1%) of the total NGOs are developed by only medical practitioners (11.6%), school teachers (19%) as well as untrained dedicated social workers (18.5%). Those NGOs operate only in urban area; 20.8 per cent and 16.7 per cent of them are promoted by medical practitioners and dedicated social workers respectively. NGOs

Table 6.16: Annual Budget of 2000-01 (in number of NGOs)

Operational Area	*Annual Budget*							*Total*
	Below 500000	500001–1000000	1000001–2500000	2500001–5000000	5000001–10000000	10000001–20000000	20000001–40000000	
Urban Area	11	1	3	2			1	18
	61.1%	5.6%	16.7%	11.1%			5.6%	100.0%
	10.4%	6.3%	14.3%	12.5%			33.3%	9.9%
Rural Area	43	8	5	6	4	3	1	70
	61.4%	11.4%	7.1%	8.6%	5.7%	4.3%	1.4%	100.0%
	40.6%	50.0%	23.8%	37.5%	33.3%	37.5%	33.3%	38.5%
Tribal Area	14	2	4	2	2			24
	58.3%	8.3%	16.7%	8.3%	8.3%			100.0%
	13.2%	12.5%	19.0%	12.5%	16.7%			13.2%
Urban & Rural Area	21	1	3	6	1	2		34
	61.8%	2.9%	8.8%	17.6%	2.9%	5.9%		100.0%
	19.8%	6.3%	14.3%	37.5%	8.3%	25.0%		18.7%
Urban, Rural & Tribal Area	17	4	6		5	3	1	36
	47.2%	11.1%	16.7%		13.9%	8.3%	2.8%	100.0%
	16.0%	25.0%	28.6%		41.7%	37.5%	33.3%	19.8%
Total	**106**	**16**	**21**	**16**	**12**	**8**	**3**	**182**
	58.2%	**8.8%**	**11.5%**	**8.8%**	**6.6%**	**4.4%**	**1.6%**	**100.0%**
	100.0%	**100.0%**	**100.0%**	**100.0%**	**100.0%**	**100.0%**	**100.0%**	**100.0%**

Source: Ibid.

Table 6.17: Backgrounds of the Promoters

Operational Area	*Promoters (in number of NGOs)*											*Total*
	Medical Practitioner	*School Teacher*	*Retd. Govt. Official*	*Political Leader*	*Freedom Fighter*	*Activist of any Movement*	*Group of Young Friends*	*Business men*	*Untrained Dedicated Social Worker*	*College or University Teacher*	*Others*	
Urban Area	5 20.8% 20.0%	1 4.2% 2.4%	1 4.2% 5.9%	2 8.3% 20%	3 12.5% 15.8%	2 8.3% 10.5%	2 8.3% 16.7%	1 4.2% 14.3%	4 16.7% 10.0%		3 12.5% 14.3%	24 100.0% 11.1%
Rural Area	5 6.5% 20.0%	24 31% 59%	7 9.1% 4.1%	4 5.2% 40%	6 7.8% 31.6%	6 7.8% 31.6%	5 6.5% 41.7%		12 15.6% 30.0%	3 3.9% 60.0%	5 6.5% 23.8%	77 100.0% 35.6%
Tribal Area	5 17.8% 20.0%	6 21.4% 15%	3 10.7% 18%		2 7.1% 10.6%	2 7.1% 10.5%	2 7.1% 16.7%		6 21.4% 15.0%	1 3.6% 20%	1 3.6% 4.8%	28 100.0% 13.0%
Urban & Rural Area	5 12.2% 20.0%	8 19.5% 20%	2 4.9% 12%	1 2.4% 10%	4 9.8% 21%	2 4.9% 10.5%	2 4.9% 16.7%	4 9.8% 57.1%	7 17.0% 17.5%	1 2.4% 20%	5 12.2% 23.8%	41 100.0% 19.0%
Urban, Rural & Tribal Area	5 10.9% 20.0%	2 4.3% 4.9%	4 8.7% 24%	3 6.5% 30%	4 8.7% 21%	7 15.2% 36.8%	1 2.2% 8.3%	2 4.3% 28.6%	11 23.9% 27.5%		7 15.2% 33.3%	46 100.0% 21.3%
Total	**25 11.6% 100.0%**	**41 19% 100.0%**	**17 7.9% 100.0%**	**10 4.6% 100.0%**	**19 8.8% 100.0%**	**19 8.8% 100.0%**	**12 5.6% 100.0%**	**7 3.2% 100.0%**	**40 18.5% 100.0%**	**5 2.3% 100.0%**	**21 9.7% 100%**	**216 100% 100%**

Source: Ibid.

who work only in rural area, maximum of them (i.e. 31%) are developed by dedicated social workers. Again, those NGOs function only in tribal area, 7.8 per cent, 21.4 per cent and 21.4 per cent of them are promoted by medical practitioners, school teachers and dedicated social workers respectively. NGOs who run programmes in urban as well as in rural area, 12.2 per cent, 19.5 per cent and 17 per cent came into existence by the help of doctors, school teachers and dedicated social workers respectively. Those NGOs carry out programmes in 'Urban, Rural and Tribal area', 10.9 per cent, 15.2 per cent and 23.9 per cent of them were promoted by the doctors, activists and dedicated social workers respectively. It is evident from the above discussions that doctors, school teachers and dedicated social workers have contributed more to promote NGOs and majority of these NGOs are located in rural areas.

8. *Present Health Programmes*

The health programmes, those are existing at present in NGOs under the study, are of various types such as awareness generation (A), occasional health camp (B), regular mobile dispensary (C), permanent clinic (D), permanent hospital (E), training of health workers (F) and R.C.H (G). Many of the NGOs have more than one of these programmes. Table 6.18 describes that only a few programmes such as A, AB, ABDF, ABF, AF, B and D are found in many of the NGOs (61.7%). Those NGOs work only in urban area, maximum (i.e. 20.8%) of them have only permanent clinic. Table also shows that some other urban-based NGOs have permanent clinic, but they run the same along with other health programmes. NGOs who operate only in rural area, 18 per cent, 16 per cent and 9.1 per cent of them have only 'awareness programme', 'awareness as well as occasional health camp' and 'awareness, occasional camp and training of health workers' respectively. These programmes are also found in other rural based NGOs, but not in significant number of organizations. NGOs running programmes only in tribal area do not project very different trends from rural based NGOs. Almost 43 per cent of them have health awareness and occasional health camp oriented programmes (i.e. A, AB and B). Those NGOs carry out programmes both in 'urban as well as rural area', thirty per cent of them continue awareness and occasional camp oriented programmes. All types of health programmes are more or less found among the NGOs who work in 'Urban, Rural and Tribal area'. On the basis of aforesaid description,

Table 6.18: Present Health Programmes

Operational Area	*Health Programmes (in number of NGOs)*												
	A	*AB*	*ABCD*	*ABCDF*	*ABD*	*ABDF*	*ABE*	*ABF*	*ABFG*	*AC*	*AD*	*ADE*	*ADF*
Urban Area		3	1		1	1	1			2		3	1
		13%	4.2%		4.2%	4.2%	4.2%			8.3%		12.5%	4.2%
		10%	16.7%		14%	7.1%	11%			22.2%		33.3%	16.7%
Rural Area	14	12	2	4	2	2	2	7	2	3	3	2	1
	18%	16%	2.6%	5.2%	2.6%	2.6%	2.6%	9.1%	2.6%	3.9%	3.9%	2.6%	1.3%
	50%	41%	33.3%	57.1%	29%	14%	22%	41.2%	33.3%	33.3%	43%	22.2%	16.7%
Tribal Area	4	5		1		3		2	3	1	1		2
	14%	18%		3.6%		11%		7.1%	10.7%	3.6%	3.6%		7.1%
	14%	17%		14.3%		21%		11.8%	50.0%	11.1%	14%		33.3%
Urban & Rural Area	6	6	1	2	3	4	3	4	1		1	1	
	15%	15%	2.4%	4.9%	7.3%	9.8%	7.3%	9.8%	2.4%		2.4%	2.4%	
	21%	21%	16.7%	28.6%	43%	29%	33%	23.5%	16.7%		14%	11.1%	
Urban, Rural & Tribal Area	4	3	2		1	4	3	4		3	2	3	2
	8.7%	6.5%	4.3%		2.2%	8.7%	6.5%	8.7%		6.5%	4.3%	6.5%	4.3%
	14%	10%	33.3%		14%	29%	33%	23.5%		33.3%	29%	33.3%	33.3%
Total	**28**	**29**	**6**	**7**	**7**	**14**	**9**	**17**	**6**	**9**	**7**	**9**	**6**
	13%	**13%**	**2.8%**	**3.2%**	**3.2%**	**6.5%**	**4.2%**	**7.9%**	**2.8%**	**4.2%**	**3.2%**	**4.2%**	**2.8%**
	100%	**100%**	**100%**	**100%**	**100%**	**100%**	**100%**	**100%**	**100%**	**100%**	**100%**	**100.0%**	**100%**

(*Contd.*)

Table 6.18 (Contd.)

Operational Area	*Health Programmes (in number of NGOs)*									
	AF	*B*	*BCE*	*BD*	*C*	*CDF*	*CE*	*CF*	*D*	*Total*
Urban Area	3 12.5% 17.6%	2 8.3% 14.3%	1 4.2% 100.0%						5 20.8% 33.3%	24 100.0% 11.1%
Rural Area	5 6.5% 29.4%	4 5.2% 28.6%		1 1.3% 20.0%	3 3.9% 42.9%	1 1.3% 100.0%	1 1.3% 100.0%		6 7.8% 40.0%	77 100.0% 35.6%
Tribal Area	1 3.6% 5.9%	3 10.7% 21.4%		1 3.6% 20.0%					1 3.6% 6.7%	28 100.0% 13.0%
Urban & Rural Area	4 9.8% 23.5%	3 7.3% 21.4%		1 2.4% 20.0%					1 2.4% 6.7%	41 100.0% 19.0%
Urban, Rural & Tribal Area	4 8.7% 23.5%	2 4.3% 14.3%		2 4.3% 40.0%	4 8.7% 57.1%			1 2.2% 100%	2 4.3% 13.3%	46 100.0% 21.3%
Total	**17** **7.9%** **100.0%**	**14** **6.5%** **100.0%**	**1** **.5%** **100.0%**	**5** **2.3%** **100.0%**	**7** **3.2%** **100%**	**1** **.5%** **100.0%**	**1** **.5%** **100%**	**1** **.5%** **100%**	**15** **6.9%** **100%**	**216** **100.0%** **100.0%**

Source: Ibid.

it is understood that permanent curative services are available more in urban-based NGOs and preventive as well as temporary health facilities are found more in rural based NGOs.

9. *Separate Health Staff*

It is understood from the Table 6.19 that 33.3 per cent of the total NGOs do not have separate health staff and 66.7 per cent NGOs have separate health staff. It is also focused from the same table that those NGOs operate only in urban area, only in rural area and only in tribal area, respectively 70.8 per cent, 70.1 per cent and 71.4 per cent of them have separate health staff. Thus, with regard to separate health staff, proportions of urban based NGOs, rural based NGOs and tribal area based NGOs are almost same. Chart 6H gives a graphical representation in this regard.

Table 6.19: Separate Health Staff (in number of NGOs)

Operational Area	*Separate Health Staff*		*Total*
	No	*Yes*	
Urban Area	7	17	24
	29.2%	70.8%	100.0%
	9.7%	11.8%	11.1%
Rural Area	23	54	77
	9.9%	70.1%	100.0%
	31.9%	37.5%	35.6%
Tribal Area	8	20	28
	28.6%	71.4%	100.0%
	11.1%	13.9%	13.0%
Urban & Rural Area	23	18	41
	56.1%	43.9%	100.0%
	31.9%	12.5%	19.0%
Urban, Rural & Tribal Area	11	35	46
	23.9%	76.1%	100.0%
	15.3%	24.3%	21.3%
Total	**72**	**144**	**216**
	33.3%	**66.7%**	**100.0%**
	100.0%	**100.0%**	**100.0%**

Source: Ibid.

Chart 6H: Distribution of NGOs as per the Separate Health Staff

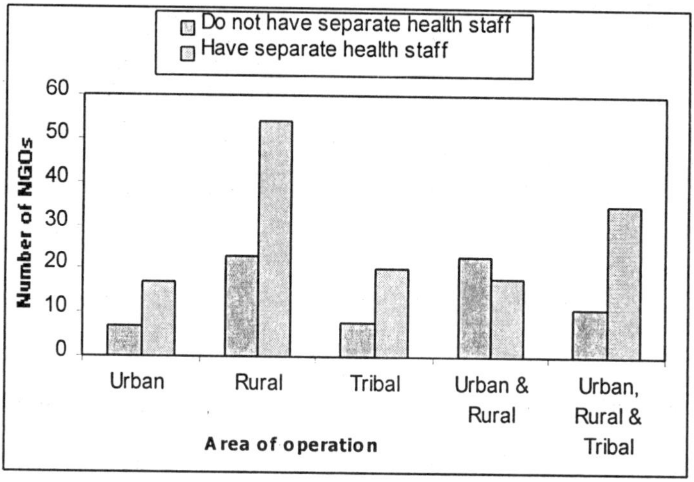

10. *Types of Health Staff*

Health staff are of various categories such as trained doctors, non-trained doctors, nurses, trained health workers, non-trained health workers, administrative staff, etc. Out of 216 NGOs, only 86 (i.e. 39.8%) organizations have trained doctors (Table 6.20). Among these organizations, many of the NGOs (i.e. 34.9%) are located only in rural area. Only 26 NGOs which works out to 12 per cent, have non-trained doctors and 50 per cent of these organizations are situated in rural area. In the present study, there are only 42 organizations who have trained nurses. Table also shows that maximum (i.e. 28.6%) of these organizations have activities in 'Urban, Rural and Tribal area'. Trained health workers are found only in. 90 (i.e. 41.6%) of the total organizations. More than one-third of these organizations (36.7%) are located only in rural area. The table also indicates that respectively 64 NGOs (i.e.29.6%) and 85 NGOs (39.3%) of the total organizations have non-trained health workers and administrative staff. Both types of staff are found more in case of rural NGOs. It is evident from the above description that rural based NGOs have the maximum capacity to utilize various types of health staff.

Table 6.20: Types of Health Staff (in number of NGOs)

Operational Area	*Health Staff*					
	Trained Doctor	*Non-Trained Doctor*	*Nurses*	*Trained Health Worker*	*Non-Trained Health Worker*	*Admn. Staff*
Urban	13 15.1%	2 7.7%	7 16.7%	13 14.4%	11 17.2%	13 15.3%
Rural	30 34.9%	13 50.0%	10 23.8%	33 36.7%	27 42.2%	32 37.6%
Tribal	11 12.8%	7 26.9%	6 14.3%	12 13.4%	8 12.5%	14 16.5%
Urban and Rural	9 10.5%	1 3.8%	7 16.7%	10 11.1%	5 7.8%	9 10.6%
Urban, Rural and Tribal area	23 26.7%	3 11.5%	12 28.6%	22 24.4%	13 20.3%	17 20.0%
Total	**86** **100%**	**26** **100%**	**42** **100%**	**90** **100%**	**64** **100%**	**85** **100%**

Source: Ibid.

11. *Health Budget*

Table 6.21 describes the health budget of the NGOs for the financial year 2000-01. Health work and health budget is nil for .9 per cent of the total NGOs and 3.7 per cent of the NGOs have health work without any separate health budget. The remaining NGOs have specific health budget and they have been classified into seven groups as per health expenditure such as up to Rs. 10,000, Rs. 10,001 to 50,000, Rs. 50,001 to Rs. 1,00,000, Rs. 1,00,001 to 2,00,000, Rs. 2,00,001 to 5,00,000, Rs. 5,00,001 to Rs. 10,00,000 and above 10,00,000. It is reflected from the table that more than half of the NGOs (i.e. 57.8%) have less amount of health budget i.e. up to Rs. 1,00,000 and only 12.1 per cent of the total NGOs have a good amount of health budget i.e. above Rs. 10,00,000. Again, those NGOs operate only in urban area, 45.8 per cent of them have health budget of below Rs. 50,001 and 25 per cent have very high amount of health activities. NGOs who function only in rural area, more than half (55.9%) of them have very limited range of health expenditure i.e. up to Rs. 50,000 only. In case of tribal area based NGOs, 46.5 per cent

Table 6.21: Health Budget of 2000-2001 (in number of NGOs)

Operational Area	*Health Budget*									*Total*
	No Health Work and Health Budget	*Health Work without Budget*	*Upto Rs. 10000*	*Rs. 10001 to 50000*	*Rs. 50001 to 100000*	*Rs. 100001 to 200000*	*Rs. 200001 to 500000*	*Rs. 500001 to 1000000*	*Above Rs. 1000000*	
Urban Area		2	5	6	1	2	1	1	6	24
		8.3%	20.8%	25.0%	4.2%	8.3%	4.2%	4.2%	25.0%	100.0%
		25.0%	10.0%	10.7%	5.3%	7.1%	5.0%	14.3%	23.1%	11.1%
Rural Area	1		22	21	8	12	7	3	3	77
	1.3%		28.6%	27.3%	10.4%	15.6%	9.1%	3.9%	3.9%	100.0%
	50.0%		44.0%	37.5%	42.1%	42.9%	35.0%	42.9%	11.5%	35.6%
Tribal Area	1	1	5	8	3	7	2	1		28
	3.6%	3.6%	17.9%	28.6%	10.7%	25.0%	7.1%	3.6%		100.0%
	50.0%	12.5%	10.0%	14.3%	15.8%	25.0%	10.0%	14.3%		13.0%
Urban & Rural Area		4	10	11	5	1	3	1	6	41
		9.8%	24.4%	26.8%	12.2%	2.4%	7.3%	2.4%	14.6%	100.0%
		50.0%	20.0%	19.6%	26.3%	3.6%	15.0%	14.3%	23.1%	19.0%
Urban, Rural & Tribal Area		1	8	10	2	6	7	1	11	46
		2.2%	17.4%	21.7%	4.3%	13.0%	15.2%	2.2%	23.9%	100.0%
		12.5%	16.0%	17.9%	10.5%	21.4%	35.0%	14.3%	42.3%	21.3%
Total	**2**	**8**	**50**	**56**	**19**	**28**	**20**	**7**	**26**	**216**
	.9%	**3.7%**	**23.1%**	**25.9%**	**8.8%**	**13.0%**	**9.3%**	**3.2%**	**12.1%**	**100.0%**
	100.0%	**100.0%**	**100.0%**	**100.0%**	**100.0%**	**100.0%**	**100.0%**	**100.0%**	**100.0%**	**100.0%**

Source: Ibid.

organizations have health budget of below Rs. 50,001 and 25 per cent NGOs fall in the category of Rs. 1,00,001 to Rs. 2,00,000. Those NGOs carry out programmes in 'urban as well as rural area', more than half of them (51.2%) show very less amount of health budget (i.e. up to Rs. 50,000). The above discussions accent two important aspects with regard to health budget. One, a major portion of the NGOs, whether located in urban area or rural area or tribal area, has very limited health activities. Two, one-fourth of the NGOs working only in urban area have a wide range of health services.

12. *Working Capacity*

Table 6.22 shows, 68 per cent of the total NGOs under the study are working at the village level. On and average each NGO covers almost 156 villages. This coverage varies from one village to three thousands five hundreds sixty-five villages. From the same table, we also understand the working capacity of NGOs at the block level, district level and state level. One may feel that NGOs of West Bengal, by and large, have more working capacity. But we get different result when this Table 6.22 is compared with Table 6.15 (total number of staff) and table 6.16 (annual budget). Since most of the NGOs have less number of staff and less amount of annual budget, covering so many villages by each NGO in order to initiate developmental activities has no meaning. This trend proves that NGOs work superficially and project themselves more than their actual contribution at the grassroots level.

Table 6.22: Working Capacity

Operational Area	*Number of NGOs*		*Mean Number*	*Minimum Number*	*Maximum Number*
	Valid	*Missing*			
Village level	147 (68%)	69	155.78 (No. of villages)	1	3,565
Block level	164 (75.9%)	52	8.84 (No. of blocks)	1	400
District level	197 (91.2%)	19	2.53 (No. of districts)	1	25
State level	200 (92.5%)	16	1.29 (No. of states)	1	12

Source: Ibid.

Distribution of NGOs also can be understood in terms of types of funding. It should not be ignored as it brings out significant issues. In the present study of 216 NGOs, 192 organizations (i.e. 88.8%) depend upon self-generated funding. This type of funding varies from one per cent to hundred per cent in each NGO. Table 6.23 shows, on and average 54.17 per cent of the total funds in each organization come from internal source (i.e. self generated source). Similarly, 34.7 per cent of the total NGOs receive funds from state government and the amount (as compared to total budget of an NGO) varies from 2 per cent to 95 per cent. In the same way, Table 6.23 describes the position of central government funding, foreign funding and Indian funding agency's (outside the government) contribution. It is understood that one-third of the total NGOs in health care in West Bengal are supported by foreign agencies. On and average 43.57 per cent of the total budget of each of these organizations come from foreign. In brief, we can point out two important aspects. One, almost 90 per cent of the total NGOs generate more than half of their required funds by their own effort (internal source). Therefore, their existence cannot be ignored. They will survive in long run. Two, one-third of the total NGOs who receive foreign support, their activeness is doubtful and they have every possibility to become sick. Because, their degree of dependency is more on external funds.

Table 6.23: Types of Funding

Funding Agencies	*Number of NGOs*		*Mean Percentage of funding*	*Minimum percentage*	*Maximum Percentage*
	Valid	*Missing*			
Self generated	192 (88.8%)	24	54.17	1	100
State Government	75 (34.7%)	141	26.12	2	95
Central Government	91 (42.1%)	125	29.74	1	100
Indian funding agencies (outside the Govt.)	44 (20.3%)	172	24.45	1	100
Foreign funding agencies	72 (33.3%)	144	43.57	1	90
Any other	41 (18.9%)	175	32.85	4	100

Source: Ibid.

In a nutshell, the chapter has illuminated the growth and distribution of NGOs in health care in West Bengal. 'Growth' has been discussed as per year of registration. It is evident that NGOs grew more in numbers in 1980s. Majority of those NGOs accentuated on developmental approach and community based activities. During that period, awareness generation programme received maximum importance and various professionals like medical practitioners, school teachers, government officials, etc. played vital role to promote NGOs. With regard to health programmes, the present study indicates that 50 per cent of the total NGOs started the same after 1985. Preventive approach in health care became a major concern for them. Again, NGOs who initiated health activities after 1985 many of them had a tendency for not having full time separate health staff and carried out health activities with limited budget. 'Distribution' of NGOs has been narrated as per the district and operational area. In the study, analysis made as per the district clearly brings out the fact that 72.19 per cent of the total NGOs are situated in Kolkata and its adjacent area (i.e. Howrah, 24 Parganas and Hoogly). It means, NGOs prefer to work in socio-economically developed area. Analysis made on the basis of responses received from the mailed questionnaires shows, except 11.1 per cent organizations, all other NGOs have either partly or fully rural based programmes. Over one-third of the total NGOs function only in rural area. The present study also points out that almost half of the NGOs are development organizations and majority of them carry out programmes in rural areas. Institutionalized services or community based services or both are available more among the rural NGOs. Again, these rural based NGOs are found to be very active in case of preventive as well as temporary health facilities, in case of use of separate health staff and in case of appointing various types of professional as well as Para-professional health staff. Therefore, it can be argued that rural based NGOs of West Bengal are acknowledgeable to a greater extent for development initiative and have a significant contribution in preventive health care. It should also be noted that these rural based NGOs are situated more in socio-economically developed districts.

PART III

Contribution of NGOs in Health Care in West Bengal

7

Profile of Selected NGOs

The present Indian society encounters many new problems and contradictions. Liberalization and globalization, through which national economy is opened up and strengthened by integrating trade investments, financial markets and consumer markets, have shown negative results. They have contributed largely in destabilizing currency, ruining the national economy and causing impoverishment of millions of people. Secondly, information and communication technology, which underpins the process of change, have adversely affected society, culture and value system. Thirdly, the 72nd and 73rd Amendments to the Constitution highlight decentralization of power at the grassroots level, in governance. But, there is a struggle to assert the federal political structure with the rise of regional force that may be reluctant to exercise decentralized power at the local level. It seeks a radical shift in the relationship of the bureaucracy with the political system. Fourthly, India continues to remain largely rural, poor, exploitative with caste and religious discrimination which is increasingly fragmenting the society. Again, polarization continues in our social structure. When we have the problem of illiteracy, high dropout in schools, universal primary education, we are crazy for human resource development and information technology. Under the above mentioned societal context present NGO sector works, which is more bewildering than what we had on the eve of Independence. Inspite of the existence of complex and multidimensional social problems, NGOs carry out their programmes in order to bring human happiness and satisfaction. NGOs of West Bengal are not exception to that.

In West Bengal, NGOs work everywhere within their jurisdiction. Though NGOs are not distributed equally across districts, they do not ignore their programmes in backward areas. West Bengal has two natural divisions. One, the Himalayan north, having some hills, comprising the districts of Darjeeling, Jalpaiguri and Cooch Behar. It is very far from the state capital and neglected by the government with respect to development activities. The Southern part, having the plain levels, which is the handiwork of many big rivers. NGOs demand that they are more efficient than government sector with regard to service delivery and immediate intervention in hilly areas, islands and the remotest corners of Bengal. In case of health care, they reach to the distant villages with doctors and medicines since people do not have access to modern health and family planning services. The population in such regions, by and large, remains outside the purview of health infrastructural facilities and hence they duly recognize the contribution of NGOs. The previous chapter has described the trends in growth and distribution of NGOs in health care in West Bengal. It did not give details regarding working of an NGO considering various aspects of programmes, staff members, beneficiaries, etc. Therefore, the present section (next four chapters) makes an effort, through case studies of three NGOs (i.e. Rural Health Development Centre, CINI Moyna Rural Health Development Centre and Southern Health Improvement Samity) located in 3 different divisions of West Bengal (Jalpaiguri, Burdwan and Presidency), to bring out the facts related to NGO's past background and present activities i.e. Profile of NGOs (present chapter), nature of programme sustainability (Chapter VIII), level of job satisfaction of the staff members (Chapter IX) and beneficiary's perception towards the working of NGOs (Chapter X). This will help to develop an understanding on how much and how long an NGO can contribute in health care. It will be useful for health planning at the state level.

PROFILE OF NGOs

A brief sketch of each of the NGOs under the study is presented here.

(A) Rural Health Development Centre (RHDC)

Background

Dr. Ratan Sarkar, present secretary and promoter of the organization was born at Baragram village under Dakshin Dinajpur district of West Bengal. His father was a farmer and owning sufficient cultivable land to maintain the family. Dr. Sarkar passed School Final (SF) examination in 1967 and Pre-University (PU) examination in 1968 from West Bengal. He was interested to serve the people and hence did a homoeopathy course (D.M.S) during the year 1969-72 under Bhagalpur University, Bihar. Having completed DMS, he did private practice at Chakulia Block (Near Kisanganj of Bihar) from 1972-73 and at Baragram (his own village) from 1973 to 1977. He took up job as Medical Officer during 1977-78 in SEED (an NGO). In the year 1979, he joined in CINI (an NGO) to work at Moyna (in Midnapore distirict of West Bengal), which was devastated by flood. During the work with CINI, Dr. Sarkar would visit his own village frequently and would discuss with local friends that an NGO could be formed to serve the villagers. In fact, it materialized in July 1983, when he came back to his native village having left CINI and developed the Rural Health Development Centre (RHDC). Dr. S.N. Choudhury, Director of CINI, encouraged all the workers at Moyna during flood relief to start work in their own village. The encouragement of Dr. S.N. Choudhury and Dr. Sarkar's zeal as well as experience in the NGO sector motivated to promote RHDC at Baragram.

Initially, RHDC did not have any legal status (registration) or officc room or accumulated fund. Mahila Samity House of the village was used as temporary office and membership fee as well as public contributions were collected to begin the work. Medical outreach programme was introduced as the first programme, which paid attention on Mother and Child Health (MCH). Patients used to pay Rs. 2 (two) as treatment fee. In order to use external funds (provided by governments or funding agencies), registration became very essential and therefore the same was done in March 1984. There was some vested land in Baragram area. Mr. Habal Das would till such type of three bighas land. With the help of local panchayat Mr. Habal Das was given some other land in some other area and these three bighas were donated to RHDC in 1984. Thus, the permanent campus came into existence. Later on, gradually one and half bighas, one bigha, and one and half bighas were purchased from the villagers in reasonable cost adjacent to the permanent campus. At present, the organization has a big campus with seven bighas of land. In the year 1985, GOAL (an international funding agency) donated (because of intervention of CINI) Rs. 12,000 to RHDC for the construction of office building. In 1986, having completed construction work, RHDC's office was shifted to its permanent and main campus from Mahila Samity House. Till today, almost all the buildings of the main campus have been made taking support from GOAL, except one big building, which is under construction with the help of general funds of the organization. RHDC has been registered under the Foreign Contribution Regulation Act in 1986. In order to spread its activities, RHDC has made another campus having purchased six kathas land at Bachamari Government Colony, Malda. Since it is situated in the town, gradually it has become a co-ordinating office for various activities spread in the entire North Bengal. As the main campus is located in a remote rural area, secretary does not like to stay there because of the communication problem. Keeping in view the ultimate target of the organization, RHDC has developed again the third campus purchasing ten kathas land at Adampur of old Malda in order to implement Community Health Programmes. Thus, RHDC functions through three different campuses in various districts of North Bengal.

Present Objectives

The major objectives of the RHDC are as follows: (a) To provide basic medical facilities to the mothers and children in the community. (b) To bring awareness among the people in general regarding hygiene, nutrition and family planning in order to improve the quality of life. (c) To introduce social, economic and infrastructure development programmes which can indirectly reduce the morbidity and mortality rate. (d) To provide welfare facilities to the destitute, deprived and neglected children for love, affection, care, education and better health. (e) To form women group and educate them for social, economic and political empowerment. (f) To rehabilitate aged, victimized and helpless women providing residential facilities in the organization campus. (g) To prepare people of vulnerable areas to combat disaster. (h) To accelerate nation's development promoting people's participation in community development programme. (i) To form a networking group of NGOs operating in North Bengal in order to strengthen voluntary action.

Area of Operation

RHDC operates in 11 villages covering 6,000 population under Harirampur block in the Dakshin Dinajpur district and 42 villages having population 60,000 (approx) under Muchia, Sahapur and Jatradanga GP of old Malda block in Malda district.

Target Groups

The Table 7.1 shows the various types of beneficiaries under the organization.

Table 7.1: Types of Beneficiaries

Sl. No.	*Actual Beneficiaries*	*Volume (2000-01)*
1.	Children (3 to 19 yrs) of BPL families	628
2.	Destitute women and girls	11
3.	Community people in general (for health)	6,000
4.	Flood victims	3,000
5.	Dai	6
6.	Aged	10
7.	NGOs	7

Organizational Structure

It is understood from the Chart 7A that Secretary of the organization is given power to control programme wing as well as administrative wing. Including all the three campuses, there are total ten programmes those are being implemented through RHDC. Under a particular programme, there are two types of staff such as programme in charge and field level worker.

Infrastructure

(a) Baragram Campus

- Office buildings 9
- Community Centres 5
- Own agricultural land – 14 bighas
- Primary School 1
- Jeep 1
- Child Resource Centres 2
- Tractor 1
- Children's Park 1
- Motor cycle 1
- Library 1
- Bicycles 6

Chart 7A: Organisational Structure of RHDC

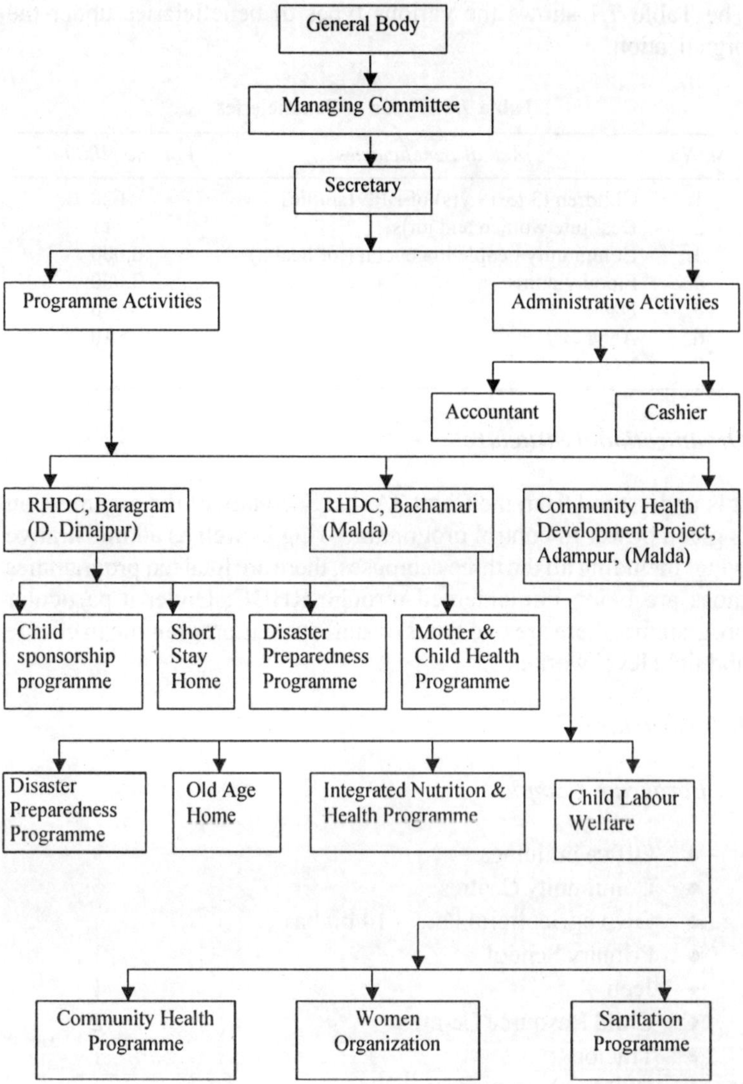

- Short Stay Home 1
- Daily outdoor clinic 1
- Big ponds for fisheries 2
- Mobile Clinic 1
- Phone connection 1
- Balwadi Centres 8
- Freeze for keeping vaccine 1
- Emergency boats 3

(b) Bachamari Campus: Adampur Campus

- Office building and old age home
- Office building 1
- Training hall 1
- Auto 1
- Jeep 1
- Bicycles 2
- Bicycles 2
- Daily outdoor clinic 1
- Computer 1
- Mobile clinic (weekly) 1
- Phone connection 1
- Van 1
- Sanitary mart 1

Programmes

(i) Community Health Programme (CHP)

It was started in November 1995 having received funds from Indian Hilfe. It is being implemented in 19 villages. The main objective of this programme is to make the people aware of herbal medicine that are available within the community, to encourage treatment of diseases domestically and finally to improve personal hygiene and community health status. CHP has total 12 components. They are as follows: (a) *Weekly Village Meeting*: There are total 39 women groups and 19 farmers groups under this programme. Each group meets weekly to carry on programme activities; (b) *Mobile Health Clinic*: It is organized on request of the group members to serve children below 12 years, mothers and aged (above 60 years) people. In this regard, village quack doctors are identified and trained; (c) *Ante-natal and post-natal care*: Monthly clinics are conducted for this purpose inviting doctors from district hospital; (d) *Immunization:* In every month, immunization programme is organized jointly by SC and RHDC; (e) *Day-night auto service* is available for the patients on cost; (f) *Referral Service*: As soon as patients of communicable diseases like TB, Leprosy, AIDS, etc. are identified, they are referred to the district hospital; (g) *Herbal garden and production centre in the campus as well as in the community*: Ultimate purpose is to produce urgent and low cost medicine. During anti-natal and post-natal clinic these medicines are provided on cost (but doctor's visit is free); (h) Women groups are motivated for maintaining *kitchen garden* in order to improve nutritional status; (i) *Awareness programme*: There are four types of groups: (i) school students; (ii) women members; (iii) farmers and (iv) staff members. They perform magic, folk song and puppet show to make awareness on health, superstition, disaster, etc; (j) *Legal aid:* Women members are getting legal aid service in case of family maladjustment, torture, divorce, etc; (k) *Removal of illiteracy*: Women and farmers groups run literacy centres to remove illiteracy; (l) *School health programme*: Students are given awareness on personal hygiene in seven primary schools and one secondary school. It is done through trained field workers and school teachers.

CHP is executed very systematically. Women and farmers groups are the whole and sole. They implement various components of the programme with the help of field workers and send monthly report to the programme co-ordinator. In the same way, when a major decision is taken in the head office, it reaches to the group by the field worker. In the year 2000-01, total budget for CHP was Rs. 1,08,000.

(ii) Integrated Nutrition and Health Programme (INHP)

INHP is in operation at old Malda block. It was started in 1998 with the help of CARE—West Bengal. The major objectives of INHP are (a) to improve health and nutritional status of women (pregnant and lactating) and children (2 years) in rural areas; (b) to form and run women's group at G.P. level for strengthening the existing ICDS centres and health centres; (c) to develop linkages among women groups and various government departments or NGOs for sustainable community level structure; (d) to enhance the number of change agents by involvement of local health service provider in order to develop positive community level health and nutritional practices. In fact, this programme is and implemented in those areas where ICDS centre's get CARE provided food. INHP has total five components, such as health awareness, nutritional awareness, women empowerment, micro-credit and take home ration. (a) *Health awareness:* With regard to baby, mothers are given awareness on breast feeding till 4 months and during respiratory infection as well as diarrhoea, introduction of solid food or supplementary food along with breast milk from 6 months, completion of immunization schedule and vitamin oil dose during 12 months (1st) month and 24 months (2nd). Mothers are also made aware of ante-natal care; (b) *Nutritional Awareness*: People are made conscious on nutritional food value, way of food preparation, low cost diet structure, essential food during pregnancy, etc; (c) *Women empowerment*: One women group is made under one ICDS centre. Members come to the group and discuss on their personal problems. At the same time, each one contributes Rs. 10 per month and develops an accumulated fund; (d) *Micro credit*: When women groups develop a good deal of amount, they open bank account. RHDC links these groups with NABARD, Gramin Bank, SBI, Animal Husbandry Department, etc. to get loan for small business; (e) *Take Home Ration (THR):* Beneficiaries get nutritious food twice in a month from the ICDS centre if they follow immunization schedule properly and pay rupees two. In the last week of month, when ration is distributed, Mother's Health Day (MHD) is celebrated discussing mother's problems.

INHP is executed in three GPs under the leadership of programme co-ordinator. In each GP, there is one programme organizer who controls four Village Level Volunteers (VLVs). Each VLV takes care of 5 or 6 villages. Thus, we can say, there is a chain, such as, *Programme Co-ordinator at the Organizational level → Programme Organizer at the GP level → VLV at the Village level.* VLVs form women groups, supervise them, aware them and build capacity to carry out programme components. INHP is integrated with various government departments such as health, ICDS, local panchayats, etc. Hence, it holds monthly meeting at the (a) *Village level* where all anganwadi workers, 2 health assistants, one representative from each women group, one VLV and one panchayat member participate; (b) *GP level* where ICDS supervisor, NGO organizer, panchayat pradhan and health supervisor participate; (c) *Organizational (RHDC) level* where CDPO, BMOH, BDO, Panchayat Samiti's representative and programme co-ordinator participate. It is found that resolution of the village level meeting comes to the organization and final decision of the organization level meeting goes back to the village level team for appropriate action. In the year 2000-01, total budget for this programme was Rs. 2,67, 881.

(iii) Child Sponsorship Programme (CSP)

RHDC has been implementing this programme in Harirampur block of Dakshin Dinajpur since 1987. It is funded by Children International, Kansus City, USA, through Sahay, Kolkata. In the year 2000-01, total 662 children of BPL families having age between 3 to 19 years were benefited from this programme. The programme has the following objectives: (a) to fulfil basic needs of the children for better future; (b) to improve the socio-economic condition of the sponsored families; (c) to provide better education to the child; (d) to facilitate health benefit to the sponsored families; and (e) to arrange various vocational training programmes for the sponsored children (who are poor in study) for a healthy future. CSP has total five components such as health, education, nutrition, material aid and assistance to the family, and value formation. These components are briefly highlighted in the following. (a) *Health*: (i) Basic health services: Running static and mobile clinics, arrangement of medicines for the clinics, in case of necessity referring child to the outside doctor, annual health check up camp for the sponsored children through child specialist, etc. come under this component; (ii) Preventive health service: It includes growing healthy habits, hygiene kit distribution (soap, brush, tooth powder, sanitary napkin, nail cutter, etc.), health education (to the adolescents, pregnant mothers and lactating mothers), health workers training, etc. (b) *Education*: (i) Primary and secondary education: It includes infrastructure development for primary and secondary schools, school supplies (books, note books, pen, pencils, geometry boxex, etc.), school uniforms, tuition and other fees, teaching aids (blackboards, tables and chairs, benches, maps, globes, etc.), etc.; (ii) Pre-school programme: This service includes construction and repairing work for balwadi centres, maintenance of balwadi teacher, pre-school supplies (slates, pencils, toys, etc.), pre-school uniform, teaching aids, training of balwadi teachers, etc; (iii) Supplemental education programme: It encompasses book supplies for the libraries, special coaching class for sponsored children and their siblings, vocational training, special coaching teacher's training, etc; (iv) Special benefits: There are two types of benefits, such as, benefit-b and benefit-e. Benefit-b is meant for clothing facility whereas benefit-e is responsible for only school uniforms; (c) *Nutrition*: Pregnant mothers, adolescent children and 0 to 5 years children get supplementary nutrition; mothers get nutrition awareness; and various balwadi centres get weight and height measurement instruments under this component; (d) *Material aid and assistance to the family:* Beneficiaries get support for home repairing, latrine construction, sanitary kits and portable water project at the community level, volunteer training (e.g. Tube well repairing), van as rickshaw purchasing (for income generation) and for buying cooking utensils; (e) *Value formation*: It includes leadership training, cultural function, tour or outing for youth, day camps, annual sports, art contest, etc. for inculcation of social values.

This programme is executed with the help of Gram Sabha, adolescents group and neighbourhood groups. As per the needs of the beneficiaries, yearly plan as well as budget is made at the organization level and get the same approved from 'Sahay' Kolkata. In every year, two letters and one photograph are sent to the sponsor through Sahay. In the same way, various gifts and letters reach to RHDC from sponsors.

(iv) Disaster Preparedness Programme (Mainly for Flood)

The disaster preparedness programme, funded by OXFAM (India), has been in operation since November 1993. The objective of this programme is to help the people to cope with disaster by reducing the loss of property as well as human resources and provide support in terms of relief. RHDC has already covered 72 villages in three districts name Malda, Uttar and Dakshin Dinajpur, through the networking of NGOs operating in North Bengal. NGOs networking have been expanded in Nepal, Assam, Bihar and Bangladesh with an object to make the people's movement stronger for reducing the damages caused by flood and at the same time to make the environment healthier. This programme has three levels of intervention, such as, pre-disaster phase, disaster phase and post-disaster phase. It has total twelve components including all the phases. They are as follows: (A) *Village level work*: (a) Community health: Preventive health care advice is given before flood. After flood, work is continued to control communicable diseases, to refer dangerous patients, etc.; (b) Pisci Culture: During flood, water and fish properties are damaged. Therefore, support is provided to reform dam in the village and to dig ponds. It helps further in pisciculture; (c) Mobile Health Clinic: Children below 12 years and aged above 60 years, who cannot go to the health centre, come to this clinic. It is conducted on request of the community people and identifying quack doctor from the villages; (d) Awareness in schools: Students are change agents for the future. They are trained regarding how to face flood; (e) Village Meeting: In the village, women groups are formed and meetings are conducted with them to discuss on pre-flood preparation (shelter identification, fuel and fodder collection, arrangement for pregnant mothers and handicapped, food and water arrangement, etc.), flood situation facing, post- flood work (road and house construction, arrangement of source of drinking water, restarting social institutions, etc.), savings, health, etc. These groups and their meetings are the actual platform for work; (f) Legal aid: During flood preparation, flood relief and rehabilitation of the flood victims, suffered women simply are not bypassed. They are linked with appropriate authority for legal aid; (g) Tree plantation: It is initiated in order to control soil erosion during flood. (B) *Central Level Work:* (a) Training: During flood, only few staff members of RHDC cannot cover the whole North Bengal for relief and rescue work. They require more manpower. Therefore, RHDC provides two types of training for flood preparation throughout the whole year i.e. (i) staff training (of other NGOs); and (ii) on call volunteers training. (b) Water testing: Bacteriological test as well as arsenic test is done quarterly for different types of sources of drinking water. (c) Field monitoring: Five community Based organizations (CBOs) carry out all the flood related activities. RHDC only co-ordinates the whole affairs. (d) Exposure visit: Staff members or volunteers are taken to the successful projects for better exposure. (e) Monthly meeting is conducted where all the CBOs come to discuss their problems and needs.

This programme is executed through chain work i.e. *Programme Co-ordinator →CBOs → Village level groups.* Programme Co-ordinator gives instructions to the CBOs and CBOs pass the same to the village level groups. In the same way group decisions and problems come to the RHDC office. During 2000-01, total budget for this programme was Rs. 11,31,200.

(v) Mother and Child Health Programme (MCH Programme)

The most vulnerable and insecure people in the community are mothers and children. The pregnant and lactating mothers suffer from poor health, lack of medical care and depend on their male counterparts throughout their whole life. Children are deprived and neglected. In order to ameliorate the health condition of mothers and children, RHDC started this programme at Baragram campus since its initial days. Now MCH clinics are held there on every Tuesday to provide ante-natal and post-natal services. The children under five years are treated through regular health check-up by trained health workers. Children are immunized against the killer diseases and Vitamin A oil is distributed to them.

(vi) Short Stay Home for the Women and Girls

Women are the most neglected and deprived human beings. We do not consider their contribution much to our community. Moreover, this is not the end of their tragic misery. They are being victimized by co-people everyday everywhere in various parts of our country.

Keeping in view the problems of women and girls, RHDC opened a Short Stay Home in 1991 at Baragram campus having taken sponsorship from CSWB. At present, there are thirteen inmates who are given free food, shelter, health care, vocational training and regular individual counselling. Inmates are helped to overcome their problems so that they can go back to their normal lives within a certain period of time. In addition, yearly excursion is arranged in order to expose them to the outer world.

(vii) Old Age Home

RHDC has been running a house for the aged persons at Bachamari Government Colony, Malda, since 1995. Its 90 per cent funds come from the Ministry of Social Justice and Empowerment, Government of India. The objective of establishing the home is to help the helpless old people with free fooding, shelter and medical care. At present, eight people are residing at home and enjoying mental peace in a healthy atmosphere. There is a committee headed by the District Social Welfare Officer for selection of inmates. Due to irregular release of funds from the Central Government, RHDC is facing problems to continue this old age home.

(viii) Child Labour Welfare

It was started in 1993 by the help of INDIEN HILFE to provide welfare service for the children engaged in paper bag making, bidi-rolling, garage (automobile), rag picking, etc. The major activities under the project are: (a) to run four educational centres at evening to promote knowledge and literacy among the working children; (b) to check up working children's health regularly and provide treatment for various diseases by the medical professionals; (c) to conduct weekly cultural programmes to inculcate values among the working children; (d) to organize picnic and tour to overcome the inferiority complex among the children; and (e) to aware the parents through meeting to take care of their children.

(ix) Women Organizations

The village women have formed groups by the active help of volunteers. These groups are engaged in various activities i.e. the campaigning on public health issues, fighting for women atrocities, involving in micro-credit programme, etc. Presently, these groups are known as Self-Help Group (SHG). So far, 39 SHGs have been formed under this programme at Adampur area.

(x) Sanitation Programme

It was started in 1996 with a purpose to create awareness for construction and use of latrines in rural and flood affected areas. Support came from UNICEF, Rural Development Department of Government of West Bengal and Malda Zilla Parishad. Families under BPL receive Rs. 200 as subsidy in order to construct latrine. So far 1925 low cost latrines have been made in Muchia, Sahapur, Mangalbari and Bhabuk Gram Panchayat under Old Malda Block. Due to devastating flood in every year, construction of low cost latrines are very much delayed.

Staff Related Information

RHDC is having total 44 full time paid staff, 26 part time paid staff, 1 honorary staff and 1,044 permanent volunteers. Characteristics of these staff members are as follows:

As far as volunteers are concerned, there is no specific organizational policy to use their help. Volunteers come from irrespective of educational statuses and have age between 15 years to 45 years.

Full time staff members of RHDC get salary as per the following pay structure: (a) Project Incharge: Rs. 4,500 to 5,500; (b) Programme co-ordinator: Rs. 3,000 to Rs 4,500; (c) Middle level staff (i.e.

Table 7.2: Characteristics of Full Time Paid Staff

Sl. No.	*Designation*	*Number*	*Sex (M & F)*	*Qualification*
1.	Project Incharge	3	M (2), F (1)	Graduate
2.	Programme Coordinator	3	M (2), F (1)	Graduate
3.	Asstt. Programme Coordinator	1	M (1)	SSC
4.	Supervisor	1	M (1)	SSC
5.	Case worker	2	M (1), F (1)	Graduate
6	Accountant	3	M (3)	Graduate
7.	Field worker	11	M (7), F (4)	VIII
8.	Health worker	5	M (1), F (4)	VIII
9.	Women organizer	1	F (1)	SSC
10.	School teacher	3	M (1), F (2)	SSC
11.	Training Organizer	1	M (1)	MSW
12.	Warden	2	F (2)	Graduate
13.	Cook	2	F (2)	Literate
14.	Care Taker	1	M (1)	VIII
15.	Driver	3	M (3)	VIII
16.	Peon	1	M (1)	VIII
17.	Craft teacher	1	F (1)	Graduate

Table 7.3: Characteristics of Part Time Paid Workers

Sl. No.	*Designation*	*Number*	*Sex (M & F)*	*Qualification*
1.	Balwadi Teacher	10	F (10)	VIII
2.	Special Coaching teacher	12	M (11), F (1)	SSC
3.	School Teacher	2	M (1), F (1)	SSC
4.	Helper for cooking	1	F (1)	Literate
5.	Sweeper	1	M (1)	Literate

Accountant, warden, craft teacher, case worker, etc): Rs. 1,500 to 3,000; (d) Lower level staff (school teacher, health worker or field worker): Rs. 700 to Rs. 1,500.

Governing Body of RHDC has developed service rules for its staff members. These are discussed below. (A) Leave rules: (i) A staff member can avail fourteen days casual leave, fourteen days medical leave and eight days special leave in a calendar year; (ii) Study leave or duty leave may be allowed as per the situation; (iii) Ninety days maternity leave at a stretch can be sanctioned. It may be allowed to a female staff twice (total 180 days) in the whole service life of RHDC; (iv) No leave can be accumulated for the next year and in case of emergency above scheduled leave rules may be cancelled. (B) RHDC's workers are treated as social workers, not as traditional employees. (C) Continuation of RHDC is subjected to availability of funds. (D) All appointments are made on temporary and contract basis. Every year contract should be renewed. (E) In case of harmful work (which is against the interest of the organization) workers will be terminated. (F) Worker may resign voluntarily with one month's prior notice. (G) One month's advance salary may be given but should be adjusted at the time of leaving this organization. (H) Canteen facility is available where wages of cook and fuel expenditure are born by the organization and fooding cost is paid by the staff members. (I) Quarter is free for emergency workers. (J) These above rules may be amended by the authority as per needs.

Financial Information

RHDC's turnover in the year 2000-01 was Rs. 1,40,00,000. During this period various sources of funds were Ministry of Social Justice and Empowerment, Central Social Welfare Board, Children International, OXFAM (India), CARE, Indien Hilfe, agricultural land, public contribution, etc. RHDC experiences problems with regard to fund raising. In government organization, harassment is more and money is not released regularly. In foreign funding agency, harassments or irregularities are not found, but sanctioning project is very difficult. They feel West Bengal is developed area.

In order to manage financial affairs, RHDC prepares annual budget considering expenditure mentioned in the project proposal, market price, last years expenditure, area needs, etc. Almost in all the programmes 5 per cent to 10 per cent money is spent for administrative purpose and 90 per cent money is used for programme activities.

Future Plans

RHDC is trying hard to start the following activities in near future: (a) community based awareness and rehabilitation for spastic children; (b) safe drinking water programme; (c) a high school at Khanjapur village (Dakshin Dinajpur); and (d) resource centre of disaster management.

In brief, various types of programmes are run by RHDC. Few of the programmes are welfare oriented, some programme focuses on relief service and rest are having developmental approach. This kind of plurality in approach has emerged as a result of socio-geographical climate of North Bengal. But, whatever may be the approach, RHDC is reformative in its operation since it tries to improve the condition of community people in general and women as well as children in particular.

(B) CINI—Moyna Rural Health Development Centre (CINI—Moyna RHDC)

Background

In 1978, there was a devastating flood in Midnapore district. Moyna block and its adjacent areas were affected very badly. Water was stagnant there for almost two months. Child In Need Institute (CINI) of South 24 parganas district went there for flood relief with a medical team comprising fourteen people (two doctors, two nurses and others trained in health care). With the help of Mr. Pulak Bera, the then MLA, flood relief camp was made in the Naichanpur area. Initially, campers provided medical treatment, distributed halogen tablets and went to spray DDT. Later on, they started distributing polythene paper, cloth and food. This relief work was continued from September 9 to December 31, 1978. Director of CINI, Dr. S.N. Choudhury, did not stop his intervention though relief work was terminated. In January 1979, he sent one doctor and three trained health workers at Naichanpur village, made a tent there and continued Mother and Child Health programme under the banner of CINI. In March 1979, Dr S.N. Choudhury sent another one doctor and one health worker in the same tent to strengthen the welfare work. Having realized the importance of work initiated by CINI, local people (i.e. Aparna Das Jalua and Madhab Chandra Jalua) donated 92 satak land to develop permanent campus of CINI in Naichanpur area. Shifting in the new campus, CINI spread its work in three GPs. Initially, it aimed to develop human resources by reducing the suffering of women and children belonging to the vulnerable segments of the population. The first programme i.e. MCH programme helped to fulfil this aim. MCH programme included care to the pregnant mothers through iron tablets, tetanus injections, referral services and services to the children through immunization as well as nutrimix food. In September 1979, CINI started office building construction in Naichanpur campus and completed the work in April 1981. Gradually, other programmes like handloom programme (in 1980), poultry training programme (in 1982), child sponsorship programme (in 1983), etc. were started in the same campus. At the time of introducing child sponsorship programme, CINI brought external funds for first time in Naichanpur campus. Since CINI was operating in Moyna block through its headquarters located at Doulatpur, South 24 parganas, i.e. 150 kms away, it was difficult to monitor staff, to supervise work and to control finance. Therefore, in 1990, CINI-Moyna Rural Health Development Centre was registered for its independent functioning. In the same year, it was completely detached from CINI, Daulatpur, South 24 parganas.

Present Objectives

The aims and objects of CINI-Moyna RHDC are as follows: (i) To develop human resources particularly with respect of children belonging to the vulnerable segments of the population; (ii) To educate the people especially the mother regarding the maintenance and improvement of the health and nutritional status of their children; (iii) To conduct classes and schools for training in matters of health, nutrition and all other allied subjects pertaining to medicine and community development; (iv) To establish and maintain hospitals, clinics and feeding centres both static and mobile, community development centres, day care centres, co-operative societies, credit union, staff welfare fund and other related service centres; (v) To incorporate or grant affiliation of social services societies with objectives similar to any or all of this society and to co-operate financially or otherwise with any person or persons in aid of and in furtherance of such objects; (vi) To act as a consignee to relief and development organization, establish in India or abroad; (vii) To established and maintain demonstration centres for disseminating knowledge on nutrition and health; (viii) To establish and maintain small scale and cottage industries for the production of processed food stuffs, commodities of daily use to generate income for the society; (ix) To receive and hold funds for carrying out the objects of the society in exchange of services rendered by the public; (x) To build, purchase, lease or otherwise acquire property both movable and immovable to carry out the aims of the society; (xi) To conduct educational programmes up to Madhyamik level for general education of the rural women, as well as other educational programmes for all age groups through schools, colleges and other educational institute; (xii) To prepare schemes for improvement of water supply, drainage, sanitary road and other measures to improve the physical environment.

Area of Operation

CINI-Moyna RHDC covers 66,000 population in 27 villages of Moyna Block under Midnapore district of West Bengal.

Target Groups

Table 7.4 shows various types of beneficiaries under the organization.

Table 7.4: Types of Beneficiaries

Sl. No.	*Actual Beneficiaries*	*Volume (2000-2001)*
1.	Children of BPL families (Age group—3 to 7 yrs)	1,337
2.	All children of below 3 yrs (for immunization)	250
3.	Pregnant and Lactating Mothers of BPL families	334
4.	Students (VI to XII attending coaching class)	1,435
5.	Patients having RTI and STD	25
6.	Community people in general (for infrastructure, water supply and sanitation facility)	44,000

Organizational Structure

The Director is the head of the organization. He exercises control over programme activities and administrative functions. Organization implements total six programmes. Except Child Sponsorship Programme, other five programmes are implemented jointly using same manpower. It may be understood from the Chart 7B. Again, it comes to our notice that there are mainly five types of staff members, such as Project Manager, Senior Project Associates, Project Associates, Project Assistants and Field workers.

Infrastructure

- Office buildings 2
- Balwadi Centres 9
- Motor cycle 1
- Handloom Section 1
- Scooter 1
- Child Resource Centres 3

Chart 7B: Organisational Structure of CINI-Moyna RHDC

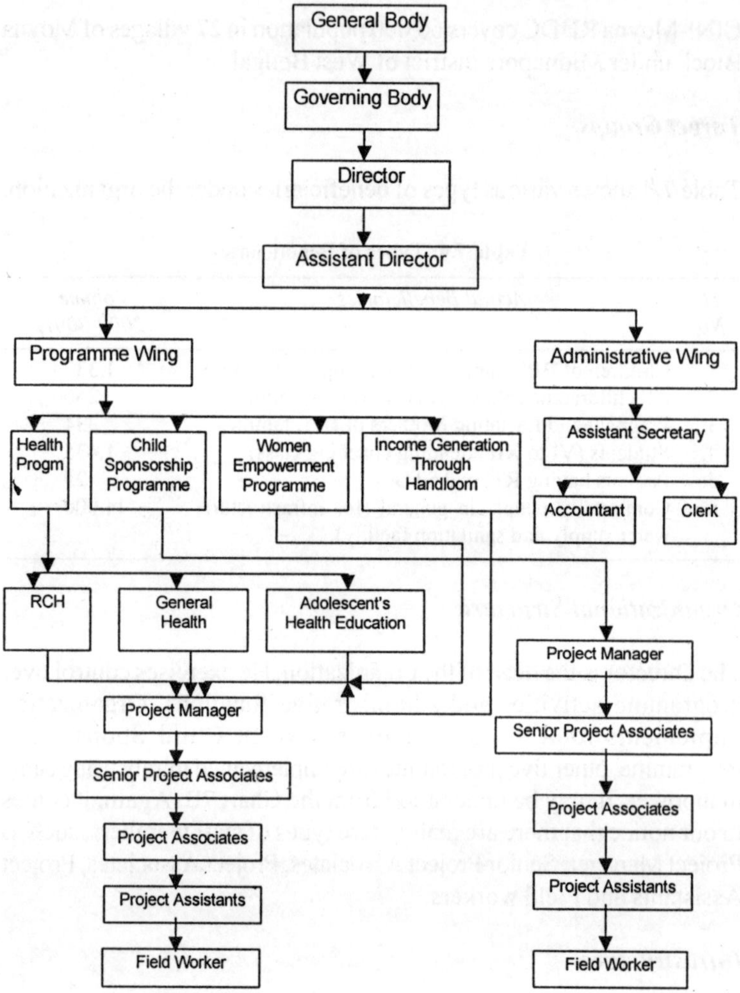

• Bicycles	12
• Children's Parks	3
• Telephone Connection	1
• Self-Help Groups	100
• Solar Units	9
• Youth Groups	29

- Community Outreach Clinic (weekly) 1
- Permanent Homoeopathic Clinic (daily) 1
- Gynaecological Clinic (weekly) 1
- Vocational Training Centre (for sponsored children) 1

Programmes

(i) Reproductive and Child Health Programme (RCHP)

It was started in May 2000 having received funds from Government of India (through M–NGO CINI). RCHP is being implemented in ten villages under three GPs and total 2,095 beneficiaries have been benefited from this programme during 2000-01. The major objectives of RCHP are: (a) to provide information with regard to reproductive system, human sexuality and marital age to the adolescents; (b) to prepare the married couple mentally and physically to have new baby; (c) to aware about Reproductive Tract Infections (RTI), family welfare and family spacing; (d) to educate the new couple regarding anti-natal and post-natal care; (e) to provide services like condoms, oral pills, folifer tablets, ORS packets, arrangements of Laparoscopic tubal operation camps, IUD, etc; and (f) to motivate the eligible couples to undergo sterilization process. In order to implement the above objectives, this programme has three major components, such as, (a) Mother and Child Care (MCH), (b) Adolescent's care, and (c) care for the RTI and STD patients. The first component includes awareness on immunization, nutrition, care for the pregnant mothers and children, personal hygiene, referral service, etc. The second component mainly encompasses awareness to adolescents for physical as well as mental changes and human sexuality. The last component provides awareness, treatment facility and referral services pertaining to RTI and STD.

RCHP is executed through a logical process. At first, health workers survey the village and submit all the data to the programme co-ordinator. Having complied all the informations, co-ordinator develops a comprehensive picture with regard to population characteristics, people's needs, community resources, etc. Then, health workers are advised to conduct 4 to 5 awareness camps per month in each village. In each camp, maximum 20 to 25 candidates are considered and topic is decided as per the beneficiaries needs. In this regard, health workers submit their monthly programme list to the head office and meet programme co-ordinator on every Friday to discuss various problems faced in the field. Apart from these camps, one central level camp is organized in every month in any one of the ten villages where programme co-ordinator, panchayat member, BMOH, visiting doctor and all the programme staff attend. In the year 2000-01, total budget for this programme was Rs. 1,39,700.

(ii) Child Sponsorship Programme (CSP)

It was started in 1983 receiving funds from Children International (through Sahay, Kolkata). CPS is being implemented in 19 villages of Moyna block and 1,337 children have been benefited under this programme in the year 2000-01. The main objectives of CSP are to make healthy, educated and self-reliant children for the future generation. This programme has already been discussed in details while described the profile of RHDC (Baragram). Various components and execution process of this programme are as same as they are in CSP of RHDC (Baragram). Therefore, same informations are not repeated here. Total budget for CSP (in CINI-Moyna RHDC) during 2000-01 was Rs. 54,43,881.

(iii) Women Empowerment Programme (WEP)

In rural areas, many of the families live below poverty line and have limited access to key productive assets like land, capital and so on. Women members of those families suffer more because of their limited employment opportunities, limited participation in rural economy, limited role in decision-making and lack of individual as well as collective strength. Hence, the present programme is designed to empower women of rural areas in Midnapore district. It is being implemented in 16 (sixteen) villages of Moyna block and the same has been able to form 100 self-help groups (SHGs) including 1,150 members. The major objectives of this programme are: (a) to link the poor women with economic activities; (b) to help the poor families to come above poverty line; (c) to initiate small trade and business in the rural areas; (d) to improve the social status and rights of women by dint of earning, etc. All the above mentioned objectives are carried out through Self-Help Groups (SHGs). A SHG under this programme has few specific characteristics, such as appropriate objectives, durability, status, unity and undivided rule, constructive attitude, leadership capacity, work culture and good communication among the mothers.

Women empowerment programme has four basic components, such as (a) income generation; (b) educational awareness; (c) health improvement and (d) participation in village panchayat. Under the first component, group members identify an area (project) for production or business, take appropriate training for efficient work in that area, collect funds either from the group savings or from the banks and develop infrastructure for better functioning of the project. The second component includes educational awareness through literacy work, sending the own children to school and encouraging the dropout children to go to the adult education centre. The third component provides health awareness to the members and motivate them for latrine construction, for following immunization schedule and family planning methods. The last component encourages the members to participate in the local panchayat.

This programme is executed with the help of field workers. They go to the villages, make the people understand regarding this programme, and create needs for SHG formation. When villagers approach to the programme co-ordinator, Self Help Groups are formed by the help of field workers having taken 15 to 20 women of BPL families. One leader as well as one secretary is identified under each group to maintain the whole affairs. Regularly women members meet to materialize various components of this programme. They hold monthly meeting to review their activities and to contribute Rs. 10 to the group's fund. In the year 2000-01, these groups accumulated Rs. 1,38,335 as savings and Rs. 6,49,975 as loan repayment amount.

(iv) Income Generation through Handloom (IGTH)

It was started in 1980 and was the most favourite income generating method for the rural poor of Moyna block. Almost all the families would be involved under this programme (from the spinning of the thread to warping, weaving, packaging and marketing). But now a days, due to heavy cost of the cotton yarn, their profits are being less and less. The poor families are reluctant to continue handloom weaving. At present, under this project, only 25 numbers of handlooms are run in four villages and each family earns on an average Rs. 400 per month. This programme has only one component i.e. producing mosquito net, towel, chawdar, bag, bed-sheet, sari, etc. and marketing them through organization's whole sale counter.

The execution process of this programme is very simple. On every Tuesday, beneficiaries come to the organization to discuss their problems, deposit the finished goods and collect raw materials for the next week. Each beneficiary gets Rs. 5.50 as remuneration for producing one square metre of cloth. Out of the total beneficiaries, half work very sincerely and other treat it as a part of their source of income. In the year 2000-01, total budget for this programme was Rs. 11,95,808.

(v) General Health Programme

Under this programme, daily homoeopathic clinic is run and propagation is made regarding homoeopathic treatment. In order to popularize homoeopathic system, organization has arranged 24 awareness camps, 2 health melas and 3 training camps in 2000-01 by the help of trained and qualified doctors. In this programme, money comes from the organization's development funds. During 2000-2001, total budget for this programme was Rs. 45,000.

(vi) Adolescent's Health Education

A group of social workers are trained from CINI (Daulatpur) in order to run this programme. These workers have selected three villages namely Laluagaria, Paschimnaichanpur and Deoly where they meet with the local panchayat members, parent's groups and adolescent boys as well as girls. Under this programme the following informations are communicated to the adolescents: (a) nutritional status during adolescence period; (b) menstrual hygiene and use of sanitary napkins; (c) mental and physical change in the body; (d) correct sexual and reproductive health information; (e) STD; (f) gynaecological diseases like leucorrhoea, vagirismus, (g) sexual abuse, etc.

In brief, 'CINI-Moyna RHDC' run total six programmes. First four programmes are full-fledged programme and contribute much to the beneficiaries. Last two programmes are supplementary in nature and do not have specific project proposal as well as staff members.

Staff related Information

CINI-Moyna RHDC is having total 30 full time paid staff, 84 part time paid staff and 600 regular volunteers. The characteristics of these staff members are as follows:

Table 7.5: Characteristics of Full Time Paid Staff

Sl. No.	*Designation*	*Number*	*Sex (M & F)*	*Qualification*
1.	Director	1	1 (M)	Graduate
2.	Asst. Director	1	1 (M)	Graduate
3.	Project Officer (manager)	4	4 (M)	Graduate
4.	Senior Project Associate	6	4 (M), 2 (F)	Graduate
5.	Project Associate	2	1 (M), 1 (F)	S.S.C
6.	Project Assistant	7	4 (M), 3 (F)	VIII
7.	Field Worker (Health Worker)	9	9 (F)	VIII

Table 7.6: Characteristics of Part Time Workers

Sl. No.	*Designation*	*Number*	*Sex (M&F)*	*Qualification*
1.	Tuition Teacher	67	42 (M), 15 (F)	Graduate
2.	Balwadi Teacher	9	9 (F)	S.S.C
3.	Balwadi Helper	8	8 (F)	IV

Regarding volunteers, there is no specific organizational policy. Services offered by the volunteers are basically used for community level work.

Full time paid staff of CINI—Moyna RHDC get salary as per the following pay structure:

(a) *Director*: Rs. 2,700–250–3,450–340–4,470
(b) *Assistant Director*: Rs. 2,200–225–2,875–295–3,760
(c) *Project Manager*: Rs. 1,800–200–2,400–250–3,150
(d) *Senior Project Associate*: Rs. 1,500–175–2,025–210–2,655
(e) *Project Associate*: Rs. 1,200–140–1,620–165–2,115
(f) *Project Assistant*: Rs. 1,000–100–1,300–115–1,645
(g) *Field Worker*: Rs. 500 (consolidated).

Along with above mentioned basic pay, staff members get 30 per cent D.A (of Basic), 15 per cent HRA (of Basic) and Rs. 100 medical allowance. Workers have P.F facility, which is deducted at the rate of 12 per cent of Basic, plus D.A. Gratuity is provided at the time of retirement and it is given 15 days per year. D.A is increased once in every 3 years constituting a committee.

Staff members are entitled to enjoy holidays sanctioned by State Government. Apart from that, they get 14 days casual leave, 15 days sick leave, 15 days earned leave and compensatory leave if work during holidays.

Financial Information

In the year 2000-01, turnover of CINI-Moyna RHDC was Rs. 95,00,000. During this period various sources of funds were central Government, Children International, Local Self Government, collection of contribution (from SHG) and internal sources (i.e. income from handloom unit, agricultural land, fisheries and public contribution). Director says regarding fund raising, problems occur more in case of government sponsorship. Government institutions have more queries, reject proposal without any enquiry, release funds through so many offices, ask bribe and after one instalment show reluctancy in fund delivery. It is also known from the director that this organization prepares annual budget considering various aspects such as specific expenditure mentioned in the project proposal, last year's expenditure, present market price and expected funds to be received.

Future Plans

CINI-Moyna RHDC has purchased a land near the sub-divisional town Tamluk. In future they would like to start there various programmes like: (a) rehabilitation for handicapped and street children; (b) adolescents health education; (c) child sponsorship programme, etc.

In brief, CINI-Moyna RHDC operates in a small area. It functions smoothly since workers are recruited locally, beneficiaries are selected through local panchayats, it has good relation with the government machineries and staff members are motivated due to appropriate salary as well as freedom of work. Problems those are encountered in the organization basically occur from external causes. For instance, due to lack of electricity, trained and highly skilled professionals do not want to come, computer cannot be used and work cannot be continued in the evening. Again, in rainy season, communication is disrupted due to mud road. Activities of the organization get stagnant almost for two months. However, the contribution of the organization is highly encouraging for promoting family welfare service, mobilizing women folk and bringing attitudinal change with regard to health and education in the local area.

(C) Southern Health Improvement Samity (SHIS)

Background

Mr. M.A. Wohab, promoter and present director of SHIS passed P.U. in 1970-71 and took admission in Susil Kar College (located at Champahati, South 24 parganas) to study B.A. Then, his father was a primary school teacher and an untrained village doctor. Financially their family was well off. According to him, in his village, people use to suffer from ignorance, illiteracy, illness and starvation. Villagers were mainly bidi sramik (labourer) and rickshaw pullers. Then, Congress party was in power in the state and was blamed by many anti-Congress people for this distressed situation. Mr. M.A. Wohab was anti-Congress and started organizing people to raise voice against Government. Since he was B.A. first year student, he had an opportunity in the college to join politics. In the year 1971, he showed his interest towards Naxalite movement which wanted to make exploitation free society. Though he was not follower of the same movement, suddenly he was identified as a Naxal. Hence, he had to abscond for 3 years. Later on, he left party politics and continued study. He passed B.A. in the year 1974 and got a job of Panchayat Secretary in 1975 in the Howrah district. In 1978, there was a devastating flood in West Bengal. Countless people were shelter-less. Relief was urgently needed for the flood victims. Government systems were pressed into service, concerned citizens were moved by the conscience and voluntary relief work was started by individuals as well as organized groups. Mr. Wohab was working as a part of the Government relief team. During his routine relief work, he observed, a fair skin lean man (perhaps a foreigner, he thought) was moving devotedly in the submerged area with a boat full of medicines, cloths, food and water. His name was Brother Gaston Dayananda—a Catholic Christian (the central figure of Dominique Lapierre's book "City of Joy"), from Switzerland. Mr. Wohab went to Brother Gaston and had a prolonged discussion on charitable activities. He told his life history to 'Brother' and wanted to know the best mechanism of serving people. Brother advised him to go back to his native village with some welfare idea for the weeping masses. In 1979, he came back to his village 'Bhangar,' and started mobilizing people as well as resources. In the next year, SHIS came into existence (without registration). An NGO called 'Seva Sangha Samity—Howrah' provided some money and five staff to start the initial work. General health clinic with special focus on tuberculosis was begun as the first programme. In the earlier days, aims and objectives of SHIS were to bring all-round development through people's own involvement and to meet the five basic needs i.e. fooding, clothing, shelter, treatment for the diseases and education. In the year 1983, SHIS was registered in order to legalize its activities and to avail public contribution, government grants and foreign sponsorships. From 1980 to 1986, organization did not have any separate office. Health clinic and other necessary meetings used to be run in a tea stall of Atihar Rahaman. In 1986, some local person donated 13,090 sq.ft. land to SHIS in order to have its own campus. With the help of nearby brick industries and public's contribution office building construction was started in the same year in main campus. Later on, other hospital buildings have been made gradually having taken sponsorship from German Doctor's Committee. In the year 1987, SHIS was shifted from Atihar Rahaman's tea stall to its own building. The organization found a hope for forthcoming days when it received foreign funds (Rs. 1,73,715) for first time in 1987 from Dominique Lapierre (France based) in order to buy medicines for general health care and tuberculosis treatment.

Present Objectives

(i) To offer opportunities for personal growth and development by providing technical and vocational skills;
(ii) To motivate and recognize each person's efforts and achievement so that one can recognize one's own worth;
(iii) To empower the poor and marginalized communities through economic and social development;
(iv) To provide on-going support system and services to the target group through efficient and readily available management information system;
(v) To reach out to the poorest and under privileged sections of society for self-reliance in health, education and economic prosperity.

SHIS's vision is to achieve a value oriented, sustainable society based on social orientation, economic growth, local capacity building and empowerment of people for a complete social transformation.

Area of Operation

SHIS now works in almost 2,000 villages of 29 blocks under four districts (South 24 parganas, North 24 Parganas, Howrah, Malda) of West Bengal. It pays attention more in Sundarban area (located in South and north 24 Parganas), which is famous for the enchanting mangrove forests and the majestic Royal Bengal Tiger. Although this area is rich in natural resources, people live in abject poverty and are disease ridden. Here frequent cyclones and floods lead large-scale destruction of lives and properties every year. The main rivers of the Sundarban area like the Matla, Bidyadhari and Piyali carry only backwaters of the sea resulting in soil salinity. As a result, people have not only been reduced to systematic impoverishment but the increased salinity of the soil has made cultivation extremely difficult. Again, continuous disasters have made the most common people to believe that they are under the curse of some "gods and goddesses". As a result, superstition is rampant and people often wear medallions or pendants to ward off from various dangers of the land, forests, rivers, nature, evil spirits, etc. It is also important to note that communication from the villages of Sundarban to Kolkata is strenuous. A large number of patients die on the way to city's hospitals.

Target Group

Table 7.7 shows the various types of beneficiaries.

Table 7.7: Types of Beneficiaries

Sl. No.	*Actual Beneficiaries*	*Volume (2000-2001)*
1.	Students (class V to X)	1,200
2.	Tuberculosis Patients	2,500 (new), 2,000 (cured)
3.	General Patients (women & children)	1,15,000
4.	Community People	2,00,000

Organisational Structure

Director is the head of the organization as per the constitution of SHIS but he takes decisions in consultation with the president. Chart 7C shows, both of them control programme as well as administrative

Chart 7C: Organisational Structure of SHIS

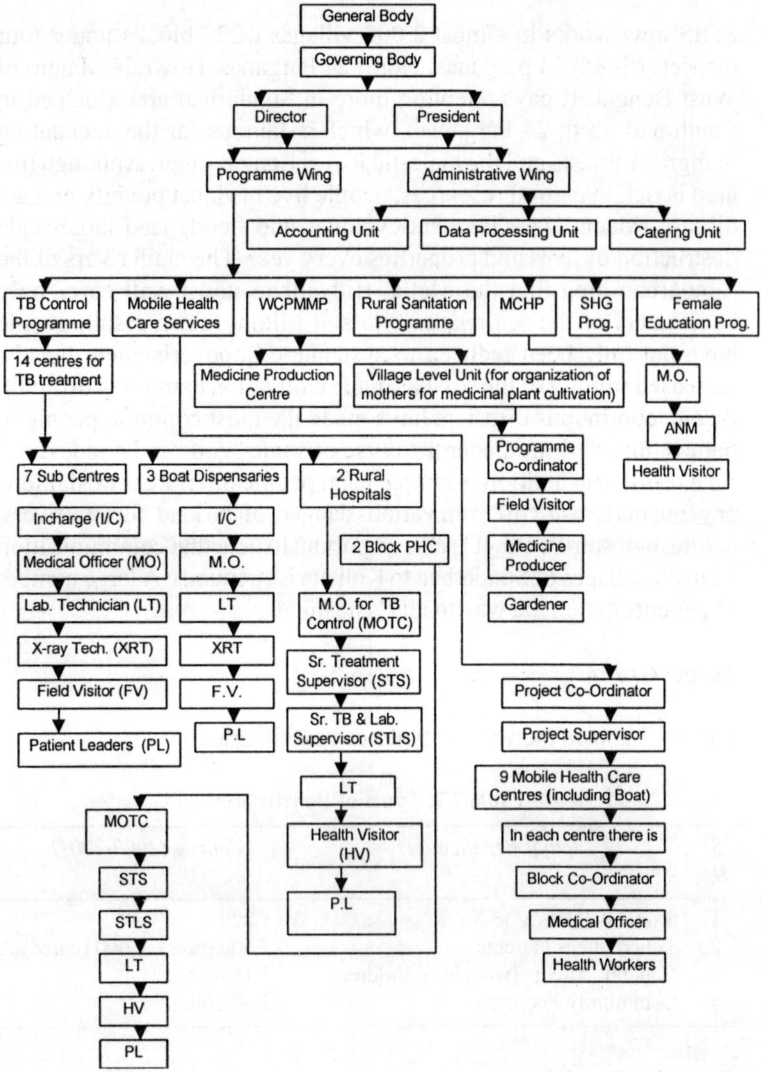

activities. Total seven programmes are being implemented in this organization. It is completely departmentalized and uses specialized personnel to perform various activities. Different types of staff are used in different programmes. More or less there are five categories of staff members. Patient leaders are not paid for their work.

Infrastructure

• Computer with Printers	4 sets
• School Vans	8
• Fax Machine	1
• X-ray Units	7 (1 big, 6 small)
• Phone Connection	1
• Pathological Labs.	27 (1 big 26 small)
• Wireless	11 sets
• Tissue Culture Lab.	1
• Ambulances	3
• Medicinal Plant (Herbal)	1
• Cars	3
• Sanitary Marts	2
• Auto	1
• Sub Centre Offices (Rented)	20
• Own buildings	4
• Dining Hall	1
• Building–	
— Administrative building	1
— Hospital building	1
— Bhabna block (Training Hall, Bank, Car Shade)	1
• Guest room	24 nos.
• Generators	10

Programmes

(i) Tuberculosis Control Programme

It has been in operation since the inception of SHIS. Now it is supported by Government of India and the author Mr. Dominique Lapierre. TB control programme has assumed large shape and size, having over 700 workers, 20 doctors, 882 short course chemotherapy centres—covering over 1,853 villages in the districts of South and North 24 Parganas, West Bengal. The major objectives of this programme are—(a) to cure 85 per cent of the existing positive TB patients; and (b) to get registered 100 per cent of new positive TB patients. All types of TB patients irrespective of income, caste, class, religion, etc. are treated under this programme. TB control programme has a total of five components. They are as follows:

- *Scheme I*—Awareness is given on concept of TB, its consequences, etc.
- *Scheme II*—Awareness is generated for prevention of TB through BCG, referring suspected cases to the nearby health centre, etc.
- *Scheme III*—Patient is referred to the diagnostic centre for testing.
- *Scheme IV*—Free treatment facility is provided to the detected cases.
- *Scheme V*—All the activities pertaining to TB are monitored regularly by tuberculosis unit.

This programme is executed at the district level by dint of a specific infrastructure. For instance, if Village Health Committee suspects a person with TB, he is sent to PHI. MO checks up and verifies it through MC. When TB is detected, free treatment is started. TC makes treatment card and sends it with required medicines to the DOT centre. DOT providers feed these medicines regularly and keep sufficient records. They go to TC

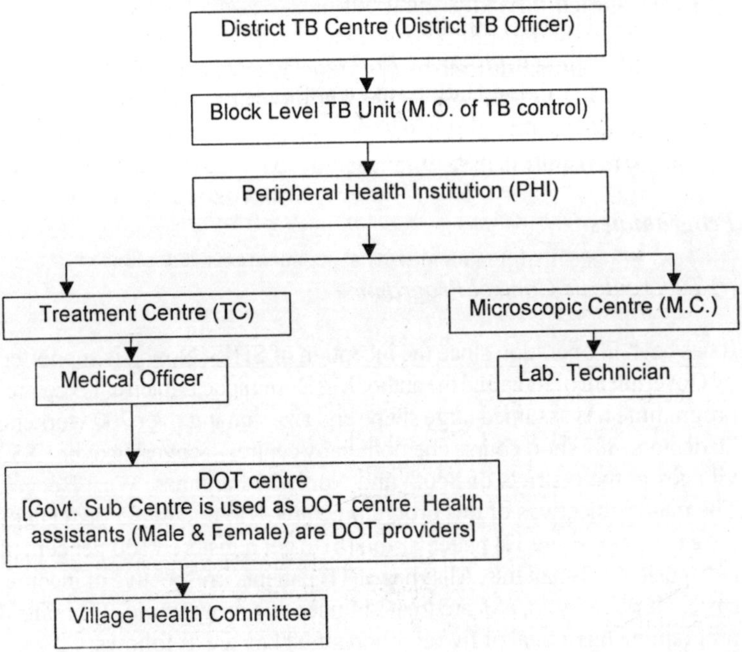

weekly during sector meeting and writes up-to-date information in another duplicate card (kept in TC). DOT providers tell all the procedures to the patient regarding when he/she has to go further for sputum test or X-ray or blood test, etc. to know the improvement. As per the results obtained from various tests, medicines are changed. Final outcome of the treatment is communicated by DOT providers to the upper level offices.

All the treatment centres are regulated by the headquarters of SHIS at Bhangar. In the year 2000-01, budget for this programme was Rs. 1,86,48,016.

(ii) Mobile Health Care Services

The infrastructural disadvantage of Sundarban is the most vital reason for its overall underdevelopment. People from far off villages of islands are deprived of basic amenities and whatever solutions as well as supports are available, these are often disrupted by the vagaries of nature. Considering the peculiar problems of Sundarban, the West Bengal government has been taking concrete steps to provide and extend the critical health care services in the remote villages of the delta. Hence, with the help of State Government and World Bank, Mobile Health Care Programme (through mechanized boat) was started in SHIS in March 1999. The major objectives were:

(a) to provide outreach health care services in remote areas of 7 blocks in South Sundarban, covering 49 villages with 90,000 population;
(b) to organize regular clinics in the project villages enabling people to avail quality medical care;
(c) to link the various village based mobile clinics through mechanized vessels, complete with diagnostic and X-ray facilities;
(d) to build a strong network of referral linkages, linking the patients from mobile health clinics to PHCs, Rural Hospitals and Hospitals of Kolkata;
(e) to build a Community Based Disease Surveillance System;
(f) to develop a comprehensive Health Information Management System with information flow from the grassroots level to project management level.

This programme has eight components, such as:

(a) Home visit (to enquire dropout patients);
(b) Awareness camp (related to family health, personal hygiene, sanitation, drinking water, child health services, etc.);
(c) Family planning services (awareness on birth control, individual counselling to eligible couples, supplying condoms and contraceptive pills, etc.);
(d) Immunization facility (to the pregnant mothers and children in association with the government health care institutions);
(e) General clinic (conducted at every week to provide primary health care facility to all sorts of patients);
(f) Special clinic (conducted periodically with the help of ENT specialist, Gynaecologist, Eye specialist, Cardiac specialist, General Physician and Orthopedic Surgeon, etc.);
(g) Ante-natal and post-natal clinic (for pregnant mothers, lactating mothers and infants);
(h) Diagnostic services (two mechanized boats equipped with X-ray and pathological facilities move around the islands as per a pre-fixed plan to provide diagnostic services);
(i) Referral services (sending patients by boat or ambulance to the city hospital) and information system (communicating field message by wireless).

This programme is executed through different types of staff members. For instance, *Programme Co-ordinator → Block Incharge → Area Incharge → Senior Health Worker*. Apart from them, there are three mechanized boats. In each boat, two doctors (MBBS, BAMS) and one laboratory technician are always on duty. Field workers organize awareness camps and immunization camps, provide family planning services, and make home visits. In the beginning of the week, each boat starts from one island and moves forward through different islands till the end of the week. Everyday, this boat conducts two clinics (two opposite sides of the river) in the morning and two clinics in the afternoon (two sides of the river). These clinics are performed as per the pre-decided schedule. When special clinics are organized, good doctors are brought from the city hospitals. Problems of the beneficiaries or field level staff reach to programme co-ordinator through proper channel and also through wireless.

(iii) Women in Cultivation, Processing and Marketing of Medicinal Plants (WCPMMP)

The present programme has two major objectives. The first is to popularize herbal medicine as a viable medical solution and the second is to promote cultivation of medicinal plants as a potential income option for women. This programme is being implemented in 11 villages directly covering 1,126 women from 962 families who have their own land. In addition, SHIS has leased out a number of land holdings in the name of women's groups. WCPMMP programme has five major components and they are as follows:

(a) *Awareness at Village Level:* To promote the women leadership, to train in agronomy practice for medicinal plants, to aware the village women for utility of herbal drugs, etc.;
(b) *Central Training Facility:* To hold the workshop on individual plant cultivation, to conduct practical training camp on drug making, to educate women on economics of the medicinal plants, to help in identifying the plants and understanding the medicinal value of the same, etc.;
(c) *Cultivation:* One hundred fifty to one hundred seventy types of plants are cultivated in SHIS nursery as well as village gardens;
(d) *Marketing*: SHIS purchases various plants from the village women and supplies to few reputed pharmaceutical companies,
(e) *Preparation of Medicine:* Medicine preparation plant is available at SHIS. These medicines are used in mobile health care programme.

In order to execute this programme, survey is conducted at the village level to understand population characteristics (i.e. number of total families, total BPL mothers, etc.).Then, women of BPL families are invited at the central level meeting and encouraged to participate in this project. Total eleven staff members are involved (i.e. one programme co-ordinator, one botanist, one pharmacist, one assistant co-ordinator, five field workers and two gardeners) to carry out the present programme. Two field workers work in the indoor production plant and the remaining three continuously visit the field and organize weekly awareness camps as per the pre-planned schedule. In every village, under the operational area, two ayurvedic clinics are conducted by the doctor (BAMS) and five mothers are given central training per month. Mother's co-operative has been formed in every village for better marketing of the plants and efforts are being made to develop a 'Central Co-operative Society' at the SHIS level. WCPMMP programme is being supported by *Terre Des Homes* (funding agency). In the year 2000-01, total expenditure for this programme was Rs. 8,79,124.

(iv) Rural Sanitation Programme

Main objective of this programme is to stop open field defecation, to provide low cost toilet facility, and to improve personal health and hygiene. This project has been initiated for three years (i.e. April 2001 to March 2004) with the help of UNICEF to cover 80,000 population. All the people of the 90 villages under South and North 24 Parganas who do not have toilet are treated as beneficiaries. This programme has four components and those are discussed below.

(a) *Village Awareness and Motivation*: Panchayat member is selected as motivator. He makes door-to-door visit for motivation;
(b) *Production of Implements of Toilet*: There is a sanitary mart to supply implements as per the demand;
(c) *Installation*: Labourer of the organization carries materials to the beneficiary's home and helps to develop low cost latrine;
(d) *Reporting*: There are two mart managers. One goes to motivators weekly to collect new orders and another person maintains official records and correspondence with Zilla Parishad in order to collect subsidy of Rs. 200 per beneficiary.

With regard to programme execution, SHIS maintains a lengthy procedure. At first, motivators are selected with the help of Gram Panchayat and they are given training for awareness work in the villages. Having become conscious and motivated, beneficiary applies to SHIS on the prescribed form with the recommendation of the panchayat. When beneficiary contributes 50 per cent of the total cost (i.e. Rs. 200), materials are sent for toilet construction. After completion of work, final bill is certified by the panchayat and SHIS takes the same to the Zilla Parishad Office to collect 50 per cent subsidy (i.e. Rs. 200).

(v) Mother and Child Health Programme (MCHP)

SHIS runs community based MCHP in 40 villages of Bhangar block, with assistance from the German Doctor's Committee. The basic programme objectives include—awareness to women on family health, ante-natal and post-natal care, immunization, nutrition, child growth and growth monitoring; health education camps in the villages; and formation of health groups for group discussion and regular meetings. A team of social workers under this programme ensure that each and every family in the target area is visited and their health status is recorded periodically. Health counselling is provided to the families including advice on family planning and welfare.

(vi) Self-Help Group (SHG)

Indebtedness and lack of opportunities are major contributing factors to poverty. Land and property of poor are forced to trade for few rupees, often resulting in trade of their own pride and dignity. The problem is so acute in the rural villages of India that whatever land a poor owns is confiscated in the name of indebtedness, in many cases for amounts as low as few hundred rupees. In the late eighties, Micro Credit was initiated as a tool to fight indebtedness and infuse motivation among people to start their own enterprise and create their own opportunities. The prelude to Micro Credit is Women's Groups, called Self-Help Groups (SHGs). Each Self-Help Group is formed by 10-20 women from village communities.

The group undergoes a series of orientation camps and workshops towards their motivation, participation and leadership in local issues. In a slow process, the group members develop mutual harmony and understanding. The Group is then motivated to save few rupees periodically. Now SHIS is having total 206 groups with 4,120 members in 12 villages.

(vii) Female Education Programme

This programme was started in 1995 and today covers 1,061 girl children, providing direct support for their education. Services like books, study materials, bags, uniforms and fees for school are being provided to the sponsored girl children, so as to provide them equal opportunities to get quality in education. SHIS has not made any parallel institution, whereas, it has entered into strategic alliance with the government run primary and secondary schools to provide quality education to children. This programme is funded by *Dr. Hacker and Sari.* During 2000-01, total budget for this programme was Rs. 5,01,322.

Staff Related Information

SHIS has total 339 full time paid staff, 15 part time paid staff, 40 honorary staff and 2,100 regular volunteers. The characteristics of these staff members are as follows:

Table 7.8: Characteristics of Full Time Paid Staff

Sl. No.	*Designation*	*Number*	*Minimum Qualification*
1.	Programme Coordinator	6	Graduate
2.	Supervisor	4	Graduate
3.	Doctor	30	Bachelor in Medical Profession
4.	Incharge	30	S.S.C
5.	Field level Health Worker	269	VIII pass

Table 7.9: Characteristics of Part Time Paid Workers

Sl. No.	*Designation*	*Number*	*Minimum Qualification*
1.	Doctor	8	Bachelor in Medical Profession
2.	Field Level Health Worker	7	VIII pass

Table 7.10: Characteristics of Honorary Staff

Sl. No.	*Designation*	*Number*	*Minimum Qualification*
1	School Teacher	6	S.S.C to M.A.
2.	Doctor	5	Bachelor in Medical Profession
3.	Field Level Health Worker	29	VIII pass

Patient leaders, birth attendants, leaders of Mahila Mandals and SHGs are used as volunteers. They come from irrespective of educational as well as social status and have age above 20 years.

The above mentioned staff members get salary as per the following pay structure:

(a) *Doctor*: Rs. 6,000–15,000
(b) *Programme Co-ordinator*: Rs 4,000–10,000
(c) *Supervisor*: Rs. 2,500–4,000
(d) *Incharge*: Rs. 2,000 to 3,500
(e) *Field Level Health Worker*: Rs. 900 to 2,000

Part time doctors get Rs. 400 to Rs. 600 per day with travelling and refreshment facility.

Financial Information

In the year 2,000-01, turnover of SHIS was Rs. 3,86,88,171. During this period various sources of funds were State Government, World Bank, Dominique Lapierre, German Doctor's Committee, SARI, Doctor Hacker, agricultural land and public contribution. Director says, with regard to fund raising, there is always tension and threat. Existing funding may be stopped by donor agencies at any time showing drawbacks in programme implementation. In the case of (WB) funding, troubles are more as WB wants that money will be spent by the organization at first and later on payment will be made to them as per the expenditure. In fact, it is a problem for the organization due to the existing financial crunch. It is also noticed in SHIS that funds of one programme are spent on other programmes; but in that case, prior approval is taken from the concerned funding agency. In order to manage financial affairs, SHIS prepares budget every year keeping in view expenditure mentioned in the project proposal, current market price and expected income in a particular year.

Future Aspirations of SHIS

SHIS is interested to start—

(i) an 'Open University' in the name of 'Titumir', which may provide educational facility to general people of Sundarban area;
(ii) a 'Research and Consultancy Wing' to provide service to the NGOs for organizational management; and
(iii) a full-fledged branch in North Bengal area.

In brief, SHIS is a family of like-minded people with its members spread all over the world. Hence, World Friendship Programme, Korean NGO Consortium, etc. have been sending a number of volunteers to SHIS. Similarly, every year numerous volunteers from Canada, France, Germany, Australia etc. spend their valuable time in SHIS. This opportunity gives great learning experience to the volunteers and to SHIS. Many leading corporate houses like TISCO, TELCO, NESTLE, SUN SECURITIES, etc. have also been involved in the movement of SHIS. In the decade of nineteen ninety, SHIS has received many awards for its popularity. For instance, Critic Circle of India Award (in 1991), Sundarban Seva Award (in 1997), Fr. Tong Memorial Award (in 1997), Hasanuzzaman Memorial National Award (in 1998), etc. But SHIS is not exception for problems in the management of its affairs. Firstly, as a result of vast operational area, it cannot control staff members properly in various sub-centres. Secondly, sometimes doctors do not attend clinic in the remote centres showing vague reasons and hence patients suffer badly. Thirdly, SHIS does not have bed facility in its hospital. Due to popularity, sometimes serious patients come to SHIS. As a result of lack of life saving medicines, oxygen and other facilities, these patients face difficulties. Inspite of these problems, SHIS has made a remarkable contribution for the people of Sundarban area.

This chapter is a discussion of different aspects (such as, past background, organizational structure, infrastructure, present activities and future plans) of a selected NGO. It is found that promoters of these NGOs are adequately experienced and interested to serve the poor people. The respective organizations have multi-dimensional programmes. Health programme is an important aspect under their wide spectrum of activities. Despite of having many difficulties, NGOs of the present study are eye opener and pathfinder for the rural masses. They prefer challenging work, have unique approach and are reformative in operation.

8

Nature of Programme Sustainability

In this Chapter, initiatives have been taken to understand the nature of sustainability of the programmes carried out by the three selected NGOs under the study. Four main programmes from each of the selected NGOs have been identified, discussed and interpreted. Researcher tries to find out how long one programme will exist; whether it will be durable for long time (more sustainable) or short time (less sustainable) or will be stopped (unsustainable) when the project duration will be over or organization will withdraw its programme from the operational area. In this regard, programmes of each NGO have been analysed on the basis of twelve factors (mentioned below). The programme, which has fulfilled all the factors, that is treated as more sustainable. If any programme lacks one or few of the factors, that programme has been understood as comparatively less sustainable. If any one does not relate to most of the factors, that has indicated unsustainability of the programme. Now programmes under each NGO are being analyzed below.

(A) RURAL HEALTH DEVELOPMENT CENTRE (RHDC)

RHDC runs total ten programmes. These programmes have already been named and briefed in Chapter 7. Out of them, four main programmes are: (i) Community Health Programme (CHP); (ii) Integrated Nutrition and Health Programme (INHP); (iii) Child Sponsorship Programme (CSP); and (iv) Disaster Preparedness Programme (DPP) [mainly for flood]. In order to understand the nature of sustainability of these programmes, we shall consider them on the basis of following factors:

(a) Capacity of the Organization

All the four programmes listed above are found appropriate and suitable for implementation as per the organization's Memorandum Association. Infrastructural conditions are also found favourable and provide a better scope. For instance, herbal garden, medicine preparation machine, static clinic and vehicle (Auto) for dropping serious patients are available in Community Health Programme; good training hall, sufficient resource persons, trained women groups, etc. help in Integrated Nutrition and Health Programme; separate office building, one static and one mobile clinic, one primary school, eight balwadi centres, one library, two child resource centres, one children's park, etc. are available for Child Sponsorship Programme; and boat as well as speed boat, zeep, trained volunteers for relief and rescue work, programme based implements for sending warning message before the disaster, etc. are seen for Disaster Preparedness Programme. With regard to programme implementation, RHDC takes decision democratically. Since workers are recruited locally and RHDC brings development in their native areas, members show their will-power and united approach in running this organization. Thus, we can assume that RHDC has sufficient capacity to carry out four main programmes such as CHP, INHP, CSP and DPP.

(b) Continuity in Funding

Community Health Programme (CHP) has been in operation since November 1995. This project will be completed very shortly and Indian Hilfe will stop funding. Under this programme, whatever money is earned having sold herbal medicine and through auto service, are deposited in the bank in order to develop a revolving fund. After the project duration is over, CHP will be continued by using this revolving fund.

Integrated Nutrition and Health Programme (INHP) has been funded by CARE for three years, which was completed in June 2001. CARE has decided to extend the duration of the same programme for another 3 years. It is found that each person, who receives ration under this programme, contributes Rs. 4 (four) per month and thus there is an alternative arrangement for fund raising.

Child Sponsorship Programme (CSP) is completely a service-oriented programme. Each child's expenditure is borne by a sponsor till 19 years. There is no alternative arrangement to continue this programme if sponsorship is stopped.

Disaster Preparedness Programme (DPP) has been receiving funds from OXFAM since 1993. Every year this project is renewed. If funding is stopped, this programme cannot be run.

So, it is evident from the above discussion that, except CHP and INHP, other programmes cannot be continued for long time without the support of funding agencies.

(c) Need Fulfilment and Ensuring Quality Service

CHP has been able to reduce birth and death rate, to motivate 100 per cent people to go for ante-natal check-up and immunization for the children, to find no death case during post-flood situation and to improve domestic treatment by using herbal medicine. Therefore, it is proved that it could fulfil needs of the beneficiaries and ensured qualitative service.

INPH is initiated to provide supplementary nutrition for better nutritional status and to bring awareness on health, nutrition, women empowerment, small savings, etc. The programme has been able to bring change at the awareness level, but it has failed to improve nutritional status. Therefore, it is clear that needs of the beneficiaries were fulfilled partially.

CSP has been able to provide basic health services (through static and mobile clinic, medicine arrangement, referral and special care), preventive health services (through health education, inculcating health habit, etc), educational facilities (through school supplies, school uniform, tuition fees, educational aids to the schools, construction of school building, etc.), supplementary education (vocational training, teacher training, etc), supplementary nutrition, material aid for domestic use (constructing latrine, repairing house, cooking utensils, etc.), community development (community hall repairing, road repairing, etc.) and value education (through youth training, field trip, day camp, art contest, etc). It is observed that this programme has fulfilled needs of the beneficiaries to a greater extent and provided very high quality service.

DPP (mainly for flood) is implemented in three phases (e.g. pre-disaster phase, disaster phase and post-disaster phase). During continuous flood in last few years, this programme could help the people very actively. Pre-disaster phase prepared the people for flood (by selecting safe shelter; collecting food, fodder and boat; making special arrangement for women, children and handicapped; etc.). Disaster phase involved in relief and rescue work in order to reduce loss of lives and properties. Post-disaster phase provided rehabilitation (constructing house and road; reforming source of safe drinking water, restarting various social institutions, starting income generation programme, etc.) to the flood victims. So, we assume that DPP fulfilled the needs of the beneficiaries.

It is evident from the above discussion that except INHP all other programmes have fulfilled the needs of the beneficiaries and maintained quality of the service.

(d) Intention of the Beneficiaries

Community Health Programme could convince the people to believe that good health was their own right. In the programme, beneficiaries understood it and expressed the same by going to Sub-Centre for immunization as well as contraceptive measures, by learning simple herbal treatment, etc. Thus, beneficiaries projected good intention.

It was found in INHP, especially at the village level women group meeting, beneficiaries expressed, by sharing their grievances, receiving safe delivery kits from the village level volunteers, taking advice of local trained *dais*, etc., that the programme was meant for them. Thus, beneficiaries divulged their good intention.

It has always been mentioned that CSP is entirely a charity-based programme. Beneficiaries always get some benefit in the form of money or material from their sponsor. This approach has spoiled the beneficiary's positive outlook and does not allow other developmental programmes to be implemented. Because beneficiaries neglect other developmental programmes without material benefit. Approach of CSP forces them to get involved with the politics to push their child under this programme. Once a child is selected, his/her all kinds of expenditures are borne by the organization. Therefore, beneficiaries are always led by self-interest and profit making motive. They do not have good intention.

DPP sensitized the beneficiaries to fight judiciously against the government administration. It was found that flood victims (only women) gave representation at the panchayat office, convinced the Pradhan and got installed a tube-well in their locality during inter-disaster phase (interval between two flood incidents). This gives evidence of good intention of the beneficiaries.

(e) Nature of People's Participation

CHP is implemented through 39 women groups and 19 farmers groups. These village level groups are called people's organizations where members are representatives of the beneficiaries. Field workers of this programme act as a via between NGOs and village groups or beneficiaries. Here, Planning is done at the NGO level and it comes to the groups for proper execution of the same. In the group meeting, needs and problems of the beneficiaries are discussed and reported to the NGO. In case of beneficiaries selection, there is an application form, which party files up and sends to RHDC through group. If group recommends the case, appropriate beneficiary is identified. Regarding treatment in outdoor as well as mobile clinic, it is noticed that beneficiaries pay for taking medicines and emergency auto service. Thus, we find that people participate in need identification, beneficiaries selection, programme implementation and in paying for the service cost. But they do not have right to participate in programme planning, monitoring and evaluation. Therefore, this situation can be treated as partial participation of the people.

We find in Part-I that INHP is implemented through village level women groups. Members of these groups are representatives of the beneficiaries. Village level volunteers (VLV) [where one VLV looks after 5 to 6 villages] form these women groups, make them aware and develop their total capacity to carry out programe implementation work. VLV is responsible for home visit, beneficiaries selection and on-going monitoring of the programme. Women's groups bear responsibility for growth monitoring of the village children, distribution of take home ration, small savings, celebration of World Health Day, Women's Day, etc. In the group meeting, women discuss their needs and problems and pass the decision on to the sub-centre level team, sector level team, block level team and district level team for taking final decision and appropriate plan. Thus, we find that beneficiaries participate in need identification, programme planning and programme implementation; but not in beneficiaries selection as will as monitoring. Therefore, we can say people's participation in this programme is partial.

In CSP, beneficiaries are selected through Gram Committee. When sponsors send some lump sum money in various occasions (e.g. Christmas) for better family atmosphere and village infrastructure development, sponsored families are called for meeting to discuss on their various physical needs and community needs. In case of community development work (e.g. Balwadi School set-up, road repairing, community hall repairing, etc.), which is an important component of the CSP, beneficiaries contribute in the form of land, labour, etc. Thus, people's participation is found in beneficiaries selection, need identification and resource contribution. They cannot participate in programme planning, implementation and monitoring. This situation is treated as partial participation of the people in CSP.

DPP is implemented through five Community Based Organizations (CBOs). Under each CBO, there are many 'on call volunteers' (rescue workers) and women groups who are the actual programme implementing agents. Members of these groups are representatives of the beneficiaries. In the pre-disaster and post-disaster periods, actual beneficiaries are selected through these groups. During disaster, badly affected victims are identified as beneficiaries by the rescue workers on the spot. With regard to needs and problems of the people, monthly meeting is conducted in various women groups and resolution is sent to the RHDC through CBO for appropriate planning. In the same way, various directions are received by the women groups (from RHDC) for execution of the objectives of the programme. Again, when DPP is monitored monthly by the programme co-ordinator, he takes into consideration opinions of the women groups. Thus, people's participation in DPP is found in beneficiaries selection, need identification, programme planning, implementation and monitoring. This can be treated as full-fledged participation.

It is manifested from the above discussion that people participate partially in CHP, INHP and CSP; but in every aspect of DPP.

(f) Recognition of the People's Participation

People's participation has been recognized duly during implementation of all the four programmes (CHP, INHP, CSP and DPP). It is done by appreciating people in the meeting, giving them more responsibility and granting their decision. In fact, doing the same is a tradition of this organization.

(g) Use of Volunteers and Continuous Liaison with Them

In CHP, there are total 800 volunteers. These volunteers are used for various activities like (a) taking class on health and hygiene in schools, (b) arrangement and maintenance of mobile clinic, (c) helping the beneficiaries to contact with various institutions for legal aid, etc. RHDC maintains continuous liaison with these volunteers through monthly meeting. Besides that, in order to keep good relation with them, RHDC organizes annual programme for herbal garden competition, baby show, women group's sports, quiz contest on health, etc. and take the volunteers for exposure visit in other NGO.

In INHP, 18 volunteers are involved permanently. They help in organizing community meeting, distributing Take Home Ration (THR), conducting mothers health day (i.e. discussing on mothers' health problems), social mapping and sometimes in home visit. Continuous liaison is maintained with them through monthly and emergency meeting.

CSP is having 105 volunteers. These volunteers are used for awareness generation in the community dewarming programme (distributing tablet to reduce worm infestation), community cleaning, etc. RHDC keeps continuous contact with them through monthly meeting.

There are total 67 volunteers in DPP. They are called 'On call volunteers'. During disaster, at the time of emergency relief, their services are used. Continuous liaison is maintained with them through field visit (when staff members go to field, meet them and maintain relation).

(h) Staff Mobility

In order to understand the nature of staff mobility, accounts of last three years (January 1999 to December 2001) have been taken into consideration. It was found that there was no staff mobility in CHP. In INHP, two VLVs left their jobs respectively in December 1999 and in March 2001. The reasons for leaving this work were (i) family pressure due to very less salary and (ii) getting married to some other area. In CSP, programme co-ordinator and one field worker left their jobs in April 1999 since they got better salaried jobs in other organizations. DPP had also witnessed the incident of staff mobility after January 1999. One field level staff left this programme in May 2001 since she was selected as ICDS worker and one training assistant resigned from his duty in June, 2001 since he was computer personnel and was not interested in this work. Thus, it is evident from the above discussion that staff mobility (since January 1999) exists in all the programmes except CHP.

(i) Innovative Component

In CHP, few innovative components are found and these components help to execute this programme in a better way. For instance, (a) Monthly central meeting is conducted in different villages in different months. Total 39 leaders of women groups, 19 leaders of farmer groups and 11 staff members (i.e. 69 people) are assembled. Having completed the meeting, each member visits one house, takes food there and shares daily life experience. This is done mainly for better health awareness generation; (b) Keeping in view the status of women's health, adolescent girls are given iron tablets as well as scope for gynaecological treatment; (c) Villagers are advised to cultivate costly medicinal plants. It helps them to generate income; (d) Women groups are linked with the public development agencies such as district hospital, bank, panchayat, police station and district court for accessibility of the facilities required in this programme.

In INHP, innovative components are also visible. For instance, (a) Mother's Health Day (MHD): INHP has a system of giving ration to the mothers. It is done in second week and last week of every month. At the last week, when mothers come for the same, MHD is celebrated on any health issue and awareness is given; (b) Counselling: During the day of ration distribution, individual counselling is given to the mothers; (c) Fund raising: During ration collection, each beneficiary contributes Rs. 2 (and thus total Rs. 4 per month). It is deposited in women group's fund and used to meet programme expenditure; (d) Health Mela: Annual Health Mela is organized for awareness generation; (e) Male group formation: Traditional Indian society does not allow village women to go out of home and to join some group. By forming male group and convincing the male members for women empowerment, barriers of women group formation and functioning are removed.

In CSP, no innovative component is found for its better existence.

With regard to disaster (mainly flood), Government spreads warning message. But this does not really reach to the people of remote area on time. RHDC has an innovative warning system under DPP. Looking at the river character, immature fruits in the market, price hike for necessary goods and receiving urgent message from the OXFAM (since it has continuous link with Bangladesh, Bihar and Assam), this organization sends warning message to the flood affected areas.

(j) Local Co-operation

CHP is carried out through Adampur campus (Old Malda). Considering the good motive of RHDC, Panchayats, Clubs, etc. extends their support in this programme as and when necessary and thus co-operation of the local people is satisfactory.

INHP as well as DPP is run by Bachamari Campus (Malda), which is located at the district town. District administration has very good connection with this campus since they use RHDC's office building in order to organize government sponsored training programmes. As a result of good relation, district administration co-operates very much to implement INHP and DPP.

CSP is implemented through Baragram Campus (Dakshin Dinajpur). Local co-operation lacks in that locality. Because, Secretary of RHDC is an active supporter of CPI (M), but local panchayat is run by Congress Party.

(k) Integrated with Other Programmes and Multi-Sectoral Activities for Better Existence

CHP is integrated with DPP and Sanitation programme. At the field level, in few cases, same workers and same daily work monitoring systems are used in these programmes to reduce wastage and to save labour. Regarding multi-sectoral activities, CHP is not an exception. In this programme, there are total 12 components and they have already been mentioned in the previous part (I). Out of them, nine components are directly related to health and nutritional aspects. Other three components (such as day-night auto service for patients, legal aid for women and removal of illiteracy) are meant to address the personal problems of women, since this programme is implemented through women groups. Because of other three components, women feel interested and regularly participate in the group sessions.

INHP is not linked with any other programme but this programme itself is having an integrated approach. It has very strong connection with Block Development Office, Primary Health Centre, ICDS Project and Panchayats for better execution. INHP is also having multi-sectoral activities. Out of its five components (mentioned in Part–I), two components such as 'Women Empowerment' and 'Micro Credit' lead to have gender equality as well as income sufficiency than health status improvement among the women. These components help to make the programme effective and enhance beneficiary's participation.

CSP is integrated with Short Stay Home and Disaster Preparedness Programme. These programmes use same Outdoor Clinic for treating common health problems and same Neighbourhood Groups (NHGs) for awareness work. With regard to multi-sectoral activities, CSP is no exception. For all-round development of the child, this programme has various components (already mentioned in Part–I) pertaining to personal hygiene, health, education vocational training, community infrastructure, domestic good, value orientation, etc.

DPP is integrated with CHP and CSP. How these programmes are interdependent to each other have already been mentioned under this factor in the preceding paragraphs. With regard to multi-sectoral activities, DPP is also important. It has total 12 components to work during pre-disaster, disaster and post-disaster period. Two components, such as mobile health clinic and legal aid services, responsible for pre-disaster work have no connection with disaster preparedness programme. These components give attraction to the beneficiaries for active participation in the programme.

Thus, it is found in the above discussion that all the four programmes have integrated approach and follow multi-sectoral activities.

(l) Regular Monitoring

CHP is monitored half yearly by a team from the funding agency. Apart from that, its activities, staff members and finances are monitored regularly in RHDC. With regard to activities, it is done monthly with the help of programme co-ordinator by checking written reports received from women groups, organizing central meeting and making surprise visit at field. Staff members are monitored everyday with the help of campus Incharge by checking attendance register. Regular monitoring with regard to finance is done quarterly through joint meeting of secretary, programme co-ordinator and accountant.

INHP is monitored quarterly by an external team sent by CARE. Apart from that, various aspects of this programme are monitored regularly in RHDC. For instance, activities are monitored monthly by programme co-ordinator through staff meeting. In this meeting, field level staff members get various documents (daily home visit diary, day to day work sheet and advanced tour diary) checked. Staff monitoring is done monthly by the programme co-ordinator through report checking and surprise field visit. Regarding finance, monitoring system is as like as practiced in CHP.

CSP is monitored half-yearly by the monitoring team of Sahay (funding agency). It is also monitored regularly by the internal members of RHDC. Regarding activities, whenever there is need, all the staff members sit and discuss on the issue. This may be weekly or fortnightly, but at least once in a month. Finance monitoring is done monthly by programme co-ordinator as per programme budget, which is made during annual budget session at Sahay (funding agency). Staff monitoring is done everyday by campus Incharge through attendance register checking.

In DPP, regular monitoring is also done. Process for activities and finances monitoring are as like as used in CHP. With regard to staff, monitoring is done suddenly or weekly with the help of programme co-ordinator by checking work plan, leave application, staff involvement and dedication, staff quality and capacity, etc.

Thus it is understood that regular monitoring is done in all the four programmes under the study.

On the basis of above analysis, it can be summarized that each programme of RHDC suffers from various problems. For instance, CHP lacks full-fledged people's participation; INHP fulfils partial needs of the beneficiaries, get low level of people's participation, and have staff mobility; CSP lacks continuity in funding, good intention of beneficiaries, people's participation, innovative components, local co-operation and is having staff mobility; DPP has staff stability, and no permanent source of funding. So, it is evident that all the four programmes (of RHDC) under the study are less sustainable.

(B) CINI-MOYNA RURAL HEALTH DEVELOPMENT CENTRE (CINI-MOYNA RHDC)

This organization executes total six programmes and they have already been discussed briefly in Chapter VII. In order to understand the nature of programme sustainability, main four of these programmes such as (i) Reproductive and Child Health Programme (RCHP); (ii) Child Sponsorship Programme (CSP); (iii) Women Empowerment Programme (WEP); and (iv) Income Generation Through Handloom (IGTH) are being analysed here on the basis of following factors.

(a) Capacity of the Organization

Having reviewed the Memorandum of Association, Researcher has found that all the above listed programmes are appropriate and within the purview of CINI-MOYNA RHDC's activities. These programmes also possess sufficient infrastructure. For instance, weekly gynaecological clinic equipments for awareness work, a central committee (comprising programme co-ordinator, BMOH, visiting doctor and all other programme staffs), etc. are seen in RCHP; one separate office building, one community outreach clinic (weekly), one outdoor clinic (daily), nine Balwadi Centres, three Child Resource Centres, two children's parks, twenty nine youth groups, one vocational training centres and twelve bicycles (for field workers) are available for CSP; one separate office room (for money transaction), Rs. 600,000 revolving fund, hundred self help groups, etc. are found in WEP; and one separate handloom section (for distributing raw materials, collecting finished goods, etc), twenty five numbers handlooms (with the beneficiaries) and one sales counter are visible in IGTH programme. During day-to-day affairs and for smooth functioning of the above mentioned four programmes, CINI-MOYNA RHDC takes various decisions democratically. It is also very interesting to note that all the staff members (from Director to Field Workers) of this organization are recruited from the local villages. Naturally they show their very strong will-power and united approach in implementing various programmes. Thus, it is evident that CINI-MOYNA RHDC has adequate capacity to run RCHP, CSP, WEP and IGTH programme.

(b) Continuity in Funding

RCHP is being funded by Government of India (through M–NGO CINI, Daulatpur). Funding will be continued for two years (i.e. 2000 to 2002) and thereafter M-NGO CINI will select another NGO to cover some other backward areas. Since CINI-MOYNA RHDC has not made any alternative arrangement regarding funding, it will be difficult to continue RCHP after completion of the project duration.

CSP is financed by 'Children International' (through Sahay, Kolkata). It is entirely a charity-based programme. Expenditure of each child is borne by a sponsor till 19 years. There is no alternative arrangement to continue this programme if sponsorship is stopped.

'GOAL,' a funding agency, has given grants of Rs. 6,00,000 to support WEP. Having used the whole amount, a revolving fund is made to extend loan facilities under this programme. Again, every group member deposits Rs. 10 per month to increase the amount of revolving fund. Whenever members take loan, they start repaying the same by dint of instalment along with monthly deposit. Therefore, it is clear that this programme will be continued unless members will show their reluctancy or group will be dissolved.

IGTH programme was started in 1980 with the help of CINI (Daulatpur). Now it is an independent and self-sufficient programme. It does not require any support from any funding agency. Here, beneficiaries collect raw materials from CINI-MOYNA RHDC, they go for production, deposit the finished goods to the CINI-MOYNA RHDC and finally receive commission for production. Organization sales these goods to the market and again buy raw materials for supplying to the beneficiaries. CINI-MOYNA RHDC goes on following the same system. If beneficiaries have interest, there will be no disruption in this programme.

It is understood from the above discussion that there will be no assurance of funding in RCHP and CSP after completion of project duration. Therefore, these programmes will be terminated or some of their components may be continued linking with other programmes. With regard to WEP and IGTH, their will be no problem in funding and no disruption in programme execution if beneficiaries show interest.

(c) Need Fulfilment and Ensuring Qualitative Service

When researcher visited CINI–MOYNA RHDC, RCHP completed one year. With its limited health workers and because of their less involvement (since poorly paid), this programme could not contribute much to the beneficiaries in one year. It had been able to provide health awareness and gynaecological treatment facilities, but quantity of service was less as compared to the number of beneficiaries. Therefore, we can say, partial needs of the beneficiaries were fulfilled.

CSP has been able to provide basic health services (through daily outdoor clinic, weekly community outreach clinic, referral and special care), preventive health services (by healthy habit formation, health education, etc.), educational facilities (through school supplies, school uniform, tuition fees, teaching aids to the schools, school building repairing and construction, etc.), training facility (vocational training, teacher's training, etc.), supplementary nutrition, family assistance, community development facility and value orientation (through youth training, outing, day camp, art contest, annual sports, etc.). It is proved that CSP has fulfilled beneficiary's needs up to maximum possible extent and provided very qualitative service.

WEP has been able to convince the women members to contest in panchayat election, to go to literacy centre, to follow immunization schedule (for children) and birth controlling methods, etc. It has also extended micro credit facility for starting small business, for purchasing foodgrains, for meeting household expenditure, etc. Thus, the present programme has fulfilled beneficiaries needs.

In order to bear the day to day expenditure, beneficiaries cannot depend only on IGTH programme. They also earn by means of cultivation of rice, pan, fish, etc. Beneficiaries treat IGTH as a part of their sources of income. Thus, it is understood that it cannot fulfil the beneficiaries needs.

From the aforesaid discussion, we find that CSP and WEP are able to fulfil the needs of the beneficiaries, but RCHP and IGTH cannot contribute much.

(d) Intention of the Beneficiaries

In order to organize awareness camp under RCHP, each health worker is supposed to take only 20 to 25 participants. Since the programme is quite helpful for the community and beneficiaries show their strong interests, number of participants increase in each camp and it reaches between 35 to 40. Again, for awareness session, beneficiaries make all arrangements (i.e. selection of time, date, spot; collection of tables, chairs, benches; message to the participants; etc.) including refreshment for the trainers. Thus, beneficiaries under this programme have good intention.

Under CSP, beneficiaries get series of benefits continuously without any cost or trouble. This has made the local people to believe that poor people are supposed to get it from the government or funding agencies through this kind of NGO (e.g. CINI-MOYNA RHDC). In fact, this is very destructive idea. It has made beneficiaries materialistic and less participative in other programmes those do not provide free hard service. Therefore, intention of the beneficiaries are not good under CSP.

Under WEP beneficiaries have the scope of small savings as well as micro credit. They also get orientation for health care, development of educational atmosphere and political empowerment. This kind of inputs really contribute towards the overall development of women. Hence, women members of the community get attracted and approach to the programme co-ordinator for joining in this scheme by forming new group. In the existing groups, members are very regular in paying monthly fees and have mutual understanding. Thus, it is noticed that beneficiaries have good intention towards this programme.

As a result of introduction of high technology, textile industries produce good quality of sari, bed-sheet, bag, towel, mosquito net, etc. in cheap cost. Naturally, handloom made goods cannot compete in the market and consequently lose demands. Hence, number of beneficiaries, under this programme are getting reduced day-by-day. This situation manifests beneficiaries negative attitude towards IGTH programme.

(e) Nature of People's Participation

RCHP is implemented at the village level through health workers. In order to organize awareness camp, beneficiaries are selected by the health worker and topic is chosen in consultation with the beneficiaries. Beneficiaries have partial role in the planning process of this camp. They cannot sanction a camp but can take decision regarding spot, time and date of a sanctioned camp. During awareness session, beneficiaries ensure their involvement by attending the programme, providing physical infrastructure (i.e. table, chair, bench, etc), controlling public gathering, arranging refreshment for the trainers, etc. When evaluation team comes from CINI (Kolkata), beneficiaries are also called to interact with that team. Thus, beneficiary's active participation is found in need identification, programme planning (partial), implementation, monitoring and evaluation. Their involvement is nil in beneficiaries selection, camp sanction, etc.

In CSP, beneficiaries are selected through Gram Committee. When special gift amount comes from the sponsor or when annual plan is made, beneficiaries are called in meeting to know their needs. In case of special gift, concerned beneficiary is asked to express domestic needs (e.g. business capital, pond excavation, almirah purchase, etc.). During annual plan, community needs are identified (e.g. tube well, culvert, school repairing, ICDS centre repairing, etc.). Under this programme, CINI-MOYNA RHDC collects contribution from the beneficiary's families in case of latrine construction (Rs. 600), Van purchasing (Rs. 600) and house repairing (Rs. 2,000). Ten per cent of the total cost is collected to ensure utilization of service. But no contribution is collected for sponsorship of the children. During community development work, beneficiaries also contribute in the form of land, labour, etc. (e.g. for balwadi centre construction). Again, in this programme, beneficiary's participation is found nil during annual planning session (at Sahay Office, Kolkata), programme implementation (i.e. to carry out various components), monitoring of work, etc. Thus, partial people's participation is manifested in CSP.

Under WEP, 100 SHGs have been formed. Members decide who will be in the group and who will go away. They contribute Rs. 10 per head per month as savings. Regularly members participate in the meeting and discuss on various community problems, loan disbursement, scope for small trade, illiteracy issue, health problems, etc. In case of programme planning and evaluation, co-ordinator, field workers, group leaders and group secretaries meet to talk on different issues. All the groups bear responsibility to implement various components of this programme. Thus, in WEP, people's participation is found at all the levels i.e. in beneficiaries selection, resource contribution, need identification, programme planning, implementation and evaluation.

In IGTH programme, beneficiaries are selected through programme staff, their needs are identified by asking them who is experienced in what production and finally they are given raw materials to develop output. Beneficiaries contribute only labour and get wages in exchange. Though these beneficiaries are the programme implementing unit, they do not participate in all the phases (from buying raw materials to selling finished goods) of the implementation. Thus, beneficiaries participate only in need identification and resource contribution. Their involvements lack in beneficiaries selection, programme planning, implementation and evaluation process.

It is evident from the above discussion that, except WEP, all other programmes (RCHP, CSP and IGTH) experience partial people's participation.

(f) Recognition of the People's Participation

People's participation, whether partial or full-fledged, is recognized duly in all the four programmes (i.e. RCHP, CSP, WEP and IGTH). It is done during the annual general meeting and various mass gatherings by encouraging the people as well as expecting the same kind of help from them in near future.

(g) Use of Volunteers and Continuous Liaison with Them

In RCHP, there are total 50 regular volunteers. They represent various local clubs, balwadi centres and ICDS centres. Services of these volunteers are utilized for spot selection, date and time fixation, propagation regarding camp, and arrangement of physical infrastructure (Table, Chair, Bench, etc). Continuous liaison is maintained with them by surprise visit of health workers (when they go to field).

In CSP, 300 volunteers are involved permanently. They help in organizing health awareness camp, day camp for community cleaning and road repairing, deworming programme, etc. Volunteers also extend support during material distribution and in writing letter (on behalf of the sponsored) to the sponsor. Continuous liaison is maintained with these volunteers through monthly meeting.

WEP has 200 regular volunteers. They are basically leaders and secretaries of self-help groups. Leaders help in organizing meeting and secretaries maintain register by taking attendance, writing resolution of the meeting, etc. In order to review programme activities, co-ordinator, field workers, all the leaders and secretaries meet in every month. Thus, through this monthly meeting, continuous liaison is maintained with the volunteers.

In IGTH programme, no volunteer is used. Thus, question of maintaining continuous liaison with the volunteers does not arise.

(h) Staff Mobility

To understand the nature of staff mobility, accounts of last three years (i.e. January 1999 to December 2001) have been considered. It is found that there is no staff mobility in all the four programmes (i.e. RCHP, CSP, WEP and IGTH) under the study.

(i) Innovative Component

No innovative component is found in RCHP. Innovative component exists in CSP. For instance, one MBBS doctor comes on every Monday and treat patients sitting at the daily outdoor clinic. This is an arrangement of special care for the sponsored children. Doctor is paid from the project fund. Those non-sponsored patients come to this doctor, very minimum fee (i.e. Rs. 10 for new patient and Rs. 2 for old patient) is collected from them. From these collected amounts, pathological facility (i.e. blood test, urine test, stool test, sperm test, etc.) is provided to the family members of sponsored children in half cost.

In IGTH programme, innovative component is also visible. For instance, under this programme, there is a sales counter to dispose of all the produced goods. Organization does not undergo any tension or find problems to market these goods. All the products are purchased by the Co-ordinator of CSP in order to provide clothing facility to the sponsored children and their family members. Thus, innovative component helps this programme to be executed in an effective way.

(j) Local Co-operation

Adolescent's education is a component of RCHP. It includes awareness on physical as well as mental changes and human sexuality. Indian society does not permit to discuss these issues openly. Therefore, in order to implement RCHP in a village, health workers first meet members of the panchayat and local club, convince them and finally conduct parents meeting with the help of these influential members. Thus, local co-operation exists very much in RCHP and without it this programme cannot be implemented.

In CSP, Gram Panchayat (for beneficiaries selection), BPHC (for preventive health care), Local Primary as well as Secondary Schools (for school health programme) and Clubs (for holding sports, awareness camps, day camps, etc.) extend full co-operation. In WEP, panchayat members or influential persons intervene if group maladjustments or conflicts occur. IGTH programme does not require and receive any local support.

It is understood from the above analysis that local co-operation exists in all the programmes (i.e. RCHP, CSP and WEP) except IGTH.

(k) Integrated with Other Programmes and Multi-sectoral Activities for Better Existence

Out of four programmes under the study, CSP is the most demanding, service oriented and active programme. It is integrated with all other three programmes (i.e. RCHP, WEP and IGTH). For instance, RCH awareness is given to the Mothers of the sponsored children. The same mothers are involved in the formation of SHG under the WEP. In IGTH programme, whenever goods are produced, those go to the 'Child Sponsorship Department' in order to provide clothing facility to the sponsored children and their mothers. This kind of inter-dependency helps in better existence of the programmes.

Again, only in CSP, multi-sectoral activities are found. For all round development of the child, this programme has various components (already mentioned in Part–I) pertaining to personal hygiene, health, education, vocational training, community infrastructure, domestic goods, value orientation, etc.

(I) Regular Monitoring

RCHP is monitored quarterly by a team of M-NGO CINI, Daulatpur. For day-to-day affairs, monitoring is done by programme co-ordinator through weekly and monthly meeting. In weekly meeting, discussion is initiated for problems related to on-going awareness camp conducting and during monthly meeting, last month's activities are reviewed, next month's plan is made and expenditure heads as well as staff attendance is checked.

CSP is monitored half-yearly by a monitoring team of Sahay (funding agency). It is also internally monitored through monthly meeting under the leadership of the programme head. All the staff members related to CSP attend the meeting and discuss on staff problems, staff regularity, expenditure as per the sanctioned budget, implemented work and future plan.

In WEP, group level activities are monitored by group leader and group secretary through monthly meeting. Group members discuss on their needs and problems joining in this meeting. In order to monitor the entire programme, monthly meeting is conducted at the organization by programme co-ordinator. All the field workers, group leaders and secretaries attend the meeting and discuss on monthly contribution collection, loan disbursement, group problems, regularity of the field workers, and future course of action.

IGTH programme is monitored weekly by programme co-ordinator. In every week, when beneficiaries come to receive raw materials and to hand over output, discussion is initiated on proper utilization of raw materials i.e. how much raw materials were given, how much goods were produced and whether there were any extra raw materials.

It is evident from the above discussion that regular monitoring is done in all the four programmes under the study.

Having made the above analysis, we understand that WEP fulfils all the required criteria and can be treated as more sustainable. Other three programmes, such as RCHP, CSP and IGTH, encounter various difficulties. For instance, RCHP lacks continuity in funding, full-fledged people's participation, innovative component and cannot fulfil beneficiaries needs. In CSP, beneficiary's participation as well as good intention is inadequate and there is no sustainable source of funding. IGTH cannot fulfil actual needs and beneficiaries have negative attitude as well as partial participation towards the programme. So, RCHP, CSP and IGTH programme under the study are less sustainable.

(C) SOUTHERN HEALTH IMPROVEMENT SAMITY (SHIS)

SHIS implements total seven programmes within its operational area. These programmes have been set out in Chapter VII. In order to understand the nature of sustainability of these programmes, four major on-going projects, such as (i) Tuberculosis Control Programme (TCP); (ii) Mobile Health Care Services (MHCS); (iii) Women in Cultivation, Processing and Marketing of Medicinal Plants (WCPMMP); and (iv) Rural Sanitation Programme (RSP) have been selected and analysed on the basis of following factors.

(a) Capacity of the Organization

It is verified by the researcher that SHIS is eligible to carry out all the four programmes cited above as per its Constitution (i.e. Memorandum of Association). Again, these programmes have and hold adequate infrastructure for appropriate implementation. For instance, one central out patient department, 882 short course chemotherapy centres, seven X-ray units, twenty seven pathological laboratories, (one big and twenty six small), sufficient medicines, etc. are found in TCP; three motor launches (well equipped with doctor, medicines and pathological facility), three ambulances, wireless (eleven sets), one auto, ENT box, dental box, eye operating instruments, etc. are visible in MHCS; medicinal plant (for production), tissue culture laboratory, SHIS nursery, village nurseries, etc. are available in the programme of WCPMMP; sanitary mart (for production of implements to construct latrine), store room, rickshaw (hired), motor cycles and adequate motivators are used in RSP. With regard to will power, all the members are united. When some instruction comes from the funding agency or external problems arise, they take active part to comply with the situation. SHIS follows democratic decision-making procedure. Director, President, Treasurer, two members of the managing committee and all the staff members meet and take major decision with regard to the functioning of SHIS. On the basis of above discussion, it is understood that SHIS is competent to execute all the four programmes under the study.

(b) Continuity in Funding

TCP is being implemented in North and South 24 Parganas districts with the funding of Government of India and Dominique Lapierre. Government of India has assured to continue this support for North 24 Parganas till 28th February, 2006. Dominique Lapierre, an author of the book titled 'City of Joy', applies different mechanism of funding. He earns a good amount of loyalty from this book and sends the same to SHIS to continue TCP in South 24 Parganas district. Thus, TCP is completely depended upon the external funds. If this support is discontinued, the present programme has to be closed down.

The project on MHCS was started in March 1999 for three years with the joint funding of State Government and World Bank. This project may be extended for few years more on request of SHIS. But, thereafter, continuity in funding will not be maintained. Hence, SHIS is in process to integrate this programme with MCHP, TCP and WCPMMP as an alternative arrangement. Using the existing infrastructure, doctors of other programmes, drugs of herbal medicinal plants and collecting cost of medicines from the patients, this project will be managed. However, this alternative arrangement cannot be assured if other programmes are discontinued. The programme on WCPMMP is sponsored by Terre Des Hommes, Switzerland. This funding will be continued till March 2003. When project duration will be over, in absence of external funding, this programme will be self-sufficient. In this regard, village nurseries will be maintained by villagers and expenditure for maintaining SHIS nursery, programme staff, manufacturing cost of medicines in the plant will be incurred from the 'General Fund' of SHIS. Having sold these herbal medicines during general clinics, special clinics, ante-natal as well as post-natal clinics and so on, income will be generated to pay back the amount of 'General Fund'.

RSP is funded by UNICEF and this sponsorship will be continued till March 2004. At the presence of UNICEF funding, beneficiaries pay 50 per cent cost of the entire service. Since SHIS has its own sanitary mart, when project duration will be over, 100 per cent service cost (i.e. Rs. 400 per latrine) will be collected from the beneficiaries to regularize this programme.

(c) Need Fulfilment and Ensuring Qualitative Services

TCP has been able to treat the patients with sincerity and regularity. All the medicines and examination facilities are provided here in free of cost. In the year 1999–2000, TCP has cured more than 2,500 TB patients. Till the year 2001 (since 1987) total number of 'Cumulative TB Patients Cured' have crossed 25,000. As a result of having regular follow up system for the patients, good quality medicines and up-to-date treatment techniques, services of this programme are treated as qualitative.

During the year 2000-01, MHCS project extended facilities in 90 villages covering 3,30,767 population. Three mechanized boats (launches) equipped with doctors, medicines and pathological facilities moved around the island villages, as per a pre-fixed plan. It had been able to conduct 2,216 general clinics (for 89,171 patients), 183 special clinics (for 13,958 patients), 277 immunization camps, 367 ante-natal and post-natal clinics (for 8,014 beneficiaries), 402 well baby clinics (for 9,940 patients), 129 awareness camps and 552 family welfare camps (for condom and pill distribution, vasectomy and tubectomy operation, etc.). This programme also provided diagnostic services for X-ray (2,380), blood (7,807), urine (3,147), sputum—AFB (2,391), ECG (326), RA factor (211), stool—OPC (2,708), serum bilirubin (162), montoux text (452), etc. during 2000-01. Beneficiaries are of the opinion that eighty per cent of the required medicines are available during clinic days and in spite of remoteness of the place service quality of this programme is very high.

Total 1,126 women were benefited under WCPMMP project during 2000–01. Beneficiaries would sale medicinal plants to the project co-ordinator per week and earn roughly Rs. 200 to Rs. 250. It helped to generate a part of their total family income. But this was not continued throughout the whole year. As per the demands in the market, organization became very choosy in purchasing plants from the women. Hence, a bulk of the total plants, those were already produced, had to be sold in very low rate. Thus, beneficiaries encountered problems and their needs were not fulfilled.

Rural Sanitation Programme, under its operational area, has been able (to some extent) to stop open field defecation and to improve family hygiene. It has fulfilled intended needs. But, many of the beneficiaries are not satisfied with the quality of service i.e. latrine construction. Because, stool reservoir or wall of latrine is not made pucca. This situation discourages and demotivates the expected and future beneficiaries.

(d) Intention of the Beneficiaries

In government health care institutions, TB patients are not treated regularly and carefully. Patients prefer to go to private doctors. Poor patients cannot afford it and come to SHIS with an intention of survival. They expect free service as per the wish and capacity of SHIS. This is not bad on the part of the patients.

MHCS project brings awareness among the masses for proper utilization of government health care institutions. It was noticed in Patharpratima and Namkhana block that people, becoming conscious, gave representation in PHC and rural hospital for irregularity of services. As a result, BMOH was transferred to reduce public pressure. This reflects good intention of the beneficiaries.

In WCPMMP programme, beneficiaries are reluctant to continue their work since there is fluctuation of demands in the market and they do not get appropriate price of the plants. Even, few of the beneficiaries do not get back their production cost. Thus, overall situation highlights beneficiaries negative attitude.

Of course, beneficiaries are not happy with the quality of service under RSP, but they have positive and realistic attitude (i.e. good intention). They create pressure on the people, who do not have latrine, by saying that latrineless people are responsible for developing unhygienic atmosphere. This sort of neighbourhood pressure compel the people to have low cost latrine.

(e) Nature of People's Participation

In TCP, there is 'Village Health Committee' (VHC) comprised of patient leaders (i.e. old TB patients), panchayat members and influential persons. Whenever members of VHC suspect somebody with TB, they send him/her immediately to treatment centre for check up. Each beneficiary contributes Rs. 5/- as registration fee during check up. Once TB is detected, treatment is provided free of cost. During treatment, old TB patients who are cured work as DOT providers.

Generally, DOT is the duty of health assistant. Village influential persons and panchayat members also intervene if DOT providers fail to feed medicines. Thus, people take part in beneficiaries selection, need identification, resource contribution (very little) and programme implementation. They have no right to participate in programme planning, monitoring and evaluation.

Under MHCS project, all categories of people (APL and BPL) get treatment facilities. In it, having discussed with Village Health Committees (VHCs), field workers inform to the programme co-ordinator to decide how many immunization camps, health awareness camps, family welfare camps, ANCs and PNCs, etc. to be conducted. What type of specialists are required and what should be the time of general clinics (morning or afternoon) are also decided as per the message received from VHC. In order to get treatment in various clinics, each patient contributes Rs. 3 as registration fee. During clinic days, local people arrange physical infrastructure (tables, chairs, benches, etc.), entertain the members of medical team, and work as volunteers to control crowd. Thus, people's participation is found at various levels except programme planning, monitoring and evaluation.

In the programme of WCPMMP, beneficiaries are selected by the programme staff after conducting survey and central level motivation meeting. Beneficiaries, under this programme, express their needs during weekly awareness camp. They use their own land for cultivation of plants and invest money for production of herbal medicines. With regard to planning, they also give ideas for various forms of cultivation, home level medicine production, marketing, when and where monthly clinic is to be conducted, etc. Without beneficiaries participation, it is impossible to implement this programme. When external evaluation team comes from the funding agency, beneficiaries help in their working process. Thus, except beneficiaries selection, people participate at all the levels of this programme.

In RSP, new latrine users explain the utility of low cost latrine construction during motivation camps and create pressure on latrineless people for making unhygienic atmosphere. This situation helps to generate beneficiaries needs. Each beneficiary, who constructs latrine, contributes Rs. 200 (per unit). Thus, people's participation is found only in case of need identification and resource contribution under this programme.

(f) Recognition of the People's Participation

There are various mechanisms for recognizing people's participation. Under TCP, yearly meeting is organized for patient leaders, influential persons and village people. Their involvement throughout the whole year is appreciated in this meeting and few active workers are given prizes. In MHCS, the very next meeting after special clinic day or family welfare camp is used for acknowledging people's support. In WCPMMP programme, from each village, when five mothers are called upon monthly to attend central training and ten mothers are invited yearly for general meeting, their participation in various phases of this programme is duly recognized. In RSP, good as well as active motivators are bucked up and awarded prizes during annual general body meeting.

(g) Use of Volunteers and Continuous Liaison with them

In TCP, patient leaders (i.e. old TB patients), panchayat members and influential persons work as volunteers. Their numbers are more than 550. These volunteers refer the suspected cases to treatment centre, help the patients in collecting medicines, as per the prescription regularly feed drugs to the beneficiaries and follow up each patient carefully. Field visitors or health visitors conduct monthly meeting with these volunteers in each month and maintain continuous liaison with them.

Under MHCS, members of local youth clubs, primary school teachers, panchayat members, etc. work as volunteers. In order to organize various camps and clinics, services of these volunteers are received. No volunteer is permanent and no specific liaison is maintained with them since off and on they insist to be employed in SHIS.

In order to implement WCPMMP programme, volunteers are not required.

In RSP, users of low cost latrine and panchayat members work as volunteers. There are total 130 volunteers under this programme. They organize poster exhibition on rural sanitation during village fair, motivate people for construction of low cost latrine, link the beneficiaries with SHIS, etc. Under the leadership of programme co-ordinator, one central level meeting is conducted quarterly where volunteers, programme staff, representatives of Block as well as Zilla Parishad attend and share views. Continuous liaison is maintained with the volunteers by dint of this meeting.

(h) Staff Mobility

With a view to comprehend the nature of staff mobility, accounts of last three years (i.e. from January 1999 to December 2001) have been considered. Under TCP, two supervisors and one health worker left job in February 2001 respectively because of less salary and better chance in other organization. In MHCS, two senior health workers discontinued their duty since January 2001 for the sake of marriage and one health worker gave up job in February 2001 as a result of family problems. No staff mobility was found in RSP and WCPMMP programme under the study.

(i) Innovative Component

In TCP, the most uncommon as well as innovative aspect is use of patients leaders. Persons who had TB and now it is cured, they are identified as patient leaders. Since TB patients get free treatment from SHIS, this organization requests the old beneficiaries (identified as patient leaders) to provide voluntary service for identification of new cases, feeding medicines to and regular follow up of the existing patients.

In MCHS, there are two considerable innovative aspects. One, this programme maintains a network with many city hospitals in order to refer serious patients from the island areas. In this regard, the present programme also extends transport facility. Two, each mechanized boat possesses and runs pathological centre for diagnostic services.

Under WCPMMP programme, herbal plants produced in village nurseries are purchased by SHIS and used for medicine preparation in its own plant. SHIS does not buy all the medicines required in MHCS project. Some of the medicines are collected from herbal medicinal plant to minimize cost. Thus, preparing medicine and supplying it to other project is an innovative aspect. In RSP, using motivators is also an innovative aspect.

(j) Local Co-operation

Co-operation of the local NGOs, clubs and panchayats is found in TCP. NGO workers show interest to work as DOT providers, club members help in identifying new cases, panchayat members facilitate by making sitting arrangement in their own locality and to convince the patients who rejects the services of SHIS.

Under MHCS, co-operation and threat both are received from the local people. Members of club, panchayat, *hari basar* (religious place) and primary school teachers actively involve during various clinics and camps. Block Primary Health Centre also fits out various technical facilities as and when require. Regarding threat, field level workers have encountered it at Hingalganj, Patharpsatima and Canning block. Local people forcefully wanted to be employed in SHIS. When SHIS expressed negative attitude, they stopped the programme activities in those areas. This problem finally was solved through intervention of the Zilla Parishad.

In both RSP and WCPMMP programme, Pradhan of Gram Panchayat, Sabhapati of Panchayat Samity and BDO encourage the beneficiaries and become instrumental to help the organization during crises.

(k) Integrated with Other Programmes and Multi-sectoral Activities

TCP is integrated with MHCS, when doctor suspects a patient with TB, he sends him/her to the pathological centre located inside the mechanized boat for examination. Once TB is detected, that patient is referred to TCP for regular treatment. Though integration is found between TCP and MHCS, treatment centres or staff members or monitoring systems exist differently.

WCPMMP programme is combined with many other programmes like SHG, MHCS, MCHP, etc. Almost 90 per cent of the mothers who cultivate herbal plants are members of SHG. Medicines those are produced in Herbal Medicinal Plant are supplied for the clinics of MHCS project and MCHP. Inspite of having integration, this programme does not share same staff or resources with other programmes.

RSP follows an independent working strategy. It has no integration with any other existing programmes of the organization.

Thus, on the basis of the above discussion, we understand, except RSP, all other programmes such as TCP, MHCS and WCPMMP follow integrated approach. Again, it is observed that none of the programmes under the study is having multi-sectoral activities.

(l) Regular Monitoring

In TCP, staff members, finances and activities are monitored regularly. Director himself monitors staff by checking attendance register and leave application everyday. Activities are monitored by programme co-ordinator through weekly meeting. Incharge of all the centres come and discuss their problems in this meeting. With regard to finance monitoring, monthly meeting is held where Director, President, Treasurer, Programme Co-ordinator and various Centre Incharges participate to discuss on the financial affairs.

MHCS programme is monitored everyday, monthly and suddenly. Everyday, informations from all the centres come to the Director (after 7 p.m) through wireless. Director enquires about the activities of the whole day, staff involvement and various expenditures. During monthly monitoring, Director, President, Treasurer, Programme Co-ordinator, Supervisors and Centre Incharges meet to review activities of the last month and to make future plan of action. In order to have suddenly monitoring, surprise visit is made by the monitoring team of SHIS. This team checks up attendance register various accounts and work schedule.

In WCPMMP programme, monitoring is done daily, weekly and monthly by programme co-ordinator. Everyday, when workers come back from the field, Co-ordinator sits with them and gets the feedback given by the beneficiaries. Staff problems, programme expenditures, progress of the work, etc. are reviewed and plan for the next week is made during weekly monitoring. In this regard, all the staff members meet at the end of the week. During monthly monitoring, five mothers who come for central training, all the programme staff, Director and President come in contact and discuss on the various agenda.

In RSP, regular monitoring for staff members, financial affairs and programme activities is found. Staff monitoring system is as like as it is practiced in TCP. Finance is monitored quarterly and a financial status report is developed by the accountant in order to send the same in Zilla Parishad Office. With regard to activities, weekly and quarterly monitoring is done. Weekly monitoring system is same as it is found in WCPMMP programme. During quarterly monitoring, representatives from Zilla Parishad, Block, SHIS and village level motivators join to share views and to regulate various activities.

It is evident from the above discussion that none of the programmes (i.e. TCP, MHCS, WCPMMP and RSP) of SHIS fulfils all the twelve requisite criteria. Each programme suffers from few bottlenecks. For instance, in TCP and MHCS, partial people's participation, staff mobility and irregularity of funding after the project duration are the major problems. Under WCPMMP programme, beneficiary's needs are not fulfilled and they have negative attitude as well as partial involvement in the entire activities. In RSP, service quality is poor and there is low level of people's participation. Hence, all the four programmes of SHIS are found less sustainable.

Thus, with regard to programme sustainability, all the three NGOs under the study show negative results. In RHDC, none of the four programmes fulfils all the twelve requisite criteria. Each programme suffers from one or more problems and thus they are less sustainable. In CINI-Moyna RHDC, only Women Empowerment Programme is more sustainable. Other three programmes do not fulfil the necessary requirements and hence they are treated as less sustainable. SHIS has the same performance like RHDC. Its all the four programmes are less sustainable.

9

Job Satisfaction of the Working Staff

The Methodology chapter has given the details regarding concept of job satisfaction, procedure of job satisfaction scale construction, criteria for selecting staff, process of data analysis and so on. This Chapter, in fact, presents data to understand the level of job satisfaction of the working staff and makes effort to explore whether there is any significant association between natures of staff and levels of satisfaction.

In this regard, thirty staff members have been taken into consideration under each NGO. A brief description of these staff members is as follows:

PROFILE OF STAFF UNDER THE STUDY

(a) Sex of Staff Members

Table 9.1: Number of Males and Females Under NGOs

Organization	*Male*	*Female*	*Total*
RHDC	16 (53.4%)	14 (46.6%)	30 (100%)
CINI-Moyna RHDC	14 (46.6%)	16 (53.4%)	30 (100%)
SHIS	24 (80%)	6 (20%)	30 (100%)
Total	**54 (60%)**	**36 (40%)**	**90 (100%)**

Table 9.1 gives an account for number of males and females under various NGOs. It highlights, number of males are found more as compared to females respectively in RHDC (53.4%) and SHIS (80%). In CINI-Moyna RHDC, more than half of the workers (53.4%) are female. Including all the three NGOs, there are total sixty per cent male and forty per cent female.

(b) Age of Staff Members

Table 9.2 shows, none of the NGOs is having staff who are below twenty-one years. Respectively in RHDC and SHIS, 46.7 per cent and 53.4 per cent of the staff members (i.e. maximum in each NGO) have age between twenty-one to thirty years. In CINI-Moyna RHDC, most of the workers (66.6%) are forty-one years and above. On the whole, out of ninety staff members maximum belong to 'Twenty one–Thirty' category.

Table 9.2: Age of Staff Members

Organization	*21 years to 30 years*	*31 years to 40 years*	*41 years and above*	*Total*
RHDC	14 (46.7%)	13 (43.3%)	3 (10%)	30 (100%)
CINI-Moyna RHDC	2 (6.7%)	8 (26.7%)	20 (66.6%)	30 (100%)
SHIS	16 (53.4%)	9 (30%)	5 (16.6%)	30 (100%)
Total	**32 (35.6%)**	**30 (33.3%)**	**28 (31.1%)**	**90 (100%)**

(c) Marital Status

Table 9.3: Marital Status

Organization	*Unmarried*	*Married*	*Widow*	*Total*
RHDC	8 (26.7%)	22 (73.3%)	0 (0.0%)	30 (100.0%)
CINI-Moyna RHDC	3 (10.0%)	26 (86.7%)	1 (3.3%)	30 (100.0%)
SHIS	12 (40.0%)	18 (60.0%)	0 (0.0%)	30 (100.0%)
Total	**23 (25.6%)**	**66 (73.3%)**	**1 (1.1%)**	**90 (100.0%)**

As per Table 9.3, in all the NGOs, most of the staff members are married. Percentage of unmarried workers is very less. Only one widow is found in CINI-Moyna RHDC.

(d) Levels of Staff

It is evident from the Table 9.4 that, in each NGO between forty to fifty per cent staff are lower level workers, between thirty-three to forty per cent are middle level staff and sixteen to twenty per cent are higher-level staff. In the methodology chapter, concepts of lower level staff, middle level staff and higher-level staff have been defined.

Table 9.4: Level of Staff

Organization	*Lower Level Staff*	*Middle Level Staff*	*Higher Level Staff*	*Total*
RHDC	13 (43.3%)	12 (40%)	5 (16.7%)	30 (100.0%)
CINI-Moyna RHDC	12 (40.0%)	12 (40.0%)	6 (20.0%)	30 (100.0%)
SHIS	15 (50.0%)	10 (33.3%)	5 (16.7%)	30 (100.0%)
Total	**40 (44.4%)**	**34 (37.8%)**	**16 (17.8%)**	**90 (100.0%)**

(e) Qualification of Staff Members

Table 9.5: Qualification of Staff Members

Organization	*V to VII*	*VIII to X*	*XI to XII*	*Bachelor Degree*	*Master Degree*	*Total*
RHDC	Nil	17 (56.7%)	3 (10.0%)	7 (23.3%)	3 (10.0%)	30 (100.0%)
CINI-Moyna RHDC	4 (13.3%)	12 (40.0%)	5 (16.7%)	7 (23.3%)	2 (6.7%)	30 (100.0%)
SHIS	Nil	6 (20.0%)	5 (16.7%)	18 (60.0%)	1 (3.3%)	30 (100.0%)
Total	**4 (4.4%)**	**35 (38.9%)**	**13 (14.4%)**	**32 (35.6%)**	**6 (6.7%)**	**90 (100.0%)**

Table 9.5 indicates, in RHDC and CINI-Moyna RHDC, more than half of the staff members have less educational qualifications i.e. between Class–V to Class–X. In SHIS, staff members are more qualified. Sixty per cent of the total numbers of staff have Bachelor Degree and more than three per cent possess Master Degree.

(f) Salary

Table 9.6: Salary of Staff Members

Organization	*Upto Rs.1000*	*Rs.1001 to Rs. 2500*	*Rs. 2501 to Rs. 4000*	*Above Rs. 4000*	*Reluctant to Disclose*	*Total*
RHDC	3 (10.0%)	20 (66.6%)	5 (16.7%)	Nil	2 (6.7%)	30 (100.0%)
CINI-Moyna RHDC	10 (33.3%)	5 (16.7%)	7 (23.3%)	8 (26.7%)	Nil	30 (100.0%)
SHIS	Nil	17 (56.7%)	6 (20.0%)	4 (13.3%)	3 (10.0%)	30 (100.0%)
Total	**13 (14.4%)**	**42 (46.7%)**	**18 (20.0%)**	**12 (13.3%)**	**5 (5.6%)**	**90 (100.0%)**

It is understood from the Table 9.6, respectively in RHDC and SHIS, 76.6 per cent and 56.7 per cent staff members get salary upto Rs. 2,500 per month. It is very less according to the cost of living. Only in CINI-Moyna RHDC, fifty per cent of the workers get salary above Rs. 2,500 per month. It has also been noticed that respectively 6.7 per cent and 10 per cent workers in RHDC and SHIS were reluctant to disclose their monthly remuneration.

JOB SATISFACTION OF THE WORKERS

(a) Variable 1: Facilities at the Job

Table 9.7 points out the worker's satisfaction pertaining to facilities available at the job (variable 1). In RHDC, respectively 3.3 per cent, 43.3 per cent and 53.3 per cent workers have very low, low and moderate satisfaction.

Table 9.7: Variable 1

Satisfaction / *Organization*	*Very Low*	*Low*	*Moderate*	*High*	*Total*
RHDC	1 (3.3%)	13 (43.3%)	16 (53.3%)	–	30 (100%)
CINI-Moyna RHDC	–	7 (23.3%)	23 (76.7%)	–	30 (100%)
SHIS	–	8 (26.7%)	21 (70.0%)	1 (3.3%)	30 (100%)
Total	**1** **(1.11%)**	**28** **(31.12%)**	**60** **(66.66%)**	**1** **(1.11%)**	**90** **(100%)**

None of the persons has high satisfaction. In CINI-Moyna RHDC, respectively 23.3 per cent and 76.7 per cent workers have low and moderate satisfaction. With regard to SHIS, none has very low satisfaction. Respectively 26.7 per cent, 70 per cent and 3.3 per cent have low, moderate and high satisfaction. It can be generalized that majority of the workers of each NGO are moderately satisfied for the facilities available at the job.

(b) Variable 2: Relationship with the Boss

Table 9.8 gives the detail for satisfaction related to 'Relationship with the boss.' Including all the NGOs, on average, 64.44 per cent of the workers are moderately satisfied and 31.12 per cent are highly satisfied. Very few staff (i.e. 4.44%) have low satisfaction.

Table 9.8: Variable 2

Organization \ *Satisfaction*	*Very Low*	*Low*	*Moderate*	*High*	*Total*
RHDC	–	1 (3.3%)	22 (73.3%)	7 (23.3%)	30 (100%)
CINI-Moyna RHDC	–	1 (3.3%)	21 (70.0%)	8 (26.7%)	30 (100%)
SHIS	–	2 (6.7%)	15 (50.0%)	13 (43.3%)	30 (100%)
Total	–	**4** **(4.44%)**	**58** **(64.44%)**	**28** **(31.12%)**	**90** **(100%)**

(c) Variable 3: Physical Condition of Working Place

From Table 9.9, we come across the degree of worker's satisfaction regarding 'Physical condition of working place.' On average, fifty per cent of the total staff are moderately satisfied and forty per cent are highly satisfied. It is evident that physical atmosphere, in each NGO, is better and tolerable as well as adjustable for the workers.

Table 9.9: Variable 3

Organization \ *Satisfaction*	*Very Low*	*Low*	*Moderate*	*High*	*Total*
RHDC	–	3 (10.0%)	16 (53.3%)	11 (36.7%)	30 (100%)
CINI-Moyna RHDC	–	3 (10.0%)	15 (50.0%)	12 (40.0%)	30 (100%)
SHIS	1 3.3%	2 (6.7%)	14 (46.7%)	13 (43.3%)	30 (100%)
Total	**1** **1.11%**	**8** **(8.89%)**	**45** **(50%)**	**36** **(40%)**	**90** **(100%)**

(d) Variable 4: Career and Self-improvement Scheme

Table 9.10 gives an account for satisfaction related to 'Career and self improvement scheme.' Including all the NGOs, on average, 65.6 per cent of the total staff have moderate satisfaction and almost one-fourth are highly satisfied. Only a few staff have low satisfaction.

Table 9.10: Variable 4

Satisfaction / *Organization*	*Very Low*	*Low*	*Moderate*	*High*	*Total*
RHDC	–	1 (3.3%)	24 (80.0%)	5 (16.7%)	30 (100%)
CINI-Moyna RHDC	–	2 (6.7%)	20 (66.7%)	8 (26.7%)	30 (100%)
SHIS	–	6 (20%)	15 (50%)	9 (30%)	30 (100%)
Total	–	**9 (10%)**	**59 (65.6%)**	**22 (24.4%)**	**90 (100%)**

(e) Variable 5: Job Security

Table 9.11: Variable 5

Satisfaction / *Organization*	*Very Low*	*Low*	*Moderate*	*High*	*Total*
RHDC	–	7 (23.3%)	23 (76.7%)	–	30 (100%)
CINI-Moyna RHDC	2 6.7%	9 (30%)	14 (46.7%)	5 (16.7%)	30 (100%)
SHIS	1 3.3%	9 (30%)	16 (53.3%)	4 (13.3%)	30 (100%)
Total	**3 3.33%**	**25 (27.78%)**	**53 (58.89%)**	**9 (10%)**	**90 (100%)**

Worker's satisfaction for 'Job security' is understood from the Table 9.11. This variable gives a different result as compared to other variables. It is found that 3.33 per cent and 27.78 per cent of the total workers respectively have very low and low satisfaction. Among the others, 58.89 per cent and 10 per cent staff have moderate satisfaction and high satisfaction.

(f) Overall Satisfaction

Having considered all the five variables, each worker's overall satisfaction has been assessed here. It is evident from the Table 9.12 that respectively 13.3 per cent and 86.7 per cent workers have low as well as moderate satisfaction in RHDC. In CINI-Moyna RHDC, 3.3 per cent, 90 per cent and 6.7 per cent workers respectively have low, moderate and high satisfaction. In SHIS respectively 10 per cent, 76.7 per cent and 13.3 per cent of the staff are lowly, moderately and highly satisfied. Including all the NGOs, it can be generalized that majority of the staff (84.44%) are moderately satisfied and a few are having low (8.89%) as well as high (6.67%) satisfaction.

Table 9.12: Overall Satisfaction

Satisfaction / *Organization*	*Very Low*	*Low*	*Moderate*	*High*	*Total*
RHDC	–	4 (13.3%)	26 (86.7%)	–	30 (100%)
CINI-Moyna RHDC	–	1 (3.3%)	27 (90%)	2 (6.7%)	30 (100%)
SHIS	–	3 (10%)	23 (76.7%)	4 (13.3%)	30 (100%)
Total		**8 (8.89%)**	**76 (84.44%)**	**6 (6.67%)**	**90 (100%)**

ASSOCIATION BETWEEN NATURE OF STAFF AND LEVELS OF SATISFACTION

'Nature' refers to essence, character, composition, sort, tendency, affections, etc. In the present context, 'Nature' indicates six characteristics of the staff, such as, sex (male and female), age (21 to 30 years, 31 years to 40 years, 41 years and above) marital status (unmarried, married and widow), levels of staff (lower level, middle level and higher level), Qualification (V to VII, VIII to X, XI to XII, Bachelor degree, Master degree) and salary (upto Rs. 1,000, Rs. 1,001 to Rs. 2,500, Rs. 2,501 to Rs. 4,000, Above Rs. 4,000) to understand them well. In the following discussion, efforts are being made to know whether any significant association exists between these characteristics and levels of satisfaction.

(a) Association between Sex and Satisfaction (Total Sample = 90)

In Table 9.13, the obtained chi-square (χ^2) value for all the workers of three NGOs under the study reveals that there is no significant association between sex of the workers and their levels of satisfaction.

Table 9.13: Association between Sex and Level of Satisfaction of Workers

Satisfaction / *Sex*	*Low*	*Moderate*	*High*	*Total*
Male	7	41	6	54
Female	1	35	–	36
Total	**8**	**76**	**6**	**90**

$\chi^2 = 5.28$, df = 2, P lies between .05 and .10.

(b) Association between Age and Satisfaction

Table 9.14: Association between Age and Satisfaction of Workers

(Total Sample = 90)

Satisfaction / *Age*	*Low*	*Moderate*	*High*	*Total*
21 to 30 years	4	25	3	32
31 to 40 years	1	29	–	30
41 years & above	3	22	3	28
Total	**8**	**76**	**6**	**90**

$\chi^2 = 3.5$, df = 4, P lies between .30 and .50

The chi-square value (3.5) calculated from the Table 9.14 reveals that no significant association exists between worker's age groups and levels of satisfaction.

(c) Association between Marital Status and Satisfaction

Table 9.15: Association between Marital Status and Satisfaction of Workers

(Total Sample = 90)

Satisfaction / *Marital Status*	*Low*	*Moderate*	*High*	*Total*
Unmarried	1	20	2	23
Married	7	55	4	66
Widow	–	1	–	1
Total	**8**	**76**	**6**	**90**

$\chi^2 = .97$, df = 4, P lies between .90 and .95

The calculated chi-square value (.97) indicates that association between marital status of the workers and their levels of satisfaction is not significant at any level of confidence.

(d) Association between Levels of Staff and Satisfaction

Table 9.16: Association between Levels of Staff and Satisfaction

(Total Sample = 90)

Levels of Staff \ *Satisfaction*	*Low*	*Moderate*	*High*	*Total*
Low	4	35	1	40
Middle	–	30	4	34
High	4	11	1	16
Total	**8**	**76**	**6**	**90**

$\chi^2 = 7.64$, df = 4, P lies between .10 and .20

Tabulated value of χ^2 for 4 df at 5 per cent level of confidence is 11.070. Since the calculated value (7.64) is less than the tabulated value, there is no significant association between levels of staff and their satisfaction.

(e) Association between Qualification and Satisfaction

Table 9.17: Association between Qualification and Satisfaction

(Total Sample = 90)

Qualification \ *Satisfaction*	*Low*	*Moderate*	*High*	*Total*
V–VII	—	4	—	4
VIII–X	3	32	—	35
XI–XII	1	12	—	13
Bachelor degree	3	23	6	32
Master degree	1	5	—	6
Total	**8**	**76**	**6**	**90**

$\chi^2 = 8.54$, df = 8, P lies between .30 and .50

Since the calculated value of χ^2 (8.54) is less than the tabulated value (15.507) for 8 df at 5 per cent level of confidence, no significant association exists between qualification and satisfaction of the workers.

(f) Association between Salary and Satisfaction

Table 9.18: Association between Salary and Satisfaction

(Total Sample = 90)

Salary (Rs.) \ *Satisfaction*	*Low*	*Moderate*	*High*	*Total*
Upto 1000	—	13	—	13
1001–2500	2	39	1	42
2501–4000	2	14	2	18
Above 4000	2	9	1	12
Reluctant to disclose	2	1	2	5
Total	**8**	**76**	**6**	**90**

$\chi^2 = 20.8$, df = 8, P lies above 0.01

The obtained chi-square value (20.8) for all the workers of three NGOs under the study reveals that association exists between salary as well as job satisfaction of the staff and this association is significant at 0.01 level of confidence. It is evident, if salary structure fluctuates, levels of satisfaction will fluctuate.

In brief, the present Chapter highlights, including all the three NGOs, 60 per cent staff are male and 40 per cent are female; 68.9 per cent have age between 21 years to 40 years; 73.3 per cent are married; 44.4 per cent are lower level staff; 57.7 per cent have educational qualification upto XII and 61.1 per cent get salary upto Rs. 2,500 (per month). The Chapter also shows that 8.89 per cent, 84.44 per cent and 6.67 per cent of the total staff members (90) respectively have *low* satisfaction, *moderate* satisfaction and *high* satisfaction. None has *very low* satisfaction. It is also found here that there is no significant association between sex and job satisfaction, age and job satisfaction, marital status and job satisfaction, level of staff and job satisfaction, qualification and job satisfaction, etc. But significant association exists between salary and levels of job satisfaction. It reveals that level of satisfaction of staff in NGOs under the study can be improved by increasing salary.

10

Perception of the Beneficiaries

Perception, at this juncture, refers to the way of seeing or understanding of beneficiaries towards the working of NGO. Since organizations under the study are health care of NGOs and their main thirst is improving the health status, beneficiaries perception pertaining to health care is our centre of attention. In this regard, four groups of beneficiaries, forming two groups from each village (one male and one female group), under each NGO have been considered. The Methodology chapter has given the details of group formation. Profile of these groups under the study has been given in Table 10.1.

In order to understand the perception, data collected from each group are being discussed below separately covering six dimensions such as: (a) health care institutions of the locality and their nature of services; (b) necessity of the NGO's health care programmes; (c) cost & quality of the NGO's health care services; (d) NGO's health care services at difficult situation; (e) staff co-operation; and (f) scope of beneficiary's participation. A brief conclusion regarding perception has been drawn at the end of discussion under each group.

RURAL HEALTH DEVELOPMENT CENTRE (RHDC)

Group 1

It was formed at nearby village named Hatnadangi with twelve male beneficiaries belonging to the scheduled caste community. Group members highlighted the various types of health care institutions, which could be utilized by the villagers. Institutions were clinics of untrained doctors of the village, RHDC's clinic (1-5 kilometres away), Sub-Centre (2 kilometres away) and Primary Health Centre (6 kilometres

Table 10.1: Profile of the Groups

Name of the NGO	*Nature of Village*	*Name of the Village*	*No. of Members of Male Group*	*No. of Members of Female Group*	*Nature of Community to which Beneficiaries belong*
Rural Health Development Centre	Nearby village	Hatnadangi	12	16	SC & very poor Muslims
	Distant village	Musan	13	13	SC & ST
CINI-Moyna Rural Health Development Centre	Nearby village	Laluagadia	10	12	SC
	Distant village	Narikeldaha	20	28	SC
Southern Health Improvement Samity	Nearby village	Ganthunirite	10	10	SC & very poor Muslims
	Distant village	West Sripatinagar	16	10	SC

away). Quack doctors would provide primary treatment having visited home. If beneficiaries would not have capacity to pay, quack doctors tried to avoid them. In RHDC, 24 hours homeopathic treatment for common illness and vehicle service for emergency patients (for going to nursing home or district hospital) were available. Sub-centre would open only one day in a week to provide services like immunization for the children, iron tablets for the mothers, contraceptive facilities, etc. PHC provided regular treatment. Beneficiaries would visit it very frequently for common fever, diarrhoea, child delivery and serious accidents. Due to heavy pressure of the patients (i.e. more number), doctor would not treat carefully. Despite of this situation, beneficiaries felt that services of PHC was better than nothing. When beneficiaries become sick, at first they went to quack doctor. If problem increased, beneficiaries respectively preferred to go to RHDC, PHC, district hospital or nursing home, etc. In fact, different kinds of health care institutes provided different sorts of services.

Beneficiaries expressed that RHDC would work in their locality with sincere effort for improvement of health and education, flood relief, etc. With regard to health, it had daily outdoor clinic for homoeopathic treatment and community outreach programme. In outreach programme, mobile clinic would be run weekly and health worker used to visit home to increase awareness and to inculcate healthy habit. Regarding education, it started and maintained balwadi as well as primary school, made special arrangement for coaching class, provided school supplies (i.e. book, note book, pen, pencil, school uniform, etc.). During floods, RHDC distributed food, medicine, halogen tablets, polythene paper, cloth, etc. Beneficiaries also indicated that RHDC extended facility for house construction, latrine construction, tube well sinking, road repairing and so on. During group discussion, three of the twelve members clearly pointed out that they treated RHDC's staff like God. Without the support of RHDC, they would not survive. One beneficiary said, "We cannot see the Government where it locates and where it operates; RHDC is our Government." The members, all of a sudden, pronounced that all-round intervention of RHDC contributed in improving health status and hence this organization was essential to them.

For health care, medicines are provided by RHDC at a nominal cost. Old and new patients collect medicines from the clinic by paying respectively one rupee and two rupees. Beneficiaries are very happy with these fees. Regarding quality of medicines, there are different opinions. Few members say, seventy-five per cent of a particular disease can be cured by taking RHDC's medicine. Many are of the opinion that this homoeopathic treatment is not suitable for all problems. It takes time to cure diseases and gives better results in case of chronic disorders. For serious problems like diarrhoea, child delivery, accidents and so on, they go to PHC; RHDC cannot help. Beneficiaries articulate that RHDC should have the facility of modern medicine.

Beneficiaries are proud of RHDC's intervention in difficult situation. Having remembered the past stories, they say that flood situations have occurred seven times after 1987. Every time, RHDC has participated in rescue operation by using a small boat. It has helped to take flood victims, their animals and various resources at the safety place. Apart from flood, beneficiaries also point out various crisis incidents. When somebody commits suicide using poison or becomes the victim of snakebite, RHDC provides primary treatment immediately and sends the patient by their vehicle to district hospital.

Beneficiaries are of the opinion that doctors, health workers and other staff members are very co-operative. Doctors listen to the patients carefully and advice meticulously. Health workers visit community regularly, talk to the people irrespective of caste as well as religion and suggest possible way out for domestic problems.

With regard to scope of participation in RHDC's activities, beneficiaries have positive view. In case of road repairing, they contribute labour, during balwadi construction, they donate land and provide materials; when evaluation team comes from the funding agency, beneficiaries sit with them to discuss on various grievances, etc. Beneficiaries also participate in selecting special coaching teacher, balwadi teacher, etc. When Gram Committee (comprised of beneficiaries) selects these teachers, everybody accepts it. But, in health care programme, beneficiaries cannot participate in selecting health staff.

In a nutshell, beneficiaries have a better perception towards the multi-dimensional activities of RHDC. Its health care programme is not very satisfactory, but of course helpful. Beneficiaries expect the facilities of modern medicines at RHDC. Local people express that RHDC's intervention is required more because of educational, flood relief and community development activities than its health care programme.

Group 2

This is a female group comprised of sixteen members. Most of the members belong to scheduled caste family and very few are poor as well as minority Muslim of nearby village named Hatnadange. Like the members of male group, members of this group have also expressed the same name of health care institutions (which could be utilized by the villagers) i.e. clinics of quack doctors, Sub-Centre, RHDC, Primary Health Centre and their nature of services.

Women members acknowledge the services of RHDC. They say, RHDC runs Disaster Preparedness Programme (for preparation of the flood, flood relief and post-flood rehabilitation), Child Sponsorship Programme (for physical, social, educational and moral development of the child), Mahila Samity (for Self-Help Group formation; family planning, better child care, health and hygiene; etc), Low Cost Cultivation Programme (providing tractor facility for land preparation in nominal charge), Short Story Home (for destitute women), Homoeopathic Treatment Centre (static and mobile—especially for mother and child) and so on. Categorically beneficiaries mention that 'Child Sponsorship Programme' is very much profitable for them. Under this programme, they may get various domestic goods (e.g. cooking utensils, winter garments for family members, etc.), facilities for latrine construction as well as house construction, community resources (like Balwadi centre, Road, etc) and the like in free of cost. Beneficiaries have confessed that they require RHDC more for its 'Child Sponsorship Programme' and 'Disaster Preparedness Programme'. When researcher asked the necessity of health care programme of RHDC, beneficiaries did not deny its importance. According to them, RHDC has been working for last eighteen years. As a result of working for long period, now awareness is more among the mothers regarding pre-natal and post-natal care, safe drinking water is available (since provided three tube wells), fifty per cent of the total population have stopped open field defecation and thus child mortality rate has come down to zero. Beneficiaries recognized the necessity of health programme and at the same time other community development programmes (e.g. tube well sinking, low cost latrine construction, etc) in improving health status.

According to beneficiaries, RHDC provides medicines free of cost. Only one rupee and two rupees respectively for regular patients and new patients are taken as registration fees. This is done to reduce the wastage of medicines and to raise some funds for better functioning of the clinic. Beneficiaries have different types of opinions regarding quality of this service. Few beneficiaries say, medicines work very slowly and we need to go to 'Doctor' three or four times to cure a particular problem. There are three doctors who attend the clinic on rotation. Few beneficiaries are very much choosy regarding doctors. When Dr. Biswanath Roy attends clinic, beneficiaries go for treatment. According to them, quality of the service has a close nexus with the quality of the doctor. Having criticized some of the beneficiaries say, question of quality of service does not arise when the most vulnerable section of the society does not get benefit. For instance, they cite that RHDC does not have any service for pregnant mothers (in case of any complication) and child delivery.

With regard to intervention of RHDC at difficult situation, this group has given the same reply like male group of Hatnadangi. They say, RHDC becomes friend during flood, serious accidents (like snakebite, suicide case, fracture of bones, etc.) and so on.

Again, regarding co-operation of the staff and scope of participation of the beneficiaries, members of this group have answered the same like male group members of Hatnadangi village.

In brief, beneficiaries have better perception towards the overall working of RHDC. This perception has been developed mainly because of 'Child Sponsorship Programme' and 'Disaster Preparedness Programme' under which free materialistic services are available. In respect of health care, beneficiaries confess the role of RHDC in improving health status since there is a positive outcome of eighteen years working. But they are not happy with the present health care services for absence of facilities of modern medicines.

Group 3

This is a male group under the distant village named 'Musan.' It is formed by taking thirteen members who belong to Scheduled Caste and Scheduled Tribe families. As per the information provided by these group members, there are four types of health care institutions which villagers use for day-to-day problems. These are clinics of quack doctors, clinic of RHDC, Sub-Centre and Primary Health Centre (PHC). Quack doctors (total four) are available at the village and they practice allopathic medicines. They have learnt it by studying books and working as compounder under a good doctor with a purpose of earning money. According to beneficiaries, these doctors charge more, inject unnecessary injections and provide lower quality medicines. Sub-centre is located four kilometres away from this village. It has been working for last eight years, but beneficiaries have come to know only two years before. It opens once in a week to provide immunization facility to pregnant mothers and children, family planning contraceptives, halogen tablets, etc. PHC is seven kilometres far from this village. These doctors work there on rotation and have twenty-four hours treatment facility free of cost. Villagers visit it very frequently for diarrhoea, child delivery, tubectomy operation, injuries and minor surgery. For common illnesses like fever, cough and cold, etc. beneficiaries prefer to go to RHDC which is two kilometres away. Beneficiaries also take their chronic problems to RHDC. RHDC runs homoeopathic programme by the help of daily outdoor clinic and weekly mobile clinic. According to beneficiaries, if somebody becomes sick, he/she first visits quack doctor. Quack doctor is easily available and accessible to them. If condition deteriorates, family members take him to district hospital or nursing home. In this regard RHDC does not play any role except vehicle provider.

As like as the female group of Hatnadangi, this group replies that RHDC runs Disaster Preparedness Programme, Child Sponsorship Programme, Low Cost Cultivation Programme, Short Stay Home and Homoeopathic Treatment Centre. Regarding health, beneficiaries are of the opinion that RHDC carries out four types of health care activities throughout the whole year. For instance, (a) yearly health check up camp is arranged for sponsored children with the help of outside doctors, (b) mobile clinic is run on every Monday and Thursday during 8 a.m. to 12.30 p.m. to provide homoeopathic treatment facility, (c) health workers survey the village yearly as well as organize awareness camp monthly, and (d) an outdoor (homoeopathic) clinic is run regularly in the permanent campus. Beneficiaries say, as a result of RHDC's intervention, their children have learnt how to speak, how to maintain personal hygiene, how to keep the environment clean, need to go to doctor, need to take medicine, need to go to school, etc. If RHDC stops working, social and educational growth of these children will be stopped. Again, beneficiaries are unhappy with the Government. Government does not extend any help during crisis. For instance, in order to get a polythene paper during flood, beneficiaries need to be involved with the politics. They say, during crisis as well as happiness, RHDC is always with them. Thus, beneficiaries require RHDC not only for health care but also for all-round growth of the future generation.

Beneficiaries express that RHDC provides medicines free of cost. It takes only registration fees respectively rupee one and rupee two for old patients and new patients (to minimize the wastage of medicines). During annual health check-up camp, those medicines RHDC cannot provide, they prescribe to buy it from outside. Regarding quality of these medicines, members do not have any comments. They say, "We do not go to RHDC, only our female counterparts go there for very common illnesses. In case of serious problems, we take our family members to PHC or district hospital." In fact, villagers overlook the services of RHDC, since it cannot give any support during serious problems.

Again, beneficiaries concede that RHDC intervenes with health facilities at the time of community crisis and family crisis. For instance, medical care during flood and after flood, primary treatment to the person who wanted to commit suicide at mid-night and referring the patient to a better hospital by own vehicle, providing treatment for snakebite, etc.

Staff members of RHDC are always co-operative with the beneficiaries in case of health care. There is no doubt in it. For instance, 'Doctors' attentively listen to the patients and advise in local language. When some patient comes to RHDC at late night, doctor does not delay to provide treatment. Health workers regularly visit community, organize camps and force the villagers to come to the outdoor clinic who suffer from various chronic diseases.

Beneficiaries say, they have no role in implementing health care programme. Though they have capacity to select balwadi teacher and special coaching teacher, they have no right to identify health worker for their own village. But, there is scope of participation in community infrastructure development. For instance, they contribute labour, land, subscription, etc. for the construction of village road, balwadi centre, culvert and so on.

At the end, we understand that beneficiaries have better perception towards the working of RHDC. Success of various programmes completed previously and existing at present have contributed to make this perception. Regarding health care, beneficiaries vent negative perception. Normally they need to go to doctor during injuries, diarrhoeal diseases, complications related to child delivery and some other serious problems. RHDC is not appropriate to handle these problems and very slow to control diseases for its homoeopathic approach. Therefore, beneficiaries overlook the services of RHDC.

Group 4

This group is comprised of thirteen female members belonging to SC/ST families of the distant village named Musan. As like as the male group of this village, members of the present group have said in reply the same names of health care institutions and their nature of services those are used by the villagers as and when necessary. These members responded a bit differently than the members of male group when researcher wanted to know where they would go during illness. Members answered back that they would approach at first to RHDC. Because RHDC was having qualified doctors and could refer the serious patients in an appropriate place unlike quack doctors because of good connection with other peripheral health care institutions.

According to beneficiaries, RHDC works in their locality in order to provide health care facility and to upgrade the condition of women as well as children. Regarding health care, it serves through homoeopathic clinics (daily outdoor clinic and weekly mobile clinic). Various health problems like cough and cold, headache, watering of eyes, ear problem, body ache and many chronic diseases are treated carefully. Beneficiaries express that RHDC runs balwadi centre to facilitate supplementary nutrition and pre-school education for children. Under Child Sponsorship Programme, it provides books, note books, school uniforms, hygiene kits (soap, brush, tooth paste, etc), cooking utensils, winter garments, etc. in free of cost. RHDC runs one 'Mahila Mandal' comprising twelve members at Musan village. It has multi-dimensional activities including family planning propagation, motivation and capacity building for income generation, preparing the people to face natural disaster, etc. This organization also becomes active during flood to extend relief. It has been observed that most of the beneficiaries are not aware of many of the programmes those are not implemented in this village. For instance, low cost cultivation facility, Short Stay Home, etc. Having highlighted the above programmes, a few of the group members say, they require RHDC for various facilities free of cost; few say that RHDC is visible as active agent of rural development during flood; almost half of the beneficiaries point out that RHDC has made very less efforts during last eighteen years in their village as compared to other localities. In fact, female beneficiaries of this village have some discontent and at the same time RHDC has negligence to deliver service due to remoteness of this area.

With regard to cost of medicines and other facilities, members of the present group replied the same like male group of this village. Regarding quality of services, beneficiaries did not raise any voice or objection. They added that it was essential to visit clinic three to four times to remove a particular health problem.

Beneficiaries say, RHDC's contribution at difficult situation is no doubt noteworthy. During flood, RHDC comes to the village by boat and distribute relief (rice, dal, medicines, polythene, halogen tablets, etc.). When floodwater goes down, it sprinkles bleaching powder or DDT to control epidemic. In case of epidemic, RHDC sends medical team to the village. Apart from that, if serious health problems or accidents occur at night time, RHDC provides first-aid and refers the patients immediately by its own vehicle to district hospital.

Regarding staff co-operation, members of the present group answered as like as male group of this village.

In view of scope of participation of the beneficiaries, members reply with satisfaction. They say, there is a 'Gram Committee' in Musan village. Being member of this committee, they participate in beneficiaries selection under Child Sponsorship Programme; take decision regarding school building repairing, road construction, culvert construction, etc; help in conducting survey; select special coaching teacher and balwadi teacher for the Musan village. They also participate for monitoring and evaluation of various programmes when external teams come from the funding agencies.

In fine, beneficiaries like RHDC for its various free services. They have a hidden anger against this organization since it serves more in other villages. It is clear that there is a contradiction between the perception of male group and the present group with regard to health care. This group is having positive perception. Members use RHDC as stepping-stone. For first aid, treatment of chronic diseases, authentic health advice and referral services, RHDC is important to them.

CINI-MOYNA—RURAL HEALTH DEVELOPMENT CENTRE (CINI-MOYNA—RHDC)

Group 1

This is a male group comprising ten members who belong to scheduled caste families under the village (nearby) named Laluagadia. Beneficiaries are of the opinion that there are five types of health care institutions, such as, quack doctor's clinic, qualified private practitioner's clinic, Sub-Centre (SC), Primary Health Centre (PHC) and CINI-Moyna RHDC which villagers use for day to day health problems. In Lalnagadia village, four quack doctors practice allopathic medicine. They have learnt it by means of health worker's training (six months). One qualified doctor (BHMS) practices homoeopathic medicine. Sub-centre is located two kilometres away from the village, which opens once in a week to provide immunization facility and contraceptive measures for family planning. PHC is situated six kilometres away where treatment is available for twenty-four hours. Patients suffering form diarrhoea, complications during pregnancy, fever for long time, etc. go to PHC. CINI-Moyna RHDC runs daily homoeopathic clinic. It operates during 9 a.m. to 4 p.m. Beneficiaries say, when they feel sick, at first they go to quack doctors for immediate treatment to get cured. Because, PHC is far, CINI-Moyna RHDC operates during office hours and qualified private practitioner is not available always. Since quack doctors use modern medicines including the facilities for stitching, saline, etc., everyone prefers to go to them at first. If people feel that quack doctors cannot control the situation, directly they go to PHC or district hospital. Beneficiaries confess that they get various types of health care services from various institutions and, therefore, all the institutions are useful to them.

According to beneficiaries, CINI-Moyna RHDC works in their locality through Child Sponsorship Programme, Reproductive and Child Health Programme, Community Development Programme and Daily Homoeopathic Clinic. Under Child Sponsorship Programme, selected children get various facilities for education, health, personal hygiene, domestic goods, winter garments, latrine construction, house construction and so on free of cost. RCH programme improves awareness among the mothers with regard to maternal and child health. Community Development Programme helps in constructing dam, repairing village road, developing balwadi centre, etc. In Daily

Homoeopathic Clinic, patients come to treat chronic problems, cough and cold, sudden fever, stomachache, body ache and so on. Beneficiaries express, having taken medicines from this clinic, sometimes diseases is cured, sometimes it is not. They are not happy with CINI-Moyna RHDC. According to them, now this organization is required for those who get benefit under child sponsorship programme. During last twenty-four years, it has helped to develop a dam for better cultivation, to sink tube well for safe drinking water and to construct latrine for better environmental health. Its previous contribution in health care is praiseworthy; but now RHDC is not much important to them.

All the children and their families who come under Child Sponsorship Programme get treatment at 'CINI-Moyna RHDC' free of cost. Non-sponsored children and their families take medicines from this clinic by paying rupees five per family per month. With regard to pathological examination, sponsored children are free but their family members require to pay half of the total cost. Non-sponsored children and their families do not get this facility (Pathological examination). Regarding quality of the medicine, beneficiaries are not very happy. According to them, it works very slowly and sometimes does not cure disease. Beneficiaries are of the opinion that 'CINI-Moyna RHDC' should keep one good qualified allopathic doctor in its permanent campus for twenty-four hours; homoeopathic doctor is not suitable always for their locality.

Beneficiaries say, 'CINI-Moyna RHDC' does not work in difficult situation always. During crisis, it responds rarely. For instance, few years before this village was affected by Cholera epidemic. Since the locality was low lying and flood affected area, cholera epidemic occurred during rainy season. Because of homoeopathic approach, it could not intervene in the situation. Again, after office hours (i.e. 9 a.m. to 4 p.m.) if some patient comes, no treatment is provided since doctor does not stay inside the campus. Off and on, when flood occurs in and around the locality 'CINI-Moyna RHDC' extends facilities by providing relief.

As far as cooperation of the staff members are concerned, no doubt it is appreciating. Medicines of this organization may fail, but doctor listens to the patients carefully and refer to the good doctors in case of emergency. Other staff members who work as health workers maintain good relation with the people and provide authentic suggestions for better health. In spite of this satisfactory cooperation, beneficiaries did not hesitate to point out the political biasness of the organization.

As per their feeling, Chief of 'CINI-Moyna RHDC' is an active supporter of CPI (M) and prefer to extend facilities to the people who belong to CPI(M) party.

In respect of scope of participation of the beneficiaries, members of the group have expressed positive view. They have opportunity to help in organizing annual sports, in constructing road (by donating land, contributing labour, removing trees from the boundary of own house, etc.), in selecting teachers for special coaching class and balwadi centre under 'Child Sponsorship Programme'. Regarding health care, they help in conducting awareness camp under RCH Programme.

On the whole, beneficiaries acknowledge the contribution of 'CINI-Moyna RHDC' for flood relief, health care, community development work and so on in its early days. Now they have negative perception towards the working of this organization due to political biasness. In health care, negative perception has been developed as a result of homoeopathic treatment facility which works very slowly, cannot be believable during emergency due to lack of life saving drugs and is not available before or after office hours. Beneficiaries demand that one MBBS doctor should be available for twenty-four hours in the campus with the facilities of modern medicines.

Group 2

It is consisted of twelve female members who belong to Scheduled Caste families under the nearby village named Laluagadia. As like as male group of this village, members of the present group have expressed the same name of health care institutions and their nature of services, which they use. Members say, when illness occurs, they go to quack doctor at first. Because, quack doctor is available always and visits home if money is paid properly. If quack doctors cannot improve the situation, beneficiaries go to PHC or district hospital.

As per the beneficiaries view, CINI-Moyna RHDC has multi-dimensional activities in this village. It implements Child Sponsorship Programme, RCH programme, Income Generation Programme and runs Mahila Samity. For health care, Child Sponsorship Programme and RCH Programme can be cited. Under Child Sponsorship Programme, annual health check-up camp for the sponsored children is conducted by bringing various specialists from outside, one daily outdoor clinic (homoeopathic) is run (during 9 a.m. to 4 p.m.) and pathological examination facility is extended. During annual Camp, doctors prescribe medicines which are purchased from outside. Beneficiaries get reimbursement for outside medicines. In outdoor clinics, sponsored and their families get free treatment and others pay rupees five per month (per family). For pathological examination, sponsored children are free, their family members need to pay half of the total cost and others do not get this facility. Under RCH programme, organization gives awareness to the adolescents, pregnant mothers and lactating mothers for family planning, reproduction and childcare. Apart from that, this organization also conducts weekly gynaecological clinic where outside doctor comes and prescribes medicines to women. In this regard, members of the group say, 'We go for check-up, get prescription, but we cannot buy medicines. Such kind of clinic with no medicine facility in this remote area has no use.' Beneficiaries feel and express that all the medical care related facilities of CINI-Moyna RHDC are basically meant for sponsored children and their families. People in general may get treatment from the daily outdoor clinic, but medicines of this clinic work very slowly due to homoeopathic approach. Therefore, members are of the opinion that health care programmes of CINI-Moyna RHDC are not very important and necessary for the common masses of this village.

In the preceding paragraph and while discussing the male group of Laluagadia village, various costs of health services have clearly been mentioned. Regarding quality of the health services, members express positive view. According to them, health services which are received by sponsored children and their family members are qualitative. These children and their families have been managing health problems for last few years based on these services. They do not go outside the CINI-Moyna RHDC for treatment.

Members of this group acknowledge that CINI-Moyna RHDC intervenes at difficult situation in order to provide health care. For instance: (a) it came into existence to provide health services in this flood-affected area. Off and on, when flood situation occurs, this organization distributes relief and provides health care and consciousness; (b) Few years before, during cholera epidemic, this organization contributed to the maximum extent by propagating the preventive measures for the problems; (c) Two years before, when cyclone took place at Daton (within the Midnapore district), CINI-Moyna RHDC went to provide relief and health care.

According to the members, health care staff are very much co-operative. Doctors listen to the patients carefully and give appropriate advice. In spite of low remuneration, health workers do not neglect their duty. They visit this village regularly, organize awareness camps and maintain good relation with the villagers. Sometimes non-sponsored families suffer from serious problems, if they ask any help to this organization, staff members make arrangement to refer that patient to the appropriate hospital at Kolkata.

Group members say, there is ample opportunity for beneficiaries to participate during programme implementation. For instance, beneficiaries help to organize nutrition camp, adolescents awareness camp, etc; in selecting special coaching teacher, balwadi teacher, etc; to hold annual sports; in external monitoring and evaluation and so on. But, they have no role in providing medical care.

In conclusion, we can say, people in general have negative perception towards the health programmes of CINI-Moyna RHDC. Because, medical care provided in this organization is basically meant for sponsored children and their families. Beneficiaries say, those services are not adequately available for the common masses. Of course, health awareness is given to all categories of people of the village, but it is not very important to them. People want curative services free of cost for twenty-four hours, which are not available at CINI-Moyna RHDC.

Group 3

This group was formed at the distant village named Narikeldaha having taken twenty male members who belonged to Scheduled Caste families. Members expressed that there were four types of health care institutions such as clinics of quack doctors, CINI-Moyna RHDC, Sub-Centre and Primary Health Centre (PHC), which villagers would use. Two quack doctors were available in the village who used to visit patient's home on call. CINI-Moyna RHDC would run daily outdoor clinic (homoeopathic) as well as weekly gynaecological clinic in the main campus and weekly mobile clinic (homoeopathic) at the present village. Sub-Centre was two kilometres away from this village. It would be opened once in a week to provide immunization facility, family planning contraceptives, water disinfectants, etc. PHC was located five kilometres far from Narikeldaha village. It had twenty-four hours treatment scope with twenty bed facilities. Patients having eye problems, gynaecological diseases, injuries, complications related to child delivery would go there very frequently. According to members of the group, all the beds in PHC would be always full. Highlighting the above health care institutions and their nature of services beneficiaries said, during illness, they would go to quack doctors at first. It happened because of better accessibility and availability of the quack doctors. If those doctors were unable to control the situation, beneficiaries directly would go to PHC or district hospital or nearby nursing home. CINI-Moyna RHDC was least preference to the beneficiaries because of remoteness from this village and inefficiency in healing a disease quickly. Beneficiaries confessed that they would use weekly mobile clinic (homoeopathic) off and on when problems were not very serious.

Beneficiaries say, 'CINI-Moyna RHDC' works in their locality to implement Child Sponsorship Programme, Community Development Programme (construction of latrine, house, sluice-gate, small bridge on the canal, tube well sinking; repairing of school building, balwadi centre; etc), RCH Programme, Income Generation Programme (handloom weaving) and run Mahila Samity as well as weekly mobile clinic (homoeopathy). Regarding health, two workers come to this village from 'CINI-Moyna RHDC' on every week. They provide health awareness to the adolescents and mothers by using Mahila Samity members, identify difficult patients and refer them to CINI-Moyna RHDC or PHC or good hospitals as per the problems. Beneficiaries are the opinion that CINI-Moyna RHDC is required to improve community infrastructure, to reinforce children's education and to get better environmental health. This organization has very minor role in curative services or in responding emergency health problems (like diarrhoea, injuries, child delivery, etc).

Regarding cost of services, variation is found in different cases. Under Child Sponsorship Programme, those sponsored families get van (for income generation) or constructed toilet they pay ten to fifteen per cent of the total cost. For treatment under daily outdoor clinic, sponsored children and their families get free service and others pay rupees five per month (per family). In case of pathological examination, sponsored are free and their family members pay half of the total cost. With regard to quality of medicines, beneficiaries have no objection. Though they go hardly to CINI-Moyna RHDC's clinic, they acknowledge the utility and soundness of that clinic's medicine if taken with sincerity and patience.

The members of the present group have replied the same like members of male and female groups of Laluagadia village regarding CINI-Moyna RHDC's intervention for health care at difficult situation.

Members express that doctors, health workers and other staff are very much co-operative. Doctors listen to the patients carefully and provide appropriate advice. Health workers maintain good relation with the people and perform their needful job. During tubectomy operation, which is sponsored by Government of India and takes place at PHC, these health workers co-operate to the maximum extent (by linking the patient for operation, being with them during operation, during discharge from PHC, etc.).

In the context of scope of participation of beneficiaries, members of the present group answered as like as participants of female group of Laluagadia village. They also added that people had no role in beneficiaries selection and organization would use political connection for the same. Since head of the organization was supporter of CPI (M) party, he preferred to select those beneficiaries who were supporter of CPI(M).

In brief, we understand that members of this group have better perception towards the working of 'CINI-Moyna RHDC', but they do not forget to highlight its political biasness. They prefer this organization for improvement of health status by developing village infrastructure. It is also felt that beneficiaries have negative perception for curative services in controlling day-to-day emergency health problems (like diarrhoea, injuries, child delivery, etc.)

Group 4

It came into existence at Narikeldaha village (distant) with active involvement of twenty-eight female participators who were members of Scheduled Caste families. Regarding types of health care institutions and their nature of services which villagers regularly use, participators answered the same name of four institutions (i.e. clinics of quack doctors, CINI-Moyna RHDC, Sub-Centre and PHC) like members of the male group of this village. They added a new problem of the locality i.e. suicide of housewives. Every year three to four housewives commit suicide as a result of family tension and conflict. In the event of crisis i.e. when a person becomes sick for attempting suicide, she is immediately taken to PHC. Members of the group are of the opinion that they go to quack doctors at first when they feel sick. If situation goes out of control, they take the patients to PHC or district hospital directly. In case of very dangerous problems, which require serious attention of experienced and good doctors, straight away they go to Velore

(Chennai). Participators do not neglect any type of health care institutions mentioned above. According to them, various types of institutions are important for various kinds of care.

According to members of the present group, CINI-Moyna RHDC works at Narikeldaha village through Child Sponsorship Programme, Reproductive and Child Health Programme, Income Generation Programme, Mahila Samity and weekly mobile clinic. As a result of intervention of this organization, during last twenty-four years, lot of changes have taken place. For instance, awareness of diarrhoea management is increased, cleanliness and sanitation system have been improved, mothers are more conscious regarding where to go and what to do during pregnancy, etc. Apart from that, school building, balwadi centre, ICDS centre, child resource centre, connecting road inside the village, culvert and so on have been constructed. Members feel and express that health care is not the only purpose for which they require CINI-Moyna RHDC. They require this organization for the development of village infrastructure, income generation, children's education, women empowerment and so on. Beneficiaries acknowledge CINI-Moyna RHDC's contribution in all-round development.

Regarding cost as well as quality of medicines and CINI-Moyna RHDC's intervention for health care at difficult situation, members of the present group replied as like as male group formed in this village.

With regard to cooperation of staff members, beneficiaries have different views. Few say, doctors are good, provide appropriate treatment and sometimes visit home if called. Others say, they have not seen doctors since they do not go to CINI-Moyna RHDC's clinic. Everybody confesses that health workers are helpful and co-operative. In this context, beneficiaries have also added that staff members of Child Sponsorship Programme are very strict and particular regarding their work.

In various programmes of CINI-Moyna RHDC, scopes of participation of beneficiaries are adequate. For instance, in RCH programme, people help to hold awareness camp by deciding time and place, by providing physical infrastructure (tables, chairs, benches, etc.), by communicating the message among the masses and so on. In Child Sponsorship Programme, Village people have right to help in selecting special coaching teacher, balwadi teacher, etc. In case of construction work at the community level (road, culvert, school building, etc.), people involve actively for planning and implementation. Apart from that, people also help in external monitoring of various programmes (done by the team of funding agencies).

In a nutshell, participants of the present group have positive perception towards the working of CINI-Moyna RHDC. Though people of this village do not depend much upon the curative health services of this organization, they do not ignore or neglect the same. They do not want the CINI-Moyna RHDC in isolation only for health care, they feel the necessity of this agency for all-round development of the community.

SOUTHERN HEALTH IMPROVEMENT SAMITY (SHIS)

Group 1

This group was formed at the nearby village named Ganthunirite having taken ten male members who belonged to scheduled caste families. Members indicated five types of health care institutions such as Clinic of Private Doctors, Nursing Homes, Nalmuri Rural Hospital, SHIS and various Hospitals of Kolkata and their nature of services, which villagers would use as per the requirement. Ghatakpukur was two kilometres away from the present village under the study and developing a small township. At Ghatakpukur, there were twenty-eight private doctors who had own clinics and would practice different systems of medicines (i.e. allopathic, homoeopathic, ayurvedic, etc.). Almost half of the doctors had professional degree (i.e. MBBS, BHMS, BAMS, etc.) and others acquired diploma or certificate. These doctors would check up the patients on payment and prescribe medicines. There were also five nursing homes at Ghatakpukur. Villagers, who were having affordability to pay, would go to nursing home during health crisis. Nalmuri Rural Hospital was four kilometres away from this village where free treatment facility was available. People would go there to control diarrhoea, to have child delivery, to perform family planning operation, to save life of patient attempted suicide and so on. SHIS was locating five kilometres away from Ganthunirite village. Within its campus, there were TB Clinic and MCH clinic where treatments were free. This organization also had pathological centre where service was available in cheap rate. Apart from that, SHIS would run monthly mobile clinic in this village and would send two health workers there to conduct awareness camps. In case of very serious problems, when nearby health care institutions couldn't control the situation, villagers preferred to go to Kolkata's hospital. Kolkata was thirty kilometres far from this place. Members of the group said if they would feel sick, at first they preferred to go to Nalmuri Rural Hospital since treatment was free. Villagers would go to SHIS if they were referred by doctor of mobile clinic or health workers.

Members express, SHIS has been working in this village for last four years. Now they run monthly mobile clinic for general health care, conduct pre-natal and post-natal awareness camp, run income generation programme and have developed 'Self Help Group' for women empowerment. As a result of continuous work of SHIS in this village, health status and general awareness of the people have been improved. Though villagers confess this contribution, they are angry with SHIS. Because, three years before this organization provided hope for construction of primary school and continuation of the same. Within three kilometres there was no primary school. On the one hand, parents had no time to drop their ward at school and on the other, they did not have dare to leave the children alone due to accident on the highway. Consequently, rate of illiteracy was increasing. Apart from the school, SHIS also wanted to develop village road, wanted to provide constructed latrine to every family free of cost and so on. Beneficiaries got neither school nor latrine nor road. One day they met the Director of Organization in this regard. Since Director denied the previous assurances, male members of the village got angry with SHIS. Due to false hope, now villagers are non-co-operative in the activities of SHIS at Ganthunirite. Local people (male) say, "We do not require SHIS. If SHIS comes and works, we shall not co-operate until and unless at least one assurance will be fulfilled."

Regarding cost of treatment at SHIS, members have answered with satisfaction. SHIS takes rupees three per patient to prepare card in mobile clinic as well as in the main campus. In mobile clinic, most of the medicines are provided free of cost. In the main campus, under MCH clinic, doctors only prescribe medicines which need to buy from outside. For tuberculosis, entire treatment is provided free of cost. In case of pathological examination, rates are reasonable. For instance, X-ray = Rs. 40, blood test = Rs 15, Stool test = Rs. 12 and Urine test = Rs. 12. With regard to quality of treatment, beneficiaries are happy. All the tuberculosis patients who take medicines from SHIS, get well very soon. Medicines, which are distributed at monthly mobile clinic, are very qualitative since they are made in the herbal medicinal plant of SHIS. In fact, quality is maintained due to good and qualified doctors. SHIS is having total thirty doctors of various systems of medicines (allopathic, homoeopathic and ayurvedic).

Beneficiaries acknowledge that most of them are illiterate and innocent about the outside world. Regarding SHIS's intervention for health care at difficult situation, members said, they did not see whether this organization provided any treatment during crisis i.e. epidemic, flood, cyclone or other natural disaster.

Beneficiaries have both good as well as bad experiences reagarding staff co-operation. They say, SHIS's clinic in the main campus operates till 3 p.m. If any patient comes from too far place after 3 p.m., staff members do not reject him/her till the time doctor stay back in campus. Again, when some serious patient seeks treatment at SHIS who requires immediate intervention, if SHIS fails to control the problem due to lack of technological facilities and life saving drugs, this organization refer the patient with their own staff and vehicle at Kolkata hospital. Apart from that, beneficiaries indicate, staff members who register names, distribute medicines, work in pathological centre and perform other technical activities are very cooperative. Regarding bad experience, members are of the opinion that doctors check up the patients hurriedly without listening carefully.

According to the members of the group, there was very less scope for male folk to participate during implementation of various programmes of SHIS. Male members would help only in conducting monthly mobile clinic. Now, they do not participate in any kind of activities of SHIS since Director has deprived them after giving assurance of school building construction, road construction and so on.

In brief, we understand that people of Ganthunirite village have negative perception towards the working of SHIS. It has been developed as a result of false assurance of this organization. Though local people acknowledge the efforts of SHIS for good quality health service at free or cheap cost, good cooperation of staff members and so on, they do not forget their anger and bitterness.

Group 2

This is a female group comprised of ten members of Ganthunirite village (nearby). Members belong to Scheduled Caste and poor Muslim families. There are total of eight hundreds people in this village and average family size is seven. Most of the people of Ganthunirite are illiterate and ignorant. Many of them do not have own land to construct house. The villagers are too poor to concentrate on health. Regarding types of health care institutions and their nature of services, which villagers use for day-to-day problems, members of the present group answered as like as male group of this village. According to them, when they feel sick, at first they go to SHIS as they are women and get free treatment at MCH clinic. During diarrhoea, child delivery, eye problem, dental problem, etc. they go to Nalmuri Rural Hospital since free treatment is available. In case of emergency problems i.e. injuries, snakebite, attempt to suicide through poisoning and so on, people prefer to go to nearby nursing homes. Kolkata's hospitals are the last options for them.

Members of the group say, SHIS is involved with so many activities of Ganthunirite village. One, it runs income generation programme by engaging mothers in herbal medicinal plants cultivation. The present organization helps them in supplying seedlings and in marketing of the produced plants. Two, SHIS has developed three Self Help Groups (SHGs) comprising fifteen, eighteen and nineteen members respectively. Each member of the Self Help Group contributes ten rupees per month. Three, it sends two health workers to this village in order to conduct weekly awareness camps for pre-natal and post-natal care. It also runs monthly mobile clinic by sending a qualified ayurvedic doctor. Four, SHIS has helped in sinking two tube wells in this locality. Beneficiaries feel and express, as a result of continuous work of SHIS during last four years, now-a-days health awareness has increased. Mothers take advice from the doctors during pregnancy, follow immunization schedule appropriately for the children, pay attention for malnourished child and there is no death from diarrhoea and the like. Beneficiaries are of the opinion that they require SHIS for both health improvement and economic upgradation. The latter one is more important to them.

Regarding cost and quality of health service, members of the present group have answered as like as male group of this village. They are very satisfied.

According to members, there was no epidemic or natural disaster during last thirty years at Ganthunirite village or its adjacent area. Therefore, they did not know whether SHIS would work at difficult situation.

Beneficiaries have mixed opinion (good and bad) regarding staff cooperation. Few say, doctors are cooperative and ask the patients to visit clinic before diseases reach to a difficult stage. Others tell, doctors are non-co-operative and spend very little time during check-up. All the members acknowledge, doctors are good because they teach the villagers to use various herbal plants for common health problems. The remaining staff members, who work in the main campus of SHIS, are also very helpful. They guide the patients during clinic hours by instructing where to stand to meet doctors, where to go to collect medicines, where to ask for pathological examination and so on. Beneficiaries rightly point out that some of the staff are very irritating. They sought and say, "Have you come here for free treatment?" Beneficiaries also add that they are thankful to the emergency staff. When SHIS fails to provide treatment to a serious patient, they refer the same by their own vehicle and emergency staff at Kolkata's hospital. These emergency staff try their level best to find out appropriate treatment facility at Kolkata.

According to participators of the present group, in this village, female members have better scope than the male folk for participation in implementation of various programmes of SHIS. Female members help in conducting weekly health awareness camp, in forming SHGs and continuing the same, in running income generation programme and so on. During monitoring and evaluation by external group, female members also participate to express their advantages and disadvantages.

In a nutshell, beneficiaries have better perception towards the working of SHIS. They are happy for women empowerment activities (SHGs, income generation, etc.) as well as health care services. Women empowerment is their first preference but the latter one is the least important issue.

Group 3

This group was formed under the distant village named West Sripatinagar with the help of sixteen male members who belonged to Scheduled Caste families. Members expressed, there were three types of health care institutions (such as clinics of quack doctors, sub-centre and SHIS's weekly clinic), which villagers would use as per the requirement. Since the present village was a part of an island and located in the remotest part of Sundarban area, use of quack doctors was very natural. There were two quack doctors at West Sripatinagar who would provide treatment by visiting patient's home. Giving first-aid, attending minor operation and treating common illnesses on payment were their major tasks. Sub-Centre would open once in a week where two health assistants (one male and one female) would be available. They would distribute family planning contraceptives, delivery kits, and tablets for common fever as well as digestion problem, water disinfectant and would extend immunization facility. SHIS was having a health centre at West Sripatinagar through which they would run weekly clinic, bi-monthly special clinic and awareness camps. According to members, when villagers would feel sick, at first they would have consulted quack doctors. Then, they would meet SHIS's doctor during weekly clinic. In case of emergency, directly villagers would have gone to Diamond Harbour or Patharpratima Hospital, which was six hours' distance by mechanized boat. Beneficiaries said, all the three types of health care institutions mentioned above would provide different types of facilities and thus all were useful to them.

Regarding the programmes of SHIS run in the present village, members highlight only health activities. It has already been mentioned that SHIS runs weekly clinic, bi-monthly special clinic and awareness camps. For weekly clinic, a medical team including manager, doctor, nurse, compounder, pathologist and record keeper comes to this village by a mechanized launch. The launch is well equipped for pathological examination. In the weekly clinic, treatment is provided for general health problems with special emphasis on mother & child health and tuberculosis. In case of pathological test, blood, urine, stool, sputum, etc. are collected by pathologist in the clinic and report is delivered in the next weekly clinic. With regard to bi-monthly special clinic, members are very happy. Eight to ten doctors specialized in various areas such as ENT, eye, heart, skin, gynaecology, neurology and so on come to special clinic. Due to the pressure of patients, treatment under this clinic is continued till 10 p.m. For awareness, two health workers come from Ramganga centre twice in a week to disseminate information on family planning, cleanliness, healthy habit formation and so on. According to beneficiaries, before coming of SHIS, the condition of health of this village was very bad and people would depend upon the quack doctors. For better treatment, they would go to Diamond Harbour or Patharpratima Hospital by hiring boat. Transport cost would go more than six hundreds and sufferings were unimaginable. As a result of intervention of SHIS, these sufferings have been reduced. If this organization stops working, again West Sripatinagar will go back to its previous days.

In the context of cost of treatment, members are very happy. SHIS takes rupees three per patient to prepare card. Most of the medicines are provided in free of cost. Medicines which are not available in the clinic are prescribed to buy from outside. For pathological test, rates are as follows: X-ray = Rs. 40; Blood test = Rs. 15 to Rs. 20; stool test = Rs. 12 and urine test = Rs. 12. In case of tuberculosis, treatment is entirely free. Regarding quality of treatment, members are also very satisfied. They express that doctors are experienced as well as qualified, staff members are adequately trained, pathological reports are reliable and medicines are quite useful. As a result of SHIS's effort during last three years, health status of the present village has been improved.

With regard to SHIS's intervention at difficult situation, members of the group have replied positively. As per their opinion, coming to the West Sripatinagar by a mechanized boat and providing health service is itself an example of work at difficult situation. Apart from that, during flood, SHIS comes to this village as well as goes to the affected areas immediately for relief distribution and medical treatment. Sometimes, in case of emergency, SHIS facilitates by giving their speedboat to take a patient to the Diamond Harbour or Patharpratima hospital.

Members say, the entire medical team of SHIS is cooperative. In every clinic, they leave the health centre having checked all the patients in spite of being late. Doctors do not treat the patients hurriedly. Due to serious problems, if any patient cannot be carried at the health centre, voluntarily doctor visits patient's home. Other staff members are also helpful. They explain regarding how to use medicines, which pathological examination is required and what to do for that and so on. In case of difficult case, who requires blood or major operation or advanced medical examination, they (staff members) refer the patient to their known place for better treatment.

Members of the group feel and indicate that local people of West Sripatinagar have scope to participate in the implementation of programmes of SHIS, who are associated with SHIS as volunteers, they make all sorts of plan during special clinic i.e. spot selection, time fixation, propagating the message to the villagers, public control during clinic and so on. When flood occurs and rescue team comes from SHIS, local volunteers help as much as possible. In case of implementation of any new programme, Director of SHIS meets with the villagers seeking local participation.

In fine, we understand that beneficiaries have better perception towards the working of SHIS. It has been possible as a result of making the affordable as well as qualitative service accessible and sincere as well as hard work of the medical team and other staff members in this remote corner of Sundarban. People say, had there been any qualified doctors permanently at SHIS's health centre, they would have been secured further.

Group 4

The present group is constituted of ten female members who reside at the distant village named West Sripatinagar and belong to Scheduled Caste families of the same area. Regarding types of health care institutions and their nature of services which local people use for day-to-day health problems, members of the group have replied as like as male group formed in this village. According to members, during sickness, at first they go to quack doctors since these doctors are easily available and accessible. Then, during weekly clinic at SHIS's health centre, they consult with the qualified doctor regarding the same problem. When condition of the patient goes out of control of the local health care institutions, villagers directly go to Diamond Harbour or Patharpartima Hospital. Participators of the present group articulate that all the three types of health care institutions indicated above are very much required for variation of services and they do not neglect any one of them.

Members say, SHIS came to West Sripatinagar for first time in 1999 in order to provide flood relief and medical service. Since then, it has been continuing health activities. Now SHIS runs weekly clinic as well as bi-monthly special clinic and organizes awareness camps for environmental cleanliness as well as inculcation of healthy habits. For weekly clinic, a medical team comes with a mechanized boat, which has pathological examination facilities. During special clinic, eight to ten doctors specialized in different fields come from Kolkata. In case of awareness camps, two health workers come to this village twice in a week. Members are of the opinion, during special clinic when gynaecologist comes, they get treatment and advice in hurried and hasty manner. Thereafter, it becomes difficult to get follow up treatment. The present group demands that the doctor who comes regularly to the weekly clinic should be a gynaecologist for their welfare. Members say, before coming of SHIS at West Sripatinagar, they would depend only upon quack doctors. It was impossible for poor people to go to Diamond Harbour or Patharpratima Hospital by hiring boat. There was no health facility for pregnant mother. Since our society was male dominated, head of the family would not feel that women should be taken to the doctor outside the village. Many pregnant mothers had died at the time of child delivery. During delivery, unhealthy techniques would be used more. For instance, nursing mother or dai would put a '*Dhama*' (a basket made of cane) on the lower abdomen to speed up the birth process. As a result of that, many women would suffer from gynaecological problem. Members of the group feel and express that due to continuous work of SHIS during last three years, awareness is created among the people to practice healthy habit. If doctor of SHIS centre advises to a pregnant mother to go for various examinations or to go to outside hospital, family members take it very seriously. Without the support of this organization, villagers feel insecured.

Regarding cost of health service, members of the present group answer as like as male group of this village. With regard to quality of treatment, members have mixed opinion. All of them feel that doctors are qualified and experienced but cannot check up a person properly due to pressure of many patients. Medical professionals of this organization take only five minutes to check up a person whereas outside doctors take at least ten to fifteen minutes. Members say, other para-professionals associated with the medical team are adequately trained. For medicines, villagers do not have any doubt regarding quality. Those are useful and up-to-date.

For SHIS's intervention at difficult situation, members of this group have answered the same like male group of West Sripatinagar.

In the context of staff cooperation, members are very happy. According to them, doctors attend clinic during 8 a.m. to 12.30 p.m. If there is pressure of patients, doctors do not work hurriedly and leave the clinic after completing check up in spite of being late. Sometimes doctors themselves give money from their own pocket to the poor patients for buying nutritious food and medicines. Co-operation is also found in case of other staff members. They help in providing advice, distributing medicines, referring difficult cases, undergoing different pathological tests and so on.

Members of the group express that local people have scope of participation in the implementation of SHIS's programmes. During weekly clinic, village volunteers convince the patients who have serious problems to come to doctor. During special clinic, local people make the overall arrangement by spot selection, time fixation, propagation, making appropriate queue at the time of clinic and so on. Apart from that, off and on, Director of SHIS meets with the villagers to know their problems and demands.

On the basis of above discussion, we understand that beneficiaries of West Sripatinagar have better perception towards the working of SHIS. Because, SHIS has been able to provide primary health care along with pathological examination facilities, to refer the serious patients to appropriate hospitals and to inculcate healthy habit among the villagers. Ultimately it has minimized the sufferings of the local people.

In brief, in this chapter, out of twelve groups, nine groups express positive perception and three groups show negative perception. By and large, beneficiaries have better perception towards the working of respective NGOs under the study. Beneficiaries say, they require an NGO more because of education, income generation, flood relief and community development (village infrastructure improvement) activities than health care programme. The health care programmes of the respective NGOs under the study are not very satisfactory to the beneficiaries, but of course helpful in improving health status. These programmes include more preventive services and less curative services than twenty-four hours curative services with all the technological facilities of modern medicines. Many beneficiaries use these NGOs as stepping-stone for better referral health services.

So, we can conclude from the case studies (discussed in Chapter VII, VIII, IX and X) that an NGO in West Bengal can help in improving health status by providing more preventive services and less curative services. Its programmes will be less sustainable after the project duration. Therefore, for continuation of a full-fledged programme, that project has to be on with adequate support. Staff mobility will not occur and affect the programme if workers are paid well.

PART IV

Conclusion

11

Discussion and Conclusion

The emphasis on the concept of 'Welfare State' was a post-Second World War phenomenon in the developed and developing countries in order to mitigate social and economic crisis in terms of mass unemployment, fall in production, political unrest, etc. As per the provisions of the Welfare State, the state invested in health care, education and other welfare programmes for enhancing productivity of labour and also reducing social inequalities. The growth period for the welfare state in the developed and developing countries was upto the early nineteen seventies. In the wake of three decades of growth of welfare state after the second world war both the developed and developing countries faced fiscal crisis. In order to overcome this crisis, many countries cut-back on spending in the welfare sectors.

Thus during the late nineteen seventies and beginning of the eighties, many developed and developing countries decided to introduce privatization, liberalization and limited the role of the state in social sector programmes. Several Third World countries who were in a crisis due to the balance of payment, cut down their budgets in the social sectors and started taking loans from International Monetary Fund (IMF) and World Bank (WB) for tiding over the fiscal crisis. The assumption that was implicit in this process was that the public sector was inefficient and markets tended to be more responsive to people's needs. Therefore, the IMF and World Bank emphasised the role of both markets and the NGOs for financing and provisioning of services. NGOs were seen as important because of their special characteristics like small size, being more participatory, less bureaucratic, more flexible, cost effective, and capable to reach vulnerable population. The World Development Report 1993, 'Investing in Health', in fact reiterated this view globally.

It is true that there is a long history of NGO activities in India. But the growth of NGOs is a phenomenon of the late nineteen seventies and eighties. This was due to a number of factors which have been discussed in greater detail in Chapter 2. Apart from certain national factors, there was an important influence of the international NGOs as well. Thus the inability of the state to invest coupled with support from donor agencies and other international NGOs provided the impetus for the expansion of this sector in India. The emphasis on the NGO sector in India was expressed through various government documents[1].

These NGOs are varied both in terms of size, levels of operation and services provided. Studies indicate that these NGOs encounter a number of problems due to lack of trained manpower and finance. In the process of development, they carry out various programmes pertaining to health, education, income generation, training, welfare of the handicapped and so on. Especially in the field of health, NGOs perform different roles. They provide clinical service, health awareness, health care training and at the same time conduct research. In India, some of the health care NGOs include the 'Parivar Seva Sanstha' in Delhi; 'Institute of Health Management-Pachod' and 'Streehitakarini' in Maharashtra; 'Society for Education Welfare and Action Rural' in Gujarat; 'Rural Unit for Health and Social Affairs' in Tamil Nadu' 'Banwasi Sewa Ashram' in UP; 'Child in Need Institute' and 'Tagore Society for Rural Development—Rangabelia Project' in West Bengal; etc. These are the larger NGOs but there are several who work at the grassroot levels. There is little information on the characteristics and distribution of NGOs at the all-India and state levels. In order to get some insights into these aspects, this study has been conducted on NGOs in health care in West Bengal. The reason for selecting West Bengal is that it is a middle ranking state with a history of a left front government that has tried to initiate policies for equity. According to experts, in West Bengal, nearly 7,000 NGOs carry out health care programmes. Review of available literature suggests that there are very few studies done on NGOs at the state level and these include Maharashtra, Andhra Pradesh and Assam (Duggal, Gupta, Jesani, 1986; Baru, 1987; and Sarkar, 1996) These studies show that NGOs are skewed in favour of socio-economically developed areas in their distribution. The study of NGOs in Assam (Sarkar, 1998) shows, there is heterogeneity among the NGOs in terms of size, ideology, organizational structure, programme and the population that they serve. These studies raise an important issue regarding to what extent NGOs actually serve the poorer areas and under privileged sections.

However, similar studies have not been initiated in West Bengal from a public health perspective on NGOs in health care. In this context, the present study has tried to examine the case of West Bengal with regard to NGOs in health care. It has made effort to understand the social basis of NGOs, their growth and distribution, contribution, etc. Ultimate aim is to locate the relative position of NGOs vis-a-vis the state in providing health care in West Bengal.

An exploratory design has been used in the present study. The study has been carried out in five phases. In the first phase, secondary data pertaining to socio-political factors influenced the rise of NGOs in West Bengal specially after independence were gathered through literature review. In the second phase, addresses of NGOs in health care were collected based on certain criteria by using the snow ball sampling technique and a comprehensive list of 705 NGOs of West Bengal was prepared. District-wise distribution of NGOs was analysed from this list. In the third phase, questionnaires were mailed to all the 705 NGOs and after three reminders were sent, there was a total of 216 responses. This was done to collect the necessary data in order to analyse the ideological motivations, the growth, distribution and characteristics NGOs in health care in West Bengal. In the fourth phase, fifteen key informants were interviewed purposively to collect much more information on the influence of socio-political factors on the rise of NGOs. In the last phase, three NGOs (i.e. Southern Health Improvement Samity, CINI-Moyna Rural Health Development Centre, and Rural Health Development Centre) were selected purposively based on certain criteria and studied in details. In each NGO, emphasis was given on historical background, administrative set-up, present activities, nature of programme sustainability, staff members and their job satisfaction, beneficiaries perception towards the working of NGOs, etc. to understand how far an NGO could contribute to health care.

Now, the important issues, which have been observed in this study, are being discussed below.

(i) Distinction Between VO and NGO

Chapter 2, while articulated the relevant literature, has discussed the distinction between VO and NGO. VOs are non-profit organizations, have voluntary service, depend on self-managing source of funding and registration is not essential for them. But, NGOs are a later phenomenon. They are non-profit organizations and provide welfare services sometimes as a part of or at the behest of government and sometimes outside it. NGOs require registration, depend on external funding and try to use professionals (where voluntarism is not entertained) for rapid and massive social development. The present study has been conducted only among the NGOs. It is found that all the NGOs under the study do not follow public health perspective i.e. do not have an integrated approach with various programmes like health care, education, nutrition, safe drinking water, sanitation, etc.

(ii) Typology of NGOs

There are different ways in which NGOs can be classified. They can be classified according to types of activities and levels of operations. In order to avoid the complexity, the present study has classified NGOs in terms of types of activities and grouped the NGOs of West Bengal into five categories such as religious organizations, service organizations, development organizations, research and consultancy agencies, and action groups. It is found that health care programmes are carried out, in most of the times, by development organizations and service organizations.

(iii) Factors influencing the Rise of NGOs

The various socio-political factors that have led to the rise of NGOs in West Bengal have been discussed in Chapter 5. In the pre-independence period, Christian missionaries, movements against casteism, Scouts and Guides movement, LIONS movement, Gandhian movement, Women's movement, etc. influenced the rise of NGOs. After independence, along with these factors, there were the Tebhaga movement and the Naxalite movement that played influential role in West Bengal. Apart from these, natural disaster like devastating flood and concerns regarding enviornmental issues, poverty, matters pertaining to the youth, handicapped, minorities, etc. were also important motivations for the growth of NGOs. As discussed in Chapter 5, except the Tebhaga movement, movement against casteism and concern regarding the reduction of poverty, all other socio-political factors contributed in initiating health care activities. Health care programme was found as a part of entire activities under most of the NGOs. It is interesting to note that some of the results found in the present study have similarity with the study conducted in Andhra Pradesh (Baru, 1987). For instance, the study of Andhra Pradesh (Baru, 1987) shows that several factors like Christian missionaries, natural disaster, etc. led the development of NGOs in Krishna and Guntur districts.

(iv) Relationship between Socio-political Factors and Nature of Programmes of NGOs

There is a relation between socio-political root and nature of programme of NGOs. For example, women organizations run development activities for women. Similarly, environmental organizations, those came into existence during the environmental movement, carry out mainly environment upgradation programmes. The action oriented groups, those originated from Tebhaga movement or Naxalite movement, have programmes pertaining to mass mobilizations or meetings or processions against social or political or economic oppression. Apart from the influence of the ideological motivations of the NGO, other factors such as financial situation or competition among NGOs compel them to initiate programmes that is contrary to their objectives.Hence, sometimes, women organizations initiate environment upgradation activities or youth organizations start aged welfare programmes because of the availability of funds. Given this incremental nature of funding and programming, very often NGOs are unable to pursue their objectives. This undermines a holistic approach to programme planning and also creates uncertainty for continuity. This clearly goes against the principles of a public health approach.

(v) Growth of NGOs

It is discussed in the Chapter 6 that NGOs have grown more in numbers in West Bengal during 1980s. Majorities of these NGOs have followed developmental approach and initiated community-based activities. It is also found that growth of NGOs, during 1980s, was reinforced by awareness generation programme and there were only few promoters like medical practitioners, school teachers and untrained dedicated social workers. These raise three important questions i.e. (a) What was the reason for rapid growth of NGOs during 1980s? (b) Why did awareness programme get importance? (c) What was the reason for more involvement of medical practitioners, school teachers and untrained social workers in NGO sector? Answers are also found in the present study. Since various documents of the Government (like National Health Policy 1983, CAARD Report–1985, Sixth Five Year Plan Report, Seventh Five Year Plan Report, etc.) expressed the need of greater involvement of NGOs in development work, there was a growth of NGOs in 1980s. The reason for focusing more on awareness programme during 1980s was mainly because of more importance on human resource development in the Sixth and Seventh Five Year Plan. Apart from that, also a paradigm shift was taking place from welfare approach to development approach in that period. With regard to promoters of NGOs, involvement of medical practitioners was more since there was availability of funds with the government for initiating health care programme in NGOs; involvement of school teachers was more as they had extra time, humanitarian attitude and efficiency for negotiation with the government as well as mobilization of Community resources; and more involvement of dedicated untrained social workers was found due to their unemployment.

(vi) Health Services provided by Government and Private Sectors are Complementary for the NGOs

The Chapter 6 also shows that half of the total NGOs (who sent back mailed questionnaires) started health care activity during the year 1985 to 2000. In that period, health awareness programme was visible more in NGOs. It raises two basic questions i.e. (a) what was the reason for more importance on health care programme after 1985? (b) Where did people go for curative services, after getting awareness from the NGOs? In fact, more involvement of NGOs in health care activity was due to favourable policy of the government (i.e. National Health Policy 1983). The answer for the second question is found in the case studies, made in three divisions (one NGO from each division) of West Bengal. After awareness, in order to get the service, people at first would go to village quake doctors; the PHC (if it was located in the nearby area) or local NGOs (if services were available) were their second preference; and district hospital or urban hospital or private nursing homes were only their last option. Thus, health services provided by the government institutions and private nursing homes were very important and complementary for the NGOs under the study.

The fact is that having received awareness from NGOs, people would go to government and private institutions for curative services. But, the quality of service that people would receive from both the public and private sectors was uneven. Uplekar's (1998) study on 'Tuberculosis Patients and Practitioners in Private Clinics in India' shows that there was lack of awareness regarding treatment procedures among the doctors who treated TB patients in their own clinics. Phadke *et al.* (1995) conducted a study on supply and use of pharmaceuticals in Satara district of Maharashtra. They found that there was a very high proportion of use of unnecessary, irrational, hazardous drugs and injections specially in the private sector. Public sector prescriptions were more rational than private sector prescriptions. Thus, we can assume from the present study that merely providing health awareness (by the NGOs) without adequate and responsive health services has serious consequences for the community.

(vii) District-wise Distribution of NGOs

In the Chapter 6, district-wise distribution of NGOs in health care in West Bengal has been analysed. This chapter has clearly brought out the fact that 72.19 per cent of the total NGOs are situated in Kolkata and its adjacent area [i.e. Howrah, 24 Parganas (South and North) and Hoogly]. It means, NGOs prefer to work in socio-economically developed areas. This kind of trend has an implication for the principle of universality, accessibility and availability. In other words, as a result of this trend, health services do not reach to all areas and sections of society. This trend also suggests that the common assumption is that NGOs work in poorer areas but the present study questions that assumption. A similar trend was observed in the study of Maharashtra, Andhra Pradesh and Assam (Duggal, Gupta & Jesani, 1986; Baru, 1987; Sarkar, 1998). In Maharashtra, NGOs are centralized in Konkan and Pune regions; in Andhra Pradesh, NGOs are skewed in favour of well developed districts like Krishna, Guntur, etc; and in Assam, more number of NGOs (63.49%) are situated in Kamrup and its adjacent districts (Barpeta, Nalbari, Marigaon, Nagaon and Darrang).

(viii) Distribution of NGOs as per the Area of Operation

It is discussed in the Chapter 6 that except 11.1 per cent NGOs, all other NGOs (who replied to mailed questionnaires) have either partly or fully rural based programmes. Over one-third (35.6%) of the total NGOs operate only in rural areas. Almost half (47.2%) of the total NGOs (who replied) are development organizations and majority of them (except 4.9%) have rural based activity. Institutionalized services or community based services or both are found more among the rural NGOs. Again, these rural based NGOs are identified as very active organizations for preventive as well as temporary health facilities, use of separate health staff and for giving appointment to different kinds of professional or para-professional health staff. Hence, it can be assumed that rural based NGOs of West Bengal have achieved very good reputation for development initiative and have significantly contributed to preventive health care. But, it should be noted that these rural based NGOs are situated more in the well-developed districts. Very few NGOs serve in remote rural area or backward districts. For instance, Cooch Behar, Dinajpur (South and North), Darjeeling, Purulia, Birbhum, etc. have very few NGOs. This kind of trend has serious consequences for availability and accessibility of services from public health perspective.

(ix) Organizational Set-up

Case Studies, in Chapter 7, bring to our notice that there is variation in organizational structures of NGOs. For instance, RHDC and CINI-Moyna RHDC have very simple or flat type of organizational structure. They have very limited coverage. But SHIS has very complex or hierarchical organizational set-up. It has very wider coverage. It tries to reach all sections of the community. As a result of this kind of plurality, it is understood that all NGOs do not contribute equally. But in public sector, there is standardisation and uniformity in the organizational set-up. For instance, district health care system (i.e. District Hospital → Community Health Centre → Primary Health Centre → Sub-Centre) is same in all the districts.

(x) Present Activities of NGOs

Case studies in the Chapter 7 also show that most of the on-going programmes of NGOs are targeted or issue based. Each programme is designed with some specific objectives. Many a time, programmes are initiated for a particular section of the people i.e. socio-economically backward class. It may be for children or mother or adolescent girls or youth or aged or so on. As a result of this trend, the principle of universality of public health approach gets undermined—since the needs of the entire population are not being addressed.

(xi) Nature of Programme Sustainability

In the Chapter 8, nature of programme sustainability of the NGOs has been discussed on the basis of twelve requisite criteria. These criteria are (details are mentioned in the methodology chapter): (a) Capacity of the organization; (b) continuity in funding; (c) need fulfilment and ensuring qualitative services; (d) intention of the beneficiaries; (e) nature of people's participation; (f) recognition of people's participation; (g) use of volunteers and continuous liaison with them; (h) nature of staff mobility; (i) innovative component; (j) local co-operation; (k) integrated with other programmes as well as multi-sectoral activities; and (l) regular monitoring. The chapter has shown negative results with regard to programme sustainability in all the three NGOs. In RHDC, none of the four programmes under the study fulfils all the twelve requisite criteria. Each programme suffers from one or more problems and thus they are less sustainable. In CINI-Moyna RHDC, only Women Empowerment Programme is more sustainable. Other three programmes do not fulfil the necessary requirement and hence they are treated as less sustainable. SHIS has the same performance like RHDC. Its all the programmes are less sustainable. In fact, it has been observed in Chapter VIII that ultimately sustainability of a programme depends on funding. If NGOs want to continue their programmes (after the project duration is over), they have to depend on beneficiaries contribution or need to integrate the programme activity with some other on-going project. As a result, felt needs of the beneficiaries will not be fulfilled appropriately. This kind of trend expresses that NGOs cannot contribute in the community for long time.

(xii) Staff and their Satisfaction

In the Chapter 9, case studies show, most of the staff members (84.44%) are moderately satisfied with their jobs. The main reason is that the terms and conditions of the job and salary structure of the staff of NGOs under the study are almost same like public sector. NGOs also provide many facilities (like public sector) to the staff members.

It is also found that the association between salary and level of job satisfaction is statistically significant and salary is a vital part. In fact, this understanding has been qualitatively proved. In NGOs under Caste study, in terms of salary structure, a large gap has been noticed between upper level staff and lower level staff. Upper level staffs are satisfied with salary but lower level staff are not. Hence, staff mobility is mainly found among the lower level staff.

This kind of trend shows that staff mobility or staff related problem is no longer a problem in NGOs if salary structure is designed properly. NGOs can contribute well if staff salary is taken care of.

(xiii) Sources of Funding

It is observed in the Chapter 6 that there is plurality in sources of funding. Self generated source, state government, central government and foreign funding agencies are the main sources. Data show that almost 90 per cent of the total NGOs generate more than half (54.17%) of their required funds by their own effort (self generated). Those NGOs depend on state government and central government, respectively 26.12 per cent and 29.74 per cent of their total budget come from state government and central government. Similarly, one-third of the total NGOs depend on foreign funds and each one receives almost 44 per cent of their total budget. This trend indicates two important aspects. (a) Since most of the NGOs depend on internal sources, their existence in West Bengal cannot be ignored. They will survive in long run; (b) Who receive foreign funds, their activeness is doubtful and they have every possibility to become 'sick'. Again, it should be noted that the reason for less dependency on the state government funding or central government funding is harassment. Government officers have more queries for funding, reject proposal without any enquiry, release funds through so many offices, ask bribe and after one instalment show reluctancy in fund delivery.

(xiv) Extent of People's Participation

The Chapter 10 shows, community participation in programme planning is very limited. People can neither be involved in fund management nor have right to know the financial status of a programme nor can intervene in top-level decision. Their view is not considered (except a few felt needs) while a project is designed. Participation of the people is sought only during programme execution or monitoring or evaluation. For instance, during health awareness camp, topic is chosen in consultation with the beneficiaries; spot, date as well as time is decided by the beneficiaries; etc. People ensure their involvement by attending the programme, providing physical infrastructure (i.e. tables, chairs, benches, etc.), controlling public gathering, arranging refreshment for the trainers, etc. But people have no right to sanction a health awareness camp, which is management level affair. It is also observed that people participate in few programmes by contributing resources or providing information to the evaluation team that comes from the funding agency. This kind of trend cannot challenge the *top-down approach* for planning, that is a criticism levelled against the public sector. It is found that government approach is replicated in NGOs.

(xv) Perception of Beneficiaries towards the Working of NGOs

By and large, beneficiaries have better perception towards the working of NGOs. They express that they need intervention of an NGO more because of community development activities (village infrastructure improvement), income generation, educational improvement, disaster relief, etc. than the health services. The health services of the respective NGOs under the case study are not very satisfactory to the beneficiaries. But, beneficiaries perceive that NGO's various health awareness camps, mobile clinics, outdoor health services, etc. contributed in improving health status during last few years. In fact, they would like to have facilities of curative services for twenty-four hours with all technological advantages of modern medicines than the temporary services during office hours only. A few of the beneficiaries are in favour of using these NGOs as stepping-stone for better referral health services.

The present study has given many new insights. It has confirmed following two hypotheses. The first hypothesis was assumed in the study of Andhra Pradesh (Baru, 1987). The second hypothesis was developed for first time in the study of Maharashtra (Duggal, Gupta and Jesoni, 1986) and was confirmed once by the study of Andhra Pradesh (Baru, 1987).

(i) Socio-political factors influence the emergence and growth of NGOs in a state.
(ii) There is an association between socio-economically developed areas and location of NGOs.

The present study has also developed two new hypotheses. These are:

(i) Contribution of NGO varies with the nature of financial sustainability of the programmes.

(ii) There is a significant relation between contribution of NGO and salary structure of the staff.

Conclusion

It is important to note that there is plurality among the NGOs in health care in West Bengal in terms of their emergence, basis of initiating programme, approach, type of service, promoter's background, source of funding, organizational set-up, nature of activity, etc. In West Bengal, NGOs prefer to work in socio-economically developed areas and cannot continue work in the community for long time due to financial unsustainability. NGOs also cannot contribute much in providing health services. They are found as suitable means to provide preventive, community based and temporary health care facilities. Ultimately people, having received the awareness from NGOs and understanding the need of health care, go to public and private sectors for better curative services. This kind of trend proves that health services provided by the government and private sectors are complementary for NGOs of West Bengal. There is a need of integration of services of government, private and NGO sectors in providing better health care. It is also important to note that the major findings of the present study will be worth for government in making plan for health care and useful for the funding agencies and NGOs to be careful in designing, implementing and monitoring various health care projects. The present study suggests that there is a need to initiate further research in the following areas: (a) Nature and extent of preventive health care of NGOs in West Bengal, (b) Extent of the requirement of public sector health care in relation to private sector considering the role of NGOs in preventive care in West Bengal, (c) Interface between Government and NGOs with regard to health care in West Bengal, etc.

NOTE

1. These government documents include the Foreign Contribution Regulation Act (1976), the National Health Policy (1983), the CAARD Report (1985) [Report of the Committee to Review the Existing Administrative

Arrangements for Rural Development], the Seventh Five Year Plan (1985-90), etc.

REFERENCES

Baru, R. 1987. 'Factors Influencing Variations in Health Services—A Study of Selected District of Andhra Pradesh'. *M.Phil Dissertation.* CSMCH, SSS, Jawaharlal Nehru University, New Delhi.

Duggal, R.; Gupta, M.; Jesani, A. 1986. *NGOs in Rural Health Care.* Foundation for Research in Community Health: Mumbai.

Phadke *et al.* 1995. *A Study of Supply and Use of Pharmaceuticals in Satara District (Part 2).* Foundation for Research in Community Health: Pune.

Sarkar, A.1998. 'Characteristics of NGOs: An Exploratory Study in Assam.' *M.Phil Dissertation.* CSMCH, SSS, Jawaharlal Nehru University, New Delhi (Unpublished).

Uplekar M. *et al.* 1998. 'Tuberculosis Patients and Practitioners in Private Clinics in India'. *International Journal of Tuberculosis and Lung Diseases.* Vol. 2, No. 4, pp. 324-329.

Appendix

Tools of Data Collection

PART-I

MAILED QUESTIONNAIRE

Sir,

I am doing research on "NGOs in Health Care in West Bengal." Hence, I am conducting a survey through 'Mailed Questionnaire'. Having considered time constraints, expenditure and communication problems, I am compelled to do so. This questionnaire, except a few questions (such as name, address, number of staffs, etc.), carries multiple-choice questions.

In this regard, I pray your necessary support and kind co-operation. Please go through the enclosed questionnaire and put tick mark (√) for right answer. A self-addressed stamped envelope is enclosed herewith for sending back the filled up questionnaire to me.

I look forward to your co-operation and an early reply.

Thanking you,

Yours sincerely

(Asok Sarkar)
Researcher

I. Identity

1. Name of the Secretary or Executive Director:
2. Name of the Organization:
3. Office address (with district, pin code and phone number).

Please put tick mark (√) in the bracket for right answer.

II. Growth and Distribution

4. Please indicate the year of registration of your organization:
5. Where does the organization operate?
   (a) Urban area [ ]
   (b) Rural area [ ]
   (c) a + b [ ]
   (d) Tribal area [ ]
   (e) Urban, Rural and Tribal area [ ]
6. How far is the organization from the district town?
   (a) At the district town [ ]
   (b) Less than 20 km [ ]
   (c) 20 to 50 km [ ]
   (d) 50 km to 100 km [ ]
   (e) Above 100 km [ ]
7. (i) Are you affiliated to any federation? Yes/No
   (ii) If yes, under whom
      (a) VHAI [ ]
      (b) Lions International [ ]
      (c) Any other, specify [ ]
8. What type of organization is this?
   (a) Religious organization [ ]
   (b) Service organization [ ]
   (c) Development organization [ ]
   (d) Research and consultancy agency [ ]
   (e) Action group [ ]
   (f) Any other, specify [ ]
9. Organization has
   (a) Institutionalized Service [ ]
   (b) Community based Service [ ]
   (c) Both [ ]
10. (i) What Programme did you initiate at the starting of this organization?
      (a) Education [ ]
      (b) Health [ ]
      (c) Income generation [ ]

(d) Environment upgradation [ ]
(e) Movement for social issues [ ]
(f) Relief [ ]
(g) Any other, specify [ ]

(ii) What was the nature of above mentioned programme at the starting of the organization?
(a) Awareness generation [ ]
(b) Service oriented programme [ ]
(c) Both [ ]

11. What was the main target group at the time of starting of this organization?
(a) Children [ ]
(b) Women [ ]
(c) Youth [ ]
(d) Aged [ ]
(e) Illiterate [ ]
(f) People below poverty line [ ]
(g) SC/ST/OBC [ ]
(h) Student [ ]
(i) Landless or marginal farmers [ ]
(j) Artisans [ ]
(k) Rural entrepreneurs [ ]
(l) Sick or ill [ ]
(m) Handicapped [ ]
(n) Community [ ]
(o) Any other, Specify [ ]

12. Please roughly indicate the percentage of source of funding:
(a) Self generated = ...%
(b) State Government = ...%
(c) Central Government = ...%
(d) Indian Funding Agencies = ...%
(e) Foreign Funding Agencies =....%

13. Health care programme
(i) Do you have health care programme? Yes/No
If yes,
(ii) When did you start health care programme?
(a) Before 1970 [ ]
(b) 1971-1975 [ ]
(c) 1976-1980 [ ]

(d) 1981-1985 [ ]
(e) 1986-1990 [ ]
(f) 1991-1995 [ ]
(g) After 1995 [ ]

(iii) What health care programme did you start initially?
(a) Awareness generation [ ]
(b) Health camp occasionally [ ]
(c) Regular mobile dispensary [ ]
(d) Permanent clinic [ ]
(e) Permanent hospital [ ]
(f) Training of health workers [ ]
(g) Any other, please mention [ ]

(iv) What is your main health care programme now?
(a) Awareness generation [ ]
(b) Health camp occasionally [ ]
(c) Regular mobile dispensary [ ]
(d) Permanent clinic [ ]
(e) Permanent hospital [ ]
(f) Training of health workers [ ]
(g) Any other, please mention [ ]

(v) How much money is allocated (fixed for spending) in the year 2000-01 for your health care programme?
(a) Less than Rs. 10,000/- [ ]
(b) Rs. 10,001/- to Rs. 50,000/- [ ]
(c) Rs. 50,001/- to Rs.1,00,000/- [ ]
(d) Rs. 1,00,001/- to Rs.2,00,000/- [ ]
(e) Rs. 2,00,001/- to Rs. 5,00,000/- [ ]
(f) Rs. 5,00,001/- to Rs. 10,00,000/- [ ]
(g) Above Rs. 10,00,000/- [ ]

(vi) (a) Do you use separate staff only for health care programme? Yes/No
(b) If yes, please indicate the number of full time paid staff engaged in health care programme.

Nature of Staff	*Doctor*		*Nurses*	*Trained Health Worker*	*Non Trained Health Worker*	*Administrative Staff*	*Total*
	Trained	*Non-trained*					

III. General Programmes

14. Please mention any five programmes that you have at present in your organization.

....

....

....

....

....

15. Please indicate the area of coverage of your programme activities:
    (a) Total number of villages:
    (b) Total number of blocks:
    (c) Total number of districts:
    (d) Total number of states:

16. Please mention the total number of full time paid staff of your organization:

....

17. Please indicate the annual budget of your organization for the year 2000-01: Rs.

....

IV. Roots

18. What was the background of the promoter who initiated this organization?
    (a) Medical practitioner [ ]
    (b) School teacher [ ]
    (c) Retired Government officials [ ]
    (d) Political leader [ ]
    (e) Freedom fighter [ ]
    (f) Activists of movement after independence [ ]
    (g) Any other specify [ ]

19. What is the story behind initiation of this organization? (Or What factors motivated to start this organization?

....

....

....

Name and designation of respondent

PART-II

(CASE STUDY)

(A) INFORMATION PROFORMA FOR NGO

I. Historical Background

1. When and what factors or issues motivated to be organized or to form this agency?

   ....

   ....

2. Who was the initial promoter of this organization (name and social background)?

   ....

   ....

3. What were the initial aims and objectives of this organization? How many times were they changed?

   ....

   ....

4. What programme was started in the beginning? (Please mention name and nature)

   ....

   ....

5. When did the organization get registered? Was there any special need for this registration?

   ....

   ....

6. How did you manage land for the organization?

   ....

   ....

7. How did you manage fund for the construction of organization building?

   ....

   ....

8. Where and how did you manage initial working shed?

   ....

   ....

9. Is there any incident of shifting campus from one place to another? If so, please mention name, place and reasons for shifting.

   ....

10. What were the sources of funds in the beginning (before getting external funds)?

    ....

    ....

11. When did you receive first time external fund and for what?

    ....

    ....

12. Various phases of work till today (year *vs.* programme) or (approach *vs.* approach).

    ....

    ....

II. Basic Information

1. Name of the Secretary or Executive Director (with Phone No.)

   ....

   ....

2. Name of the organization:

   ....

   ....

3. Office address (with district and pin code):

   ....

   ....

4. Philosophy, mission and vision of the organization:

   ....

   ....

5. Present objectives of the organization:

   ....

   ....

6. Area of operation: No. of states: ....
   No. of districts: ....
   No. of blocks or wards: ....
   No. of villages or slums: ....
7. Target group:

Sl. No.	*Actual Beneficiaries*	*Volume*

8. Organizational set-up:

9. What kind of infrastructural capacity do you have in order to carry out different programmes?

Infrastructure	*Different Programmes*

10. How is the will-power of the members of the organization? Do the members work in a united way or there are sub-groups among them?

....

....

....

11. How do you take decision in the organization? Is it taken democratically?

....

....

....

III. Programme Related Information

1. Programmes completed previously:

Sl. No	*Name of the Programme*	*Duration*	*Target Group*	*Budget*	*Sources of Fund*	*Nature of Activities & System of Service Delivery*

2. Current programmes:

Sl. No	*Name of the Programme*	*Duration*	*Target Group*	*Budget*	*Sources of Fund*	*Nature of Activities & System of Service Delivery*

IV. Financial Information

1. Please indicate the turnover of your organization for the year 2000-2001.
2. What are the sources of funds of your organization?
   [Please put (√) mark].

   ☐ Central Government
   ☐ State Government
   ☐ Central Social Welfare Board
   ☐ CAPART
   ☐ Non-government Funding Agencies (Indian)
   ☐ Foreign Funding Agencies
   ☐ Local Self Government
   ☐ Public Donation
   ☐ Collection of Contribution
   ☐ Internal Sources
   ☐ Any other, please specify
3. What problems or barriers do you find in financing?
4. What is your organizational policy pertaining to fund raising?

   ....
5. (a) Do you prepare annual budget? Yes/No
   (b) If not, how do you manage?
   (c) If yes, how?

   ....

   ....

(d) What criteria do you use for allocation of funds among the different programmes?

....

....

(e) How do you allocate funds for various aspects within a particular programme?

....

....

V. Information Related to Staff

1. Please indicate the total number of workers:
   (i) No. of full time paid staff:
   (ii) No. of part time paid staff:
   (iii) No. of honorary staff:
   (iv) No. of volunteers:
2. Please indicate the characteristics of full time paid staff:

Sl. No.	*Desig- nation*	*No.*	*Age*	*Sex (M & F)*	*Qualifi- cation*	*Experience*	*Salary*

3. If you use part time worker, please indicate the categories and numbers:

Sl. No.	*Category*	*No. of Part Time Worker*	*Amount per Person per Month*

4. Please indicate the following characteristics of part time worker.

Sl. No.	*Designation*	*Nos.*	*Age*	*Sex*	*Qualification*	*Job*

5. Does your agency have a policy to use the services of volunteers? Yes/No. If yes, please make a brief statement of this policy.

....

....

6. What are the jobs in your agency for which services of volunteers could be utilized? (Please specify the jobs of volunteers except in health care programme).

....

....

VI. Monitoring

1. (a) Do you monitor your programme activities, finance and staff? Yes/No.
   (b) If yes, please indicate time, person and process involved in monitoring activities (for each programme except health).

....

....

VII. Other Information

1. Please indicate the various strengths, weaknesses, opportunities and threats of the organization in terms of administrative work, programme implementation, finance, staff, beneficiaries, ideological issues and so on.

....

....

- Please collect the following documents from the office of the NGO: (1) Audited Statement of Account for last three years, (2) Annual Report for last three years, and (3) Constitution of the organization.

(B) INTERVIEW SCHEDULE IN UNDERSTANDING NATURE OF SUSTAINABILITY OF HEALTH CARE PROGRAMME*

1. Title of the programme: ....
2. Objectives of the programme: ....
3. Target group(s) of the programme:

Target Group(s)	*Beneficiaries*	*Eligibility*	*Process of selection (Role of target groups)*	*Volume & Distribution*

4. Various components of the programme:

Sl. No	*Various Components*	*Nature of Work*

5. Programme execution process:
   (Beginning with launching the programme till the completion—Each different components—responsibility of the different units of the organization at various phases)
   ....
   ....
6. Duration of programme: ....
   Starting month and year: ....
   Completion month and year: ....
7. Area of operation of this programme:
   No. of states (if applicable) ....
   No. of districts ....
   No. of blocks (or wards) ....
   No. of villages (or slums) ....

---

* Programme refers to activities having specific project proposal, programme staff and budget allocation.

8. Does this programme provide service free of cost? If not, how does it provide?

. . . .

9. (a) What are the resources (e.g. Manpower, Medicines, Instruments, Working shed, Vehicle, etc.) utilized in this programme? How do you arrange (collect) this resource? Please specify total budget and annual budget for this health care programme.

Types of Resources	*Process of Resource Arrangement*	*Annual Budget*	*Total Budget*

(b) Can you arrange this resource continuously for long time?

. . . .

. . . .

10. Have you made any alternative arrangement for resource collection after the project duration is completed? If so, what is the arrangement?

. . . .

. . . .

11. (a) Are the health care needs of the beneficiaries fulfilled by this programme? If yes, how do you say it?

. . . .

. . . .

(b) Are the health care services qualitative? If so, how do you say it?

. . . .

. . . .

. . . .

12. Is there any component in the health care programme, which makes the people understand that good health is their own right? If so, do the people really understand health right? If so, do they fight judiciously for better health care services? If so, how?

. . . .

. . . .

. . . .

13. How do you make plan in this health care programme? (Top down approach or bottom up approach—please make me understand with suitable example).

. . . .

. . . .

14. Please highlight the nature of actual participation of the beneficiaries at various levels of programme.

Sl. No	*Various Levels of Programme*	*Nature of Participation*
1.	Need identification	
2.	Resource contribution and resource collection	
3.	Programme planning	
4.	Beneficiaries selection	
5.	Programme implementation	
6.	Programme monitoring	
7.	Programme Evaluation	

15. Do you recognize the people's contribution to the programme? If so, how (please give an example)?

. . . .

. . . .

16. Do you create people's organization (such as SHG, sub-village, Mahila Samiti, Club, etc.) to represent people's interest or to mobilize community resource for this particular programme? If so, please give details.

. . . .

. . . .

17. Do you provide support to people's organization to link with public development agencies (c.g. Panchayats, Banks, PHC, etc.) for accessibility of the resources required for this programme? If so, please give details.

. . . .

. . . .

18. Do you hand over responsibility to carry out the programme to the target group? If so, what is the process of doing it?

19. (a) Do you use volunteers for health care programme? If so, what jobs are performed by them?

. . . .

. . . .

(b) How many volunteers do you have for health care programme? Do you maintain continuous liaison with them? If so, how?

. . . .

. . . .

20. Please discuss the nature of staff mobility highlighting the numbers of staff left and reasons for the same in last year and this year.

Year	*Month*	*Sl. No.*	*Designation*	*Nos. Left*	*Reasons for Leaving Job*
1999-2000		1			
		2			
		3			
		4			
		5			
2000-2001		1			
		2			
		3			
		4			
		5			

21. Do you select health care staff from the community? If so, how? Which are the levels for which staff are recruited from the community?

. . . .

. . . .

. . . .

22. What staff related difficulties do you find in your NGO in implementing this health care programme? (Difficulties in recruitment, competency of staff, turnover, conflict, etc.)

. . . .

. . . .

. . . .

23. (a) Is there any innovative component (e.g. Promotion of low cost health care, use of polyclinic as referral service and income generation, etc.) in your health care programme? If so, please specify and discuss its nature.

. . . .

. . . .

. . . .

(b) How does this innovative component or initiative or incentive help to sustain level of motivation of the community people?

. . . .

. . . .

24. Please describe the co-operation of local people, influential persons and other organizations of the community to execute this programme in a better way.

. . . .

. . . .

25. Do you find any threat to carry out programme from political parties or opponent groups whose interests are not met? If so, please explain with some example.

. . . .

. . . .

. . . .

26. Do you integrate the health care programme with other multi-sectoral programmes (e.g. Income generation programme, agriculture programme, social forestry programme, etc) for its better existence? If so, please explain how and what other programmes are integrated in this regard?

. . . .

. . . .

. . . .

27. Please describe the health care expenditure under different heads for last year (2000-2001).

Heads	*Expenditure* (*Rs.*)	*Availability* (*Rs.*)	*Source*	*Deficit* (*Rs.*)	*Surplus* (*Rs.*)
Fly. Planning Medicine Vaccines Nutrition Salary & Allowances Travelling Administration					

28. Is there any component in your health care programme to play the role of advocacy? If so, please give details.

. . . .

. . . .

29. Is this health programme associated with any other programme for which same resources are used, common staff are involved and same monitoring system is followed? If so, please give details.

....

....

....

30. Is this programme dependent on any aspects like donor agency, willingness of the staff members, etc.? If so, please mention.

....

....

....

31. Can the health care activities be continued when project duration will be over? If so, how?

....

....

....

32. Do you monitor or regularly follow up your health care programme? If so, please mention person, period and process involved in monitoring or regular follow up of health care programme

....

....

....

33. Investigator's observation:

(Sustainable component of the activities, sustainable outlook of the staff or beneficiaries or community people)

....

....

....

Name and Designation of the respondent (with date)

(C) INFORMATION PROFORMA FOR HEALTH CARE STAFF

1. Please indicate the total number of health care staff of your organization:

   (i) Number of full time paid staff:

   ....

   (ii) Number of part time paid staff:

   ....

   (iii) Number of honorary staff:

   ....

2. Please indicate the following characteristics of health care staff (to be collected from the office).

Nature of Staff	*Sl. No.*	*Designation*	*Number*	*Qualification Required*	*Nature of Job Responsibility*	*Salary Rs.*
(a) Full time staff	1					
	2					
	3					
	4					
	5					
	6					
(b) Part time staff	1					
	2					
	3					
	4					
	5					
	6					
(c) Honorary staff	1					
	2					
	3					
	4					
	5					
	6					

(D) JOB SATISFACTION SCALE FOR FULL TIME HEALTH CARE STAFF

Sir,

In this booklet there are some statements pertaining to job satisfaction of the full time paid health care staff. Each statement has five alternative answers, such as, strongly disagree, disagree, undecided, agree and strongly agree. Please read carefully and indicate your response, which one of the five answers you feel correct, by putting a tick mark (√) against each statement. Your reply will be kept secret and used only for research purpose.

Thanking you,

Asok Sarkar
Researcher

Staff Identity

Serial No: ....Name of the Organization: ....
Name of the Staff:..............................Age:............ Sex:............
Marital Status:........... Educational Qualification: ....
Experience: .... Designation:...........Nature of Work.............

Sl. No.	*Statements*	*Response Category*				
		Strongly Disagree	*Disagree*	*Undecided*	*Agree*	*Strongly Agree*
		(1)	(2)	(3)	(4)	(5)
1.	My present job is as per my ability/qualification and experience.					
2.	Comparing the salary for a similar job in other organizations (NGOs) I feel my pay is better.					
3.	Taking up this job does not involve risks as it guarantees fair amount of security.					

(Contd.)

(Contd.)

Sl. No.	*Statements*	*Response Category*				
		Strongly Disagree	*Disagree*	*Undecided*	*Agree*	*Strongly Agree*
		(1)	(2)	(3)	(4)	(5)
4.	My supervisor keeps me informed about all policies or happenings of the organization.					
5.	My colleagues like me and give due respects at the working place.					
6.	My job has helped me to learn some new skills.					
7.	I often feel that my employer will not terminate me if I commit a mistake.					
8.	My supervisor increases team spirit in the work group.					
9.	My supervisor behaves properly (have cordial relation) with me.					
10.	This job (of NGOs) helps for my professional growth.					
11.	We often face problems because there is crowding in our room (we are too many people in our room).					
12.	Physical condition of my room (such as lack of furniture or fan or sufficient light, etc.) gives maximum trouble to work during summer season.					
13.	If for certain specific reason I do not reach at my working place on time, I do not get threat to leave this work.					
14.	I have often felt that at our organization we have inappropriate leave rules.					
15.	My supervisor takes into account my wishes as well as work done.					
16.	Physical condition of my room leads to health problems during monsoon as it becomes damp or moist.					

(Contd.)

(Contd.)

Sl. No.	*Statements*	*Response Category*				
		Strongly Disagree	*Disagree*	*Undecided*	*Agree*	*Strongly Agree*
		(1)	(2)	(3)	(4)	(5)
17.	This organization has career advancement scheme. Whenever there is possibility, it sends us for further education and training.					
18.	I am really not interested to this job but circumstances force me to continue with it.					
19.	There is no facility related to social security provision or provident fund or gratuity or pension etc. in my job.					
20.	My organization provides good housing facilities to its employees.					
21.	I am satisfied with the medical facilities (for staff) provided by the organization.					
22.	On the whole, I have good prospects for advancement in my job.					
23.	If I get similar job with good pay in any other organization, I would like to quit this job.					
24.	Hard work as well as better performance is appreciated in my organization, which I like most.					
25.	The activities of my supervisor are governed by self-interest.					
26.	My co-worker does not create any tension or conflict talking too much on working problems (of this organization). He helps me in my work to reduce tension or conflict.					
27.	I often find myself disadvantaged at my working place due to lack of technical information.					
28.	My job (of this NGO) does not help to increase prestige or social recognition.					

(Contd.)

(*Contd.*)

Sl. No.	*Statements*	*Response Category*				
		Strongly Disagree	*Disagree*	*Undecided*	*Agree*	*Strongly Agree*
		(1)	(2)	(3)	(4)	(5)
29.	I am not interested to continue this job, as I usually feel tired at the end of the day's work.					
30.	Promotions are made as per qualifications and experiences in this organization. I have been getting it.					
31.	When my 'Boss' throws his temper at me I feel like protesting it to set him right.					
32.	Drinking water facilities are satisfactory and usually provided at work place.					
33.	My job does not provide opportunity for independent thought and use of my talents.					
34.	Recreational facilities are negligible in my organization.					
35.	My all the abilities are not utilized fully in my present job.					
36.	Canteen or kitchen facilities are well at working hours in this organization.					
37.	I seldom watch the clock when I am at office as time passes smoothly.					
38.	Childcare facilities (like Day Care Centre or Crèche) are very good in our organization to provide support to the working mothers (employees of this organization).					

(E) INTERVIEW SCHEDULE FOR GROUP DISCUSSION*

Group Identity

1. Name of the organization: ....
2. Name of the village: ....
3. Nature of village: ....Nearby/Distant ....
4. Nature of group: .... Male/Female ....
5. Total number of group members: ....

Health Care Programmes of the Locality

1. What kind of health care institutions are available in your area? How far are they?

   ....

   ....

2. How does government institution work in your locality?

   ....

   ....

3. Where do you go when you feel sick? Why?

   ....

   ....

4. Are you getting same service from different organizations free of cost in your area?

   ....

   ....

   ....

Necessity of the NGO's Health Care Programme

1. Is this NGO working in your locality? If so, what activities are being done by them?

   ....

   ....

* This is used to understand perception of beneficiaries towards the working of NGOs in health care.

2. Does it help in health care activities? If so, who comes for the help and what do they do (i.e. what service you get)?

   ....

   ....

3. Is this health care programme of NGO need based in the locality? If so, please justify the ultimate necessity of this health care programme?

   ....

   ....

4. What was the health condition of this locality before reaching this NGO?

   ....

   ....

Service Cost and Quality of the NGO's Health Care Programme

1. Do you get the service free of cost? If not, do you pay for the service? If so, is this cost reasonable or are you happy with the cost?

   ....

   ....

2. What kind of services are 'Pay Services'?

   ....

   ....

3. As per your understanding, what should be the actual cost?

   ....

   ....

   ....

4. What is your feeling regarding the quality of medicines, doctors, staff members, medical instruments, etc. of this organization? Are you happy with this quality of service?

   ....

   ....

   ....

5. Do you get all sorts of medicines from the organization prescribed by their doctors? If not, how do you manage?

   ....

   ....

   ....

NGO's Health Service in Difficult Situation

1. Does it provide any health services in remote rural area? If so, how and what services are provided?

   ....

   ....

2. What kinds of services are provided by this organization during epidemic within its operational area?

   ....

   ....

3. When natural disaster takes place (like flood, cyclone, drought, etc.) within its own or nearby area, how does this NGO respond? Does it reach late when epidemic starts?

   ....

   ....

4. Having done journey for two or three hours when some serious patients (like delivery case or accident case) come from vary far off place, how does the organization treat them? Does it reject the patient due to lack of bed or medicine facility in spite of availability of good doctors?

   ....

   ....

Staff Co-operation

1. What is your opinion regarding co-operation of the doctors in order to get treatment?

   ....

   ....

2. Do you find nurses and health care staff are co-operative? If so, how?

   ....

   ....

   ....

3. Do you find other staff members are co-operative within the hospital or dispensary or clinic? If so how?

   ....

   ....

   ....

4. In case of paid services, when you are unable to pay, do you find the co-operation of the health care staff for making alternative arrangement or for some other suggestion?

   ....

   ....

5. Please mention any other co-operation that you get from the staff members.

   ....

Beneficiary's Participation

1. Do you participate in the planning process of the health care programme? If so, how?

   ....

   ....

2. Do you participate in providing physical infrastructure (like place, furnitures, manpower, money, etc.) to organize health camp and clinic in the community? If so, what and how?

   ....

   ....

3. Do you take part in executing, monitoring and evaluation of the programme? If so, how?

   ....

   ....

4. Does the organization select health care staff from the community? What is the actual process of health care staff selection?

   ....

   ....

Bibliography

REPORTS

Central Social Welfare Board. 1961. *Report of the Grants in Aid Care Committee.* Ministry of Welfare: New Delhi.

Committee for Economic Development (CED). 1995. *Building Inner-City Communities: A New Approach to the Nation's Urban Crisis.* Author: New York.

Government of India. 1946. *Report of the Health Survey and Development Committee—Bhore Committee.* New Delhi.

Government of India. 1958. *State Assistance to Voluntary Organizations.* Planning Commission: New Delhi.

Government of India. 1959. *Report of the Study Team on Social Welfare and Welfare Board of Backward Classes.* Planning Commission: New Delhi.

Government of India. 1961. *Report of the Health Survey and Planning Committee—Mudaliar Committee.* Ministry of Health: New Delhi.

Government of India. 1966. *Report of the Rural Urban Relationship Committee.* Ministry of Health: New Delhi.

Government of India. 1977. *Health Care Service in Rural India Draft Plan.* Ministry of Health: New Delhi.

Government of India. 1978. *Study of the Working of the Aided Voluntary Agencies in Social Welfare Programmes. Planning Commission: New Delhi.*

Government of India. 1978. *Report of the Committee on Panchayati Raj Institutions. New Delhi.*

Government of India. 1981. *Recommendations of the Seventh Joint Conference of the Central Council of Health and Central Family Welfare Council.* Ministry of Health and Family Welfare: New Delhi.

Government of India. 1981. *Report of the Working Group on Health for All By 2000 AD.* Ministry of Health and Family Welfare: New Delhi.

Government of India. 1982. *Statement of National Health Policy.* Ministry of Health and Family Welfare: New Delhi.

Government of India. 1985. *Report of the Committee on the Existing Administrative Arrangements for Rural Development and Poverty Alleviation Programme.* Ministry of Agriculture: New Delhi.

Government of Bangladesh. 1985. *Report on Responding to the Challenge of Rural Poverty in South Asia: Role of NGOs.* Dhaka.

Government of India. 1952. *First Five-Year Plan.* Planning Commission: New Delhi.

Government of India. 1956. *Second Five-Year Plan.* Planning Commission: New Delhi.

Government of India. 1961. *Third Five-Year Plan.* Planning Commission: New Delhi.

Government of India. 1974. *Fifth Five-Year Plan.* Planning Commission: New Delhi.

Government of India. 1984. *Sixth Five-Year Plan—Midterm Appraisal.* Planning Commission: New Delhi.

Government of India. 1985. *Seventh Five-Year Plan.* Planning Commission: New Delhi.

Government of India. 1992. *Eighth Five-Year Plan.* Planning Commission: New Delhi.

Government of India. 1997. *Ninth Five-Year Plan.* Planning Commission: New Delhi.

Government of India. *Economic Survey 1999-2000.* Ministry of Finance: New Delhi.

Government of India. *Economic Survey 2000-2001.* Ministry of Finance: New Delhi.

Government of India. *Statistical Abstract India 1999.* Ministry of Statistics and Programme Implementation: New Delhi.

Government of India. *India 2001—A Reference Annual.* Ministry of Information and Broadcasting: New Delhi.

Government of India. *Annual Health Report 1989-90.* Ministry of Health & Family Welfare: New Delhi.

Government of India. *Annual Health Report 1991-92.* Ministry of Health & Family Welfare: New Delhi.

Government of India. *Annual Health Report 1997-98.* Ministry of Health & Family Welfare: New Delhi.

Industrial Development Bank of India. *Report on Development Banking in India 1999-2000.* Mumbai.

National Institute of Health and Family Welfare. 1978. *An Evaluation of Community Health Workers Scheme—A Collaborative Study.* New Delhi.

Tata Energy Research Institute (TERI). *TERI Energy Data Directory and Year Book 1995-1996.* New Delhi.

Tata Energy Research Institute (TERI). *TERI Energy Data Directory and Year Book 2000-2001.* New Delhi.

The World Bank. *World Development Report 1993.* Oxford University Press: New York.

UNDP. *Human Development Report—1993.* Oxford University Press: New York.

UNDP. *Human Development Report—1996.* Oxford University Press: New York.

UNDP. *Human Development Report—1998.* Oxford University Press: New York.

BOOKS

Alliband, T. 1983. *Catalysts of Development: Voluntary Agencies in India.* Kamarian Press: West Hartford.

Allsop, J. 1984. *Health Policy and the National Health Service.* Longman: London.

Antia, N.H & Bhatia, K. 1993. *People's Health in People's Hand.* FRCII: Mumbai.

Aves, G. 1969. *The Voluntary Workers in the Social Services.* Allen and Unwin: London.

Ball, C. and Dunn, L. 1995. *Non-Governmental Organizations: Guidelines for Good Policy and Practice.* The Common Wealth Foundation: London.

Bava, N. (ed). 1997. *Non-Governmental Organization in Development: Theory and Practice.* Kanishka Publishers and Distributors: New Delhi.

Beveridge, W. 1949. *Evidence for Voluntary Action.* Allen and Unwin: London.

Beveridge, L. 1949. *Voluntary Action: A Report on Methods of Social Advance.* Allen and Unwin: London.

Beveridge, W. 1979. *Voluntary Action in a Changing World.* Allen and Unwin: London.

Bhatt, A. 1988. *Development and Social Justice.* Sage: New Delhi.

Bourdilon, A.F.C. 1945. *Voluntary Social Service—Their Place in Modern State.* Methuen: London.

Carroll, T.F. 1992. *Intermediary NGOs: The Supporting Link in Grassroots Development.* Kumarian Press: West Hartford.

Cannon, L. 1999. *Life Beyond Aid: Twenty Strategies to Help Make NGOs Sustainable.* Initiative for Participatory Development: Johannesburg.

Chin, S. 1991. *PVOs in Health Programmes: Prospects for Sustainability.* USAID.

Chandhoke, N. 1995. *State and Civil Society: Explorations in Political Theory.* Sage: New Delhi.

Chatterjee, M. 1998. *Implementing Health Policy.* Manohar: New Delhi.

Choudhury, D.P. 1962. *Social Welfare Administration Through Voluntary Agencies.* Atma Ram & Sons: Delhi.

Choudhury, D.P. 1971. *Voluntary Social Welfare in India.* Starling Publisher: New Delhi.

Choudhri, R. (ed). 1989. *Conflict, Development and NGOs.* Best Books: Kolkata.

Choudhury, B.L. 2000. *Communication Strategy of NGOs for Rural Development.* Assam University: Silchar.

Chuke, P.O. 1996. *Innovative Health Care Financing Scheme.* WHO: Geneva.

Clark, J. 1990. *Democratizing Development: The Role of Voluntary Organizations.* Kumarian Press: West Hartford.

Cole, G.D.H. 1945. *Voluntary Social Services.* Methuen: London.

Combe, S. 1987. *The Indigenous Voluntary Agency Sector and Rural Change in India.* Department of Town and Country Planning: University of Sydney.

Dasgupta, S. 1973. *Voluntary Organization in Rural Development.* Society for Developing: New Delhi.

Dayal, P. 1986. *Gandhian Approach to Social Work.* Gujarat Vidyapith: Ahmedabad.

Desai, A.R. 1967. *Social Background of Indian Nationalism.* Popular Book Stall: Mumbai.

Djukanovic, V. and Mach, E.P. 1975. *Alternative Approaches to Meeting Basic Health Needs in Developing Countries.* WHO: Geneva.

Dube, S.C. 1976. *Social and Cultural Factors in Development.* Abhinav Publications: New Delhi.

Dutt, R.R. 1965. *Rural Health Services in India: Primary Health Centres.* Central Health Education Bureau: New Delhi.

Edwards, M. and Hulme, D. (eds). 1996. *Beyond the Magic Bullet: NGO Performance and Accountability in the Post-Cold War World.* Kumarian Press: West Hartford.

Edwards, M. and Hulme, D. (eds). 1996. *Making a Difference: NGOs and Development in a Changing World.* Earthscan Publications: London.

Etzioni, A. 1975. *A Comparative Analysis of Complex Organizations.* The Free Press: New York.

Evelyn, H. 1955. *Voluntary and Private Welfare Agencies in India.* Technical Co-operation Mission in India: Delhi.

Eyden, J. 1975. *The Welfare Society.* The National Council of Social Service: London.

Fort, C. 1991. *Promoting NGO Sustainability: The Lessons of Enterprise.* The Enterprise Project: Arlington.

Frankel, F. 1978. *India's Political Economy 1947-77.* Princeton University Press: New Jersey.

Freedman and Smith. 1972. *Voluntary Associations: Perspective in the Literature.* Harvard University Press: Cambridge.

Friedlander, A. 1975. *International Social Welfare.* Prentice Hall Inc: New Jersey.

Goel, S.L. 1980. *Health Care Administration: Ecology Principles and Modern Trends.* Sterling Publishers: New Delhi.

Green, A. 1992. *An Introduction to Health Planning in Developing Countries.* Oxford University Press: Oxford.

Green, A. and Matthias, A. 1997. *Non-Governmental Organizations and Health in Developing Countries.* Macmillan Press: London.

Heredia, R. 1988. *Voluntary Action and Development: Towards a Praxis for Non-Government Agencies.* Concept: New Delhi.

Heyzer, N.; Riker, J. and Quizon, A. 1995. *Government—NGO Relations in Asia.* APDC: Kuala Lumpur.

Hiscock, I.V. 1954. *Community Health Organization.* Harvard University Press: Cambridge.

Hulme, D. and Edwards, M. 1997. *NGOs, States and Doctors: Too Close for Comforts.* St. Martin's Press: New York.

Jagannadham, V. 1967. *Social Welfare Organization.* The Indian Institute of Public Administration: New Delhi.

Janowitz, B.; Jamil, K. *et al.* 1996. *Productivity and Costs for Family Planning Service Delivery in Bangladesh: The NGO Programme.* Family Health International: Arlington.

Jain, R.B.(ed). 1995. *NGOs in Development Perspective.* Friedrich Ebert Stiftung: Delhi.

Jeffery, R. 1988. *The Politics of Health in India.* University of California: Berkeley.

Johnson, N. 1981. *Voluntary Social Service.* Basil Blackwell & Martin: Oxford.

Kibna, T. 1992. *Health Care Financing in Kenya: Private Sector and NGO Development.* Ministry of Health: Kenya.

Kohli, M. 1984. *Voluntary Action in India, Some Profiles.* NIPCCD: New Delhi.

Korten, D.C and Alphonso, F.B. (ed). 1980. *Bureaucracy and the Poor: Closing the Gap.* McGraw Hill: Singapore.

Kothari, R. 1970. *Politics in India.* Little Brown & Company: Boston.

Kulkarni, V.M. 1969. *Voluntary Action in a Developing Society.* Indian Institute of Public Administration: New Delhi.

Madan, G.R. 1973. *Indian Social Problems, Vol. II.* Allied Publishers: New Delhi.

Maheshwari, S. 1995. *Rural Development in India—A Public Policy Approach.* Sage: New Delhi.

Malayala Manorama. 1999. *Manorama Year Book 1999.* Kottayam.

Malayala Manorama. 2002. *Manorama Year Book 2002.(Bengali Version).* Kottayam.

Maskay, B.K. 1998. *NGOs in Development.* Modern Printing Press: Kathmandu.

March, G. and Simon, A. 1958. *Organization.* John Wiley & Sons: New York.

Mathur, K. 1996. *Development Policy and Administration: Readings in Indian Government and Politics.* Sage: New Delhi.

Mathias, E. and Raj, S.L. 1998. *People's Power and Panchayati Raj—Theory and Practice.* Indian Social Institute: New Delhi.

McLennan, G. 1990. *The Idea of the Modern State.* Open University Press: Philadelphia.

Mess, H.A. 1974. *Voluntary Social Services Since 1918.* KTTC: London.

Mishra, M.S. 1982. *Directory of Organizations in Rural Development, Vol. 1.* Indian Institute of Management: Kolkata.

Mishra, R. 1984. *The Welfare State in Crisis.* Harvester Press: Sussex.

Naik, J.P.(Ed). 1977. *An Alternative System of Health Care Service in India.* Allied Publishers: Mumbai.

Nayyar, D. 1993. *Economic Liberalization in India: Analysis, Experiences and Lessons.* Orient Longman: Kolkata.

Omen, T.K. 1972. *Stability and Change: An Analysis of Bhoodan and Gramdan Movement in India.* Thomson: New Delhi.

Pachauri, S. 1994. *Reaching India's Poor-Non-Governmental Approaches to Community Health.* Sage: New Delhi.

Pandey, S.R. 1978. *A Profile Study of Selected Voluntary Projects in India.* ICSSR: New Delhi.

Park, K. 1995. *Park's Text Book of Preventive and Social Medicine.* Banarsidas Bhanot Publishers: Jabalpur.

Paul, S. 1982. *Managing Development Programmes: The Lessons of Success.* West View Press: Boulder.

Pfiffner, J.M. and Sherwood, F.P. 1968. *Administrative Organization.* Prentice Hall of India: New Delhi.

PRIA. 1999. *Civil Society and Governance—An Overview of Issues and Trends in India.* Participatory Research in Asia: New Delhi.

Pulley, C. *et al.* 1993. *Endowments as a Tool for Financial Sustainability: A Manual for NGOs.* PROFIT: Arlington.

Rao, T.V. 1996. *Human Resources Development: Experiences, Interventions and Strategies.* Sage: New Delhi.

Rohde, J. *et al.* 1993. *Reaching Health for All.* Oxford University Press: London.

Ron, A. *et al.* 1990. *Health Insurance in Developing Countries: The Social Security Approach.* ILO: Geneva.

Rooff, M. 1957. *Voluntary Societies and Social Policy.* Routledge and Kegan Paul: London.

Sachdeva, D.R. 1993. *Social Welfare Administration in India.* Kitab Mahal: New Delhi.

Sahni, A. *et al.* 1990. *Community Participation in Health and Family Welfare: Innovative Experiences in India.* Indian Society of Health Administrators: New Delhi.

Sengupta, A. 1997. *High Tide and Low Tide in Seventies and Eighties (Joar Bhatay Shat Sottor).* Pearl Publishers: Kolkata.

Sen, A.C. 1971. *Introducing Voluntary Agencies in India.* Impex India: Delhi.

Shah, G. 1997. *Public Health and Urban Development: The Plague in Surat.* Sage: New Delhi.

Shah, A.M. 1979. *Neighbourhood and Social Networks in Urban India: South Indian Voluntary Association in Delhi.* Marwah Publication: New Delhi.

Sills, D.L. 1957. *The Volunteers: Means and Ends in a National Organization.* The Free Press: Illinois.

Singh, R.D.E. 1993. *The Story of B.P.* Bharat Scouts and Guides: New Delhi.

Siwal, B.R. 1984. *All India Directory of Voluntary Agencies in Rural Development.* NIPCCD: New Delhi.

Smith, C. and Freedman, A. 1972. *Voluntary Associations: Perspective on the Literature.* Harvard University Press: Cambridge.

Smiley and Gould. 1952. *Your Community's Health.* Macmillan Company: New York.

Sundaram, I.S. 1986. *Voluntary Agencies and Rural Development,* B.R. Publishing Corporation: Delhi.

Sur, A.K. 1992. *History and Culture of Bengal.* Best Books: Kolkata.

The Central Institute of Research and Training in Public Cooperation. 1967. *A Study on Voluntary Services in India.* New Delhi.

Uddin *et al.* 1996. *NGO—Donor-Government Relationships.* Voluntary Health Services Society: Bangladesh.

Union of International Organization. 1978. *Year Book on International Organizations.* UIO: Brussels.

Werner, D. 1996. *Disabled Village Children.* VHAI: New Delhi.

World Commission on Environment and Development. 1987. *Our Common Future.* Oxford University Press: New Delhi.

Wolfenden, S. 1977. *Future of Voluntary Organizations.* Croom Helm: London.

PUBLISHED RESEARCH STUDIES

Ahlawat, N.1995. *Women Organizations and Social Networks.* Rawat Publications: New Delhi.

Charyulu, U.V.N. and Natarajan, V.K. 1980. *A Case Study of Cuddapah District.* NIRD: Hyderabad.

Dave Sen, P. 1997. *Case Studies of Mosque and Church Clinics in Cairo, Egypt.* Data for Decision Making Project: Cambridge, MA.

Dave Sen, P. and Berman, P. 1990. *The Costs and Financing of Health Care: Experiences in the Voluntary Sector, Case Study 1—The Voluntary Health Services, Madras.* The Ford Foundation: New York.

Dave Sen, P. and Berman, P. 1990. *The Costs and Financing of Health Care: Experiences in the Voluntary Sector, Case Study 2—Sewa Rural Jhagada.* The Ford Foundation: New York.

Dave Sen, P. and Berman, P. 1990. *The Costs and Financing of Health Care: Experiences in the Voluntary Sector, Case Study 3—Parivar Seva Sanstha, New Delhi.* The Ford Foundation: New York.

Dave Sen, P. and Berman, P. 1990. *The Costs and Financing of Health Care: Experiences in the Voluntary Sector, Case Study 4—Ashish Gram Rachna Trust, Pachod.* The Ford Foundation: New York.

Duggal, R. Gupta, M. Jesani, A. 1986. *NGOs in Rural Health Care.* FRCH: Mumbai.

Duggal, R. and Amin, S. 1989. *Cost of Health Care: A Household Survey in an Indian District.* The Foundation for Research in Community Health: Mumbai.

Franda, M. 1983. *Voluntary Associations and Local Development in India.* Young Asia Publications: New Delhi.

Indian Institute of Management, Ahmedabad. 1987. *Study of Health Care Financing in India: Based on Case Studies in Maharashtra and West Bengal.* Asian Development Bank: Manila.

Kapoor, A.K. and Singh, D. 1997. *Rural Development Through NGOs.* Rawat Publications: New Delhi.

Kapoor, U. 1995. *Women and Welfare—A Study of Voluntary Agencies.* Indus Publishing Company: New Delhi.

Kamal, A. 1989. *Survey of Community Health Care Financing Existing Projects in Bangladesh: Cost Recovery Systems Implemented in Primary Health Care.* Government of Bangladesh: Dhaka.

Lalitha, N. 1975. *Voluntary Work in India.* NIPCCD: New Delhi.

Mishra, S. 2000. *Voluntary Action in Health and Population—The Dynamics of Social Transition.* Sage: New Delhi.

Prasad, A. 1997. *Voluntary Action and Rural Reconstruction.* Inter-India Publications: New Delhi.

Private Initiatives for Primary Health Care Project. 1997. *A Case Study of Rxiin Tnamet, Guatemala: An Organizational Transformation into an Indigenous NGO, A Summary.* John Snow Inc: Arlington, VA.

Rich *et al.* 1998. *Collaborating to Reduce Poverty: City Halls and Community Based Organizations Working Together to Revitalize Neighbourhoods.* National League of Cities: Washington D.C.

Sachchidananda *et al.* 1994. *Tribal Development and Voluntary Action.* Inter-India Publications: New Delhi.

Society For Participatory Research in Asia. 1991. *Voluntary Development Organization in India.* New Delhi.

Tendler, J. 1982. *Turning Private Voluntary Organization into Development Agencies: Questions for Evaluation.* USAID: Washington D.C.

Wirsing, R.C. 1977. *Sociologist, Society and Free Enterprise Politics: A Study of Voluntary Associations in Urban India.* Vikash: New Delhi.

Wiesgrau, M. 1997. *Interpreting Development: Local Histories, Local Strategies.* University Press of America: New York.

SPECIAL ISSUES

————. 1984. Special Issue on 'Voluntary Organizations.' *Yojana.* Vol. 28, No. 20/21.

————. 1987. Special Number on 'Voluntary Organizations and Development—Their Role and Functions.' *The Indian Journal of Public Administration.* Vol. 33, No. 3.

————. 1996. Special Issue on 'Voluntary Organizations.' *Social Action.* January to March.

————. 1999. Special Issue on 'NGO, Development and Technology.' *Social Action.* January to March.

————. 2001. Special Issue on 'Year of Volunteers.' *Yojana.* Vol. 45, December.

ARTICLES

Alexander, K.C.1981. 'The Dynamics of Peasant Organizations in South India.' *Social Action.* Vol. 31, No. 1.

Ali, A. and Sisodia, P. 1995. 'Health Profile of India: An Overview.' *Health For The Millions.* Vol. 21, Souvenir.

Amin, R. *et al.* 1989. 'Community Health Services and Health Care Utilization in Rural Bangladesh.' *Social Science and Medicine.* Vol. 29, No. 12.

Antrobus, P. 1987. 'Funding For NGOs: Issues and Options.' *World Development.* Vol. 15, Supplement.

Babchuk, N. *et al.* 1965. 'Voluntary Associations and the Integration Hypothesis.' *Sociological Inquiry.* Vol. 35, Spring.

Banton, M. 1968. 'Anthropolitical Aspects and Voluntary Association.' *International Encyclopedia of Social Sciences.* Vol. 16.

Baig, T.A. 1985. 'Voluntary Action: Retrospect and Prospect.' *Mainstream.* January 12.

Baru, R. 1998. 'Structural Adjustment and Health: Changing Role of NGOs.' *Paper Presented at International Seminar on Global Governance and Social Policy.* Baltic Sea Centre: Kellokeski.

Bandyopadhyay, D. 2001. 'Tebhaga Movement in Bangal: A Restrospect.' *Economic and Political Weekly.* October 13.

Benjamin, J. 1986. 'Voluntary Bodies and Rural Development.' *Mainstream.* July 19.

Berman, P. *et al.* 1996. 'Experiences in Paying For Health Care in India's Voluntary Sector.' *International Journal of Health Planning and Management.* Vol. 11.

Bhattacharjee, A. 1985. 'Voluntary Agencies: Identity Crises.' *Mainstream.* pp. 23-48.

Bhushan, B. 1986. 'Depoliticising NGOs: Meaning of New Code of Conduct.' *The Times of India.* July 15.

Bose, A. 2000. 'The National Population Policy and After.' *Health For the Millions.* Vol. 26, No. 4.

Boyce, W. 1994. 'CBR NGO Relationships with Donors and the State.' *ICACBR.* Queens' University: Kingston.

Brinkerhoff, D. *et al.* 1992. 'Promoting the Sustainability of Development Institutions: A Framework for Strategy.' *World Development.* Vol. 20, No. 3.

Brett. 1993. 'Voluntary Agencies as Development Organizations.' *Development and Change.* No. 24.

Chad, S. 1985. 'Limitations of Voluntarism.' *Mainstream.* May 15.

Choudhury, K. 1980. 'Village Reconstruction Organization.' *Voluntary Action.* Vol-22, No. 1

Choudhury, N. 1981. 'Micro Action at the Grassroots.' *Voluntary Action.* Vol-23, No. 1.

Chatterjee, M. 1998. 'Women's Struggle Against Poverty: the SEWA Story.' *Health for the Millions.* Vol. 24, No. 6.

Conn, C. *et al.* 1996, 'Strengthening Health Management: Experience of District Teams in the Gamibia' *Health Policy and Planning.* Vol. II, No. 1.

Coston, J. *et al.* 1998. 'A Model and Typology of Government—NGO Relationships.' *Non-profit and Voluntary Sector Quarterly.* Vol. 27, No. 3.

Cumper, G. 1986. 'The Changing Role of NGOs: No Longer the Eunuch in the Harem?' *Health Policy and Planning.* Vol. 1, No. 4.

Das, A.N. 1988. 'Politics Without People: Role of Voluntary Agencies.' *The Times of India.* January 12.

Dave Sen, P. 1991. 'Community and Self-Financing in Voluntary Health Programmes in India.' *Health Policy and Planning.* No. 6.

Dey, S.K. 1985 'Voluntary Action or Collusion.' *Kurukshetra.* October.

Deo, J.M. 1987. 'Voluntary Agencies vis-à-vis Government.' *Yojana.* Vol. 31, No. 4.

Desai, M.M. 1960. 'Voluntary Workers and Rehabilitation of Women.' *The Indian Journal of Social Work.* Vol. 21, No. 1.

De Winter, E. 1993. 'Which Way to Sustainability? External Support to Health Projects in Developing Countries.' *Health Policy and Planning.* Vol. 8, No. 2.

Dharmadhikari, C.S. 1985. 'Role of Voluntary Action Groups'. *Redesigning India for 21st Century.* November 1.

Dogra, B. 1991. 'Government and Voluntary Agencies.' *The Tribune.* June 11.

Drabek, A.G. 1987. 'Development Alternatives: The Challenge for NGOs—An Overview of the Issues.' *World Development.* No. 15.

Duggal, R. 1988. 'NGOs, Government and Private Sector in Health.' *EPW.* March 26.

Eldridge, P. *et al.* 1988. 'Voluntary Organizations and Popular Movements in Bihar.' *Lokayan Bulletin.* Vol. 6, No. 4.

Fiedler, J. 1990. 'Organizational Development and Privatization (A Bolivian Success Story).' *International Journal of Health Planning and Management.* No. 6.

Fiedler, J. and Day, L. 1997. 'A Cost Analysis of Family Planning in Bangladesh.' *International Journal of Health Planning and Management.* Vol. 12, No. 4.

Franco, F. 1999. 'Poverty Reduction: Challenges and Opportunities.' *Social Action.* Vol. 49, No. 4.

Gangrada, K.D. 1987. 'Development of Voluntary Action.' *Encyclopaedia of Social Work.* Ministry of Welfare, Government of India, New Delhi.

Garain, S. 1993. 'Towards a Measure of Organizational Effectiveness for NGOs.' *The Indian Journal of Social Work.* Vol. LIV, No. 2.

Garain, S. 1994. 'Government-NGO Interface in India: An Overview.' *The Indian Journal of Social Work.* Vol. LV, No. 3.

Gavett, J.W. and Mushlin, A.I. 1996. 'Calculating the Cost of Training in Primary Care.' *Medical Care.* Vol. 24, No. 4.

Ghosh, S. 1994. 'Health Delivery Strategies: Lessons From the NGO Experience.' *Reaching India's Poor-Non-Governmental Approaches to Community Health.* Sage: New Delhi.

Gilson, L.; Sen, P.D.; Mohammed, S. 1994. 'The Potential of Health Sector Non-Governmental Organizations: Policy Options. *Health Policy and Planning.* Vol. 9, No. 1.

Government of India. 1996. 'Deepalaya on the Road to Sustainability.' *NGOs Newsletter Sampark.* Vol. 2, No. 2.

Green, A. 1987. 'The Role of NGOs and the Private Sector in the Provision of Health Care in Developing Countries.' *International Journal of Health Planning and Management.* Vol. 2.

Green, A. and Matthias, A. 1996. 'How Should Governments View Non-Governmental Organizations?' *World Health Forum.* Vol. 17.

Guha, R. and Gadgil, M. 1994. 'Ecological Conflicts and the Environmental Movement in India.' *Development and Change.* Vol. 25.

Gupta, J. 1988. 'Lonely Path of the Voluntary Sector.' *The Statesman.* Kolkata.

Hearn, J. 1998. 'The NGO-isation of Kenyan Society: USAID and the Restructuring of Health Care.' *Review of African Political Economy.* No. 75.

Institute for Motivating Self-Employment. 1981. 'A New Type of Social Movement.' *News Bulletin.* Vol. 1 No. 1.

Islam, N. and Khan, A.N. 1996. 'NGOs in Bangladesh: A Commentary.' *Journal of Rural Development.* Vol. 15, No. 4.

Jain, L.C. 1984. 'Grass Without Roots: Rural Development Under Government Auspices.' *Mainstream.* October 13.

John, J. 1982. 'A Critique of Action Groups.' *The Marxist Review.* Vol. 16, No. 2.

Johnson *et al.* 1996. 'NGOs, Health Providers, and Universities: Collaboration in CBR.' *ICACBR.* Queen's University: Kingston.

Karat, P. 1984. 'Action Groups/Voluntary Organization: A Factor in Imperialist Strategy.' *The Marxist.* Vol. 2, No. 2.

Karat, B. 1997. 'Year of Independence and the Multiple Struggles of Women.' *Frontline.* October 3.

Kothari, R. 1986. 'Masses, Classes and the State.' *Alternatives.* Vol. 11.

Kothari, R. 1986. 'The NGOs, the State and World Capitalism.' *Social Action.* Vol. 36, October–December.

Korten, D.C. 1980. 'Community Organization and Rural Development: A Learning Process Approach.' *Public Administration Review.* Vol. 40, No. 5.

Korten, D.C. 1987. 'Third Generation NGO Strategies: A Key to People Centred Development.' *World Development.* No. 15, July–December.

Korten, D.C. 1990. 'Development as Transformation: Voluntary Action in the 1990s.' *Development.* Vol. 3, No. 4.

Kulkarni, P.D. 1978. 'The Central Social Welfare Board—Promise and Performance.' *Social Welfare.* Vol. XXV, No. 5-6.

Kulkarni, P.D. 1979. 'Voluntary Action for Social Development.' *The Indian Journal of Social Work.* Vol. XXV, No. 4.

Kulkarni, P.D. 1983. 'Voluntary Action: Myth and Reality.' *J.B.M. Lecture. NIPCCD:* New Delhi.

Kulkarni, M. 1985. 'Bunkar, Baxi and Voluntary Sector.' *Mainstream.* June 5.

Kulkarni, S. 1986. 'VOLAGS and the New Policy.' *Lokayan Bulletin.* Vol. 3, No. 4.

Kurien, C.T. 1987. 'Poverty.' *Encyclopaedia of Social Work in India.* Vol. II.

Lafond, A. 1995. 'Sustainability in the Health Sector: The Research Study.' *Health Policy and Planning.* No. 10, Supplement.

Lorgen, C.C. 1998. 'Dancing with the State: The Role of NGOs in Health Care and Health Policy.' *Journal of International Development.* No. 10.

Manimekalai *et al.* 2000. 'Empowerment of Women Through SHGs.' *MARGIN.* Vol. 32, No. 4.

Mahajan, G. 1999. 'Civil Society and its Avatars: What Happened to Freedom and Democracy?' *Economic and Political Weekly*. May 15.

Matthias, A.R. *et al.* 'The Comparative Advantage of NGOs in the Health Sector—A Look at the Evidence.' *World Hospitals.* Vol. 30, No. 1.

Martina, V. 1994. 'The New Popularity of NGOs—Will the Enthusiasm Last?' *D+C.* No. 30.

Mburu, F.M. 1989. 'NGOs in the Health Field: Collaboration, Integration and Contrasting Aims in Africa.' *Social Science Medicine.* Vol. 29, No. 5.

McPherson, J.M. 1982. 'Hyper Network Sampling: Duality and Differentiation Among Voluntary Organization.' *Social Networks.* No. 3.

Mehta, J. 1987. 'Voluntarism Can Hold Its Own.' *People's Action.* Vol. 1, No. 5.

Melchior, S.X. 1985. 'Voluntary Agencies.' *The Indian Express.* February 9.

Muricken, A. 1982. 'Again on Action Groups—Agents of Change for Revolution.' *The Marxist Review.* Vol. XVI, No. 4.

Narayana, K.V. 1991. 'Political Economy of State Intervention in Health Care.' *EPW.* October 19.

Owens, R.L. 1975. 'Organizational Growth and Organizational Participation: Voluntary Association in a West Bengal City.' *Contribution to Indian Sociology.* Vol. IX, No. 1.

Panini, M.N. 1987. 'Voluntarism and Voluntary Organization in India: A Sociological Assessment.' *People's Action.* January.

Patnaik, S. 1987. 'Political Economy of Involving Voluntary Sector in the Path of Development (Unpublished).' *A Paper Presented at Indian Social Science Congress, Mysore.*

Perlman, J. 1979. 'Grass rooting the System.' *Social Policy.* Vol. 7, No. 2.

Priya, R. 1986. 'Voluntary Action for an Alternative Health System.' *Lokayan Bulletin.* Vol. 4, No. 3/4.

Priya, R. 1993. 'Town Planning, Public Health and Urban Poor: Some Exploration, from Delhi.' *Economic and Political Weekly.* April 24.

Prasad, K. 2000. 'Poverty Alleviation: Shift in Paradigms.' *Kurukshetra.* Vol. 49, No. 1.

Quadeer, I. 1985. 'Health Services System: An Expression of Socio-Economic Inequalities.' *Social Action.* Vol. 35, July–September.

Rao, D.N. 1999. 'Social Sector and Development Planning.' *Employment News.* Vol. XXIV, No. 1.

Rao, Y.V. 2000. 'TRYSEM Through NGOs.' *Kurukshetra.* Vol. 48, No. 9.

Rajasekhar, D. 2000. 'NGOs in India: Opportunities and Challenges.' *Journal of Rural Development.* Vol. 19, No. 2.

Ravallion, M. and Datt, G. 1996. 'India's Chequered History in Fight Against Poverty: Are There Lesson for the Future?' *Economic and Political Weekly.* Vol. XXXI, No. 35-37.

Radhakrishna. 1987. 'Sarvodaya Movement in India.' *Encyclopaedia of Social Work in India.* Vol. III.

Ranade, S.N. 1965. 'Social Welfare Administration Through Private Agencies.' *The Indian Journal of Social Work.* Vol. XXVI, No. 2.

Rahnema, M. 1985. 'NGOs: Shifting the Wheat From the Chaff.' *Development*. No. 3.

Reddy, G.N. 1986. 'Women's Movement: The Indian Scene.' *The Indian Journal of Social Work*. Vol. XLVI, No. 4.

Ritchie, M.A. *et al.* 1995. 'Roles and Approaches of NGOs in Health Development.' *World Health Forum*. No. 16.

Roy, S. 1982. 'NGOs in Changing Role.' *Seminar*. May.

Satia, J.K. 1994. 'Upscaling Successful Innovations: Role of NGOs.' *Reaching India's Poor—Non-Governmental Approaches to Community Health*. Sage: New Delhi.

Sethi, J.D. 1991. 'A General Theory of Voluntary Action in a Decentralized Polity.' *Man and Development*. Vol. XIII, No. 2.

Sethi, H. 1985. 'Wither Voluntary Action?' *Seminar*. May.

Sen, A. 1996. 'Economic Reforms, Employment and Poverty: Trends and Options.' *Economic and Political Weekly*. Vol. XXXI, No. 35 to 37.

Shah, K. 1988. 'Voluntary Agencies, The State and The Society.' *Seminar*. August.

Shanker, D. 1981. 'Is The Voluntary Sector Viable?' *Voluntary Action*. Vol. 24, No. 2.

Sharma, S.K. 1991. 'NGOs Must Unite.' *The Tribune*. June 28.

Sivasubramanian, M.A. 1999. 'Credit Based Poverty Alleviation Programme: Innovative Approach.' *Kurukshetra*. Vol. 48, No. 2.

Smith, K. 1989. 'NGOs in the Health Field: Collaboration, Integration and Contrasting Aims.' *Social Science and Medicine*. Vol. 29, No. 3.

Soeters, R. *et al.* 1994. 'Primary Health Care Training Companies for Sustainable Development.' *World Health Forum*. No. 15.

Srivastava, T.N. 1982. 'Voluntary Sector in a Welfare State.' *Social Welfare*. Vol. XXX, No. 5.

Stefanini, A. 1995. 'Sustainability: The Role of NGOs.' *World Health Forum*. No. 16.

Stefanini, A. *et al.* 1992. 'Managing Externally Assisted Health Projects for Sustainability in Developing Countries.' *International Journal of Health Planning and Management*. No. 7.

Streefland, P. *et al.* 1990. 'The Long Term Role of Non-Government Development Organizations in Primary Health Care: Lessons from Bangladesh.' *Health Policy and Planning*. Vol. 5, No. 3.

Stremlau, C. 1987. 'NGO Co-ordinating Bodies in Africa, Asia and Latin America.' *World Development*. No. 15.

Streeten, P. 1987. 'The Contribution of NGOs to Development.' *Development.* No. 4.

Tandon, R. 1992. 'Civil Society in the First Sector.' *Development.* No. 3.

Tandon, R. 1991. 'Government-NGO Relations in India.' *Social Action.* Vol. 41, No. 2.

Tandon, R. 1994. 'Where are the People? Community Participation in Health.' *Reaching India's Poor—Non-Governmental Approaches to Community Health.* Sage: New Delhi.

Thakur, S.G. 1995. 'Women, Poverty and Empowerment.' *The Administrator.* Vol. XL, No. 4.

The Asia Foundation and Horizons. 2001. 'Assessment of Anti-Trafficking Efforts Finds Disunity Among NGOs.' *Horizon Report.* Spring.

The Commonwealth Foundation. 1995. 'NGOs: Guidelines for Good Policy and Practice.' CF: New Delhi.

Tiwari, N.D. 1982. 'Voluntary Agencies in a Welfare State.' *Social Welfare.* Vol. XXIX, No. 5.

Tongsawate, M. and Tips, W. 1988. 'Coordination Between Government and Voluntary Organizations in Thailand's Rural Development.' *Public Administration and Development.* Vol. 8.

Uphoff. 1993. 'Grassroots Organizations and NGOs in Rural Development.' *World Development.*

Valkin, H. 1984. 'Action Group—Beginning or End of a Drama.' *Social Action.* No. 2.

Vishwanathan, L.S. 1985. 'People's Organization for Rural Development.' *Mainstream.* July 27.

Walley, J. *et al.* 1991. 'Integrating Health Services: The Experience of NGOs in Ethiopia.' *Health Policy and Planning.* Vol. 6, No. 14.

Wishwakarma, R.K. *et al.* 'Organizational Effectiveness of Urban Basic Services Programme in Slums of Delhi'. *Nagarlok.* Vol. 27, October–December.

Wolleback, D. and Selle, P. 2002. 'Does Participation in Voluntary Associations Contribute to Social Capital? The Impact of Intensity, Scope and Type.' *Nonprofit and Voluntary Sector Quarterly.* Vol. 31, No. 1.

NEWSPAPER CLIPPING

'A Vision for Progress.' *The Hindu.* New Delhi. 18 April, 1999.

'Basu Stresses on NGO's Role in Health Care.' *The Statesman.* Kolkata. 23 July, 2000.

'Code for Contributions.' *The Pioneer*. New Delhi. 2 November, 2000.

'Caution Against Giving Grants to Bogus NGOs.' *The Times of India*. Mumbai. 9 May, 2000.

'Foreign Funding of NGOs.' *The Hindu*. New Delhi. 29 October, 1999.

'Grassroots Touch.' *The Telegraph*. Kolkata. 17 September, 1996.

'Government and NGOs—Similar Goals but Contrasting Styles.' *The Times of India*. New Delhi. 10 March, 1999.

'Health Care: Gujarat Fails to Rope in NGOs.' *The Indian Express*. New Delhi. 7 January, 2001.

'Issues Facing Voluntary Bodies in the North East.' *The Sentinel*. Guwahati. 14 September, 1996.

'It is Boom Time for NGOs.' *The Pioneer*. New Delhi. 19 September, 1999.

'Indian Health Institute Makes An Impact in US.' *The Times of India*. New Delhi. 16 June, 2000.

'Indian Health NGO Wins Accolades in US.' *The Times of India*. Mumbai. 16 June, 2000.

'Misappropriation of Funds by NGOs Alleged.' *The North East Times*. Guwahati. 10 January, 1996.

'Ministries Issued Strict Rules to Monitor NGOs.' *The Times of India*. New Delhi. 13 December, 1997.

'Naxalites in the Guise of NGOs.; *The Sunday Observer (Weekly)*. New Delhi. 11 April, 1999.

'Nepali, Indian NGOs Lock Horns.' *The Indian Express*. New Delhi. 1 September, 1996.

'Night Census For the Houseless.' *The Deccan Herald*. Bangalore. 8 January, 2001.

'Not Even Half of Slum Health Project Target Met in Delhi.' *The Hindu*. New Delhi. 15 April, 1999.

'NGOs: Need For a Code of Ethics.' *The Hindu*. Chennai. 19 January, 1999.

'NGOs Don's Want Any Scrutiny.' *The Pioneer*. New Delhi. 6 August, 1999.

'NGOs and the Fifth Column.' *The Indian Express*. New Delhi. 6 October, 1999.

'NGO to Take BCCI to Court.' *The Indian Express*. New Delhi. 2 September, 1996.

'NGOs Join Hands to Find Answer to N-E Problems.' *The Times of India*. New Delhi. 5 January, 1997.

'NGOs Take WB Officials to Task.' *The Pioneer*. Hyderabad. 23 June, 2000.

'NGOs Need to Mobilize the Youth.' *The Pioneer*. New Delhi. 4 September, 2000.

'NGOs Doctors Declare War Against Abortion Drug.' *The Statesman*. New Delhi. 1 November, 2000.

'NGOs Attempt to Educate Sex Workers on AIDS.' *The Deccan Chronicle*. Hyderabad. 2 July, 2000.

'NGO Seeks Clear Cut Policies on Earth Cutting in City.' *The Assam Tribune*. Guwahati. 12 February, 1997.

'NGOs Pick Charity Flaws.' *The Telegraph*. Kolkata. 11 September, 1997.

'NGOs Movement Not Viewed With Scepticism.' *The Hindu*. New Delhi. 8 May, 1997.

'NGOs Resolve to Tackle Prostitution.' *The Hindu*. New Delhi. 10 May, 1997.

'Orissa Plan to Monitor NGOs.' *The Hindu*. Bhubaneswar. 18 December, 2000.

'Rights Body Urges Rebels to Set NGO Official Free.' *The Telegraph*. Kolkata. 12 July, 1997.

'Role of NGOs.' *The Hindu*. New Delhi. 18 May, 1997.

'Spirit of Voluntarism—Building Greater Institutional Capacities.' *The Times of India*. New Delhi. 18 September, 1999.

'Sixteen NGOs Lose Ministerial Sanctions.' *The Pioneer*. New Delhi. 19 May, 2000.

'Senior Citizens Anguished Over Discrimination.' *M.P. Chronicle*. Bhopal. 21 August, 2000.

'Taming Helms and NGOs.' *The Hindustan Times*. New Delhi. 28 July, 1997.

'The Other Side of Conflict.' *The Hindu*. New Delhi. 10 October, 1999.

'UP Government Bans NGOs for Funds Misuse.' *The Indian Express*. Lucknow. 22 February, 2000.

'Voluntary Agencies and Their Role.' *The Indian Express*. New Delhi. July, 1985.

'Voluntary Action: Case Studies.' *The Hindu*. New Delhi. 12 October, 1999.

'Voluntarism and Political Action.' *The Indian Express Magazine*. 20 June, 1989.

'Voluntary Agencies: Leave Them Alone.' *The Indian Express*. New Delhi. 31 October, 1986.

'Will The State Crush NGO Obscurantism?' *The Pioneer*. New Delhi. 11 November, 1999.

'Women's Organizations Misused Funds.' *The Hindu*. New Delhi. 26 April, 1997.

UNPUBLISHED DOCUMENTS

Dissertations

Baru, R. 1987. 'Factors Influencing Variations in Health Services.' *M.Phil. Dissertation*. Centre for Social Medicine and Community Health, School of Social Sciences, Jawaharlal Nehru University, New Delhi.

Bhattacharjee, S. 1996. 'NGO Approaches to Health and Development in India: Strategies and Sustainability.' *M.A. Dissertation*. Prins Leopold Instituut Voor Tropische Genceskunde: Belgiam.

Patnaik, S. 1988. 'Voluntarism and Development—A Social Science Focus on Health.' *M.Phil. Dissertation*. Centre for Social Medicine and Community Health, School of Social Sciences, Jawaharlal Nehru University, New Delhi.

Sarkar, A. 1996. 'An Exploration into Sustainable Development Efforts of a Selected NGOs.' *M.A. Dissertation*. Department of Medical and Psychiatric Social Work, Tatā Institute of Social Sciences, Mumbai.

Sarkar, A. 1998. 'Characteristics of NGOs: An Exploratory Study in Assam.' *M.Phil. Dissertation*. Centre for Social Medicine and Community Health, School of Social Sciences, Jawaharlal Nehru University, New Delhi.

Seshagiri, S. 1999. 'Role of the Indian State and NGOs in Public Health.' *M.Phil. Dissertation*. Centre for Political Studies, Jawaharlal Nehru University, New Delhi.

Files

Voluntary Health Association of India. 2002. *Files on NGOs and Development*. VHAI: New Delhi.

West Bengal Voluntary Health Association. 2002. *Files on NGOs in West Bengal*. WBVHA: Kolkata.

Index